AF327504

Drug-Induced Movement Disorders

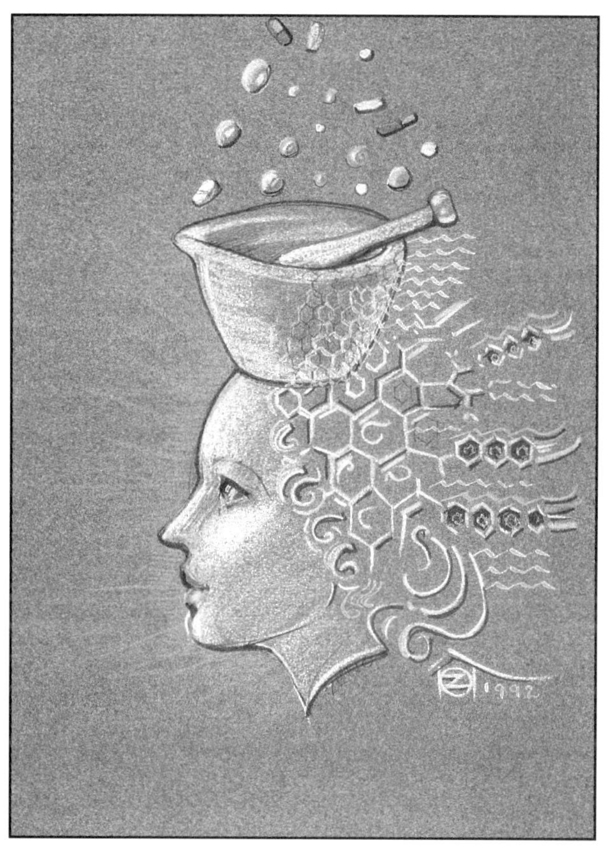

edited by

Anthony E. Lang, M.D.

William J. Weiner, M.D.

Drug-Induced Movement Disorders

edited by

Anthony E. Lang, M.D.
Director, Movement Disorders Clinic
Associate Professor
Division of Neurology
Toronto Hospital, Western Division
University of Toronto
Toronto, Ontario, Canada

and

William J. Weiner, M.D.
Director, Movement Disorders Clinic
Professor of Neurology
University of Miami School of Medicine
Miami, Florida

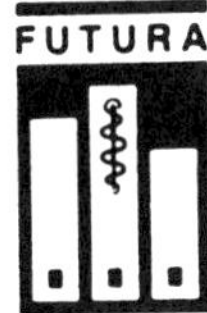

Futura Publishing Co., Inc.
Mt. Kisco, NY

Library of Congress Cataloging-in-Publication Data
Drug-induced movement disorders / edited by Anthony E. Lang and
    William J. Weiner.
        p.   cm.
    Includes bibliographical references and index.
    ISBN 0-87993-525-1
    1. Movement disorders—Etiology.   2. Drugs—Side effects.
3. Antipsychotic drugs—Side effects.   4. Neuroleptic malignant
syndrome.   5. Antiparkinsonian agents—Side effects.   I. Lang,
Anthony E.   II. Weiner, William J.
    [DNLM: 1. Dyskinesia, Drug-Induced.   WL 390 D794]
RC385.5.D78   1992
616.8'3—dc20
DNLM/DLC
for Library of Congress   91-34678
                                                               CIP

Copyright 1992
Futura Publishing Company, Inc.

Published by
Futura Publishing Company, Inc.
2 Bedford Ridge Road
Mount Kisco, New York 10549
LC #:   91-34678
ISBN #:   0-87993-525-1

Every effort has been made to ensure that the information in this
book is as up to date and as accurate as possible at the time of publication. However, due to the constant developments in medicine, neither the author, nor the editor, nor the publisher can accept any
legal or any other responsibility for any errors or omissions that may
occur.

Printed in the United States of America.

This book is printed on acid-free paper.

To the memory of
Maxine and Leonard Weiner
– gone too soon.
(WJW)

To Tom and Lina, Art and Jane,
with love, affection, and
gratitude.
(AEL)

Contributors

Lenard A. Adler, M.D.
Psychiatry Service, New York VAMC, and Department of Psychiatry, New York University School of Medicine, New York, New York

Burt Angrist, M.D.
Psychiatry Service, New York VAMC, and Department of Psychiatry, New York University School of Medicine, New York, New York

Robert E. Burke, M.D.
Associate Professor, Department of Neurology, Columbia University, New York, New York

Daniel E. Casey, M.D.
Chief, Psychiatric Research and Psychopharmacology, VA Medical Center, Professor of Psychiatry and Associate Professor of Neurology, Oregon Health Sciences University, Portland, Oregon; Collaborative Scientist, Oregon Regional Primate Research Center, Beaverton, Oregon

Michael F. Egan, M.D.
Senior Staff Fellow, NIMH Neuroscience Center at St. Elizabeth, Washington, DC

Stewart A. Factor, D.O.
Assistant Professor of Neurology, Albany Medical College, Albany, New York

Joseph H. Friedman, M.D.
Neuropsychiatric Research and Training Center, Cranston, Rhode Island; Associate Professor of Clinical Neurosciences, Brown University Program in Medicine, Providence, Rhode Island

Thomas M. Hyde, Ph.D., M.D.
Director, Neurology Consultation Services, Clinical Brain Disorders Branch, Chief, Neuropsychiatry Branch, NIMH Neuroscience Center at St. Elizabeth, Washington, DC

Vikram Khot, M.D.
Guest Researcher, NIMH Neuroscience Center at St. Elizabeth, Washington, DC

Roger Kurlan, M.D.
Associate Professor of Neurology, University of Rochester School of Medicine, Rochester, New York

Anthony E. Lang, M.D., F.R.C.P.
Director, Movement Disorders Clinic, Associate Professor, Division of Neurology, Toronto Hospital, Western Division, University of Toronto, Toronto, Ontario, Canada

John G. Nutt, M.D.
Professor of Neurology, Departments of Neurology and Pharmacology, School of Medicine, Oregon Health Sciences University, Portland, Oregon

Christopher O'Brien, M.D.
Instructor in Neurology, University of Rochester School of Medicine, Rochester, New York

David E. Riley, M.D.
Director, Movement Disorders Center, Mount Sinai Clinic, Cleveland, Ohio

John Rotrosen, M.D.
Psychiatry Service, New York VAMC, and Department of Psychiatry, New York University School of Medicine, New York, New York

Juan Sanchez-Ramos, M.D., Ph.D.
Associate Professor in Neurology, Associate Director of Clinical Research, Comprehensive Drug Research Center, University of Miami School of Medicine, Miami, Florida

Carlos Singer, M.D.
Assistant Professor of Neurology, University of Miami School of Medicine, Miami, Florida

William J. Weiner, M.D.
Director, Movement Disorders Clinic, Professor of Neurology, University of Miami School of Medicine, Miami, Florida

Richard Jed Wyatt, M.D.
Chief, Neuropsychiatry Branch, NIMH Neuroscience Center at St. Elizabeth, Washington, DC

Preface

Side effects of pharmacological agents have been intimately related to both the development of the subspecialty field of "movement disorders" as well as subsequent progress in the area. Initially, this began with the occurrence of parkinsonism induced by reserpine, which stimulated a revolution in the understanding of neuropharmacology. Subsequently, dopamine receptor-blocking antipsychotic agents were found to have a broad spectrum of motor complications, and levodopa therapy for Parkinson's disease resulted in an astounding array of abnormal movements. These and other drug-related movement disorders have provided considerable insights into brain function in both health and disease. To date, there has been no single work that has attempted to address in detail this area, which at the same time is both a broad and a somewhat restrictive field.

Currently, drug-induced movement disorders are a common source of referral to both neurologists and psychiatrists. An extremely broad range of pharmacological agents has been described to cause these side effects, although certain classes of drugs, such as the antipsychotics, are still much more commonly implicated than others. Indeed, this side-effect profile is a major impetus driving the revolution in dopamine pharmacology as well as encouraging the development of "atypical" neuroleptics devoid of these problems.

In this volume, we have attempted to bring together scholarly up-to-date reviews covering the entire field of pharmacologically induced movement disorders. Each chapter addresses such issues as history, clinical features, epidemiology, pathophysiology, management, and future trends in research. Although we have coordinated and interrelated this material, each chapter is a definitive review of the topic and can be read in isolation. The introductory chapter provides a common ground of definitions of various abnormal movements, the broad differential diagnosis which must be considered when faced with these problems, and an approach to their investigation. Chapters 2 through 7 deal with the wide range of movement disorder-related complications of antipsychotic drugs. Chapter 8 deals with the general topic of antidepressant therapy and movement disorders. Chapter 10 considers dyskinesias induced by antiparkinson drugs, while Chapter 11 deals with movement disorders associated with other dopaminergic compounds, particularly stimulants. The final chapter discusses movement disorders occurring with numerous other miscellaneous agents. For the most part, we have limited the discussion to prescription pharmaceuticals, avoiding the large area of toxins (e.g., MPTP) and heavy metals (e.g., manganese poisoning). However, certain commonly used nonproprietary pharmacological agents such as alcohol (Chapter 12) and cocaine (Chapter 11) are discussed. Given the common occurrence of movement disorders in patients treated for psychiatric illnesses, we felt that it was important to include a discussion of motor disorders seen in psychiatric disease unrelated to pharmacological intervention (Chapter 9). One final "anomaly," included because of its widespread therapeutic use in psychiatric patients, is a discussion of electroconvulsive therapy (ECT) and movement disorders (Chapter 8). We have consciously chosen to avoid a separate discussion of the extensive and complicated medico-legal issues surrounding these topics. Although this is an extremely important aspect of the field, the general appeal of this work, which extends across geographic borders as well as medical disciplines, would make it difficult to adequately consider the unique features of the different judicial systems involved.

We are indebted to our collaborators who have contributed material of the highest quality to this book. We believe that a broad spectrum of readers including students, residents, clinicians, particularly neurologists and psychiatrists, as well as clinical and basic scientists will all find something of interest here.

Anthony E. Lang, M.D.
William J. Weiner, M.D.

Acknowledgment

We would like to thank the members of our respective research and clinical groups, the Parkinson's Disease Research Group and the Movement Disorders Center at the University of Miami School of Medicine and the Toronto Western Movement Disorders Clinic as well as the National Parkinson Foundation (WJW) for their support during this project. Raiza Perez, Shelley Malton, and Lisa Hatton were particularly helpful in the preparation of the manuscripts. We are also indebted to Dr. Juan Sanchez-Ramos for producing the cover figure which highlights the topic in striking fashion.

Contents

1

Movement Disorders:
Approach, Definitions, and Differential Diagnosis

Anthony E. Lang, M.D.

Introduction

Movement disorders are an important component of any neurological practice. Prescription drugs and illicit pharmaceutical agents are common causes for almost all types of movement disorders. Neurologists and general physicians should have an awareness of these potential complications. The common occurrence of movement disorders, complicating treatment of mental illness in particular, emphasizes the need for this awareness, especially by psychiatrists.

The accurate diagnosis of a movement disorder complicating the use of a specific drug requires some basic understanding of the general classification of types of movement disorders. Occasionally, reports in the literature utilize terms such as chorea, tics, and myoclonus without conforming to accepted definitions of these disorders. Review of the original case report may reveal significant confusion or inaccuracy. However, the report may have been cited multiple times and the described association widely accepted despite poor or inappropriate documentation. An appreciation of the broad differential diagnosis of movement disorders is also necessary when attempting to implicate a specific drug as causative. A lack of this awareness often accounts for case reports of a specific drug causing abnormal movements when better explanations are readily available. Unfortunately, the literature is rife with examples of such reports. Another important potential source of confusion is the possibility that certain neurological diseases can present first with "non-neurological" symptoms. Treatment prescribed for these symptoms may be wrongly implicated when a movement disorder eventually develops due to the primary disease process. Probably the most common example of this would be the use of neuroleptic drugs for the initial psychiatric manifestations of certain neurological disorders. We have seen this sequence of events result in significant delays in diagnosis of such disorders as Wilson's disease, Huntington's disease, and systemic lupus erythematosis. Another potential source of diagnostic error is that certain brain disorders (occult or overt) can predispose to the development of movement disorders as a consequence of specific drugs. Occasionally the underlying disorder will require treatment in its own right quite distinct from the need for withdrawal of the agent that precipitated the obvious movement disorder.

The purpose of this introductory chapter is to define the descriptive terms that are used repeatedly in this text and to present the reader with an approach to the patient with a movement disorder. Multiple tables are provided outlining the broad differential diagnoses that must be considered when faced with these clinical problems.

Definitions and Differential Diagnoses

The analysis of patients with movement disorders involves an additional step to the standard clinical neurological approach of "where" and "what." Prior to deciding "where" in the nervous system the disease process is located, and then "what" that process is, the clinician must first observe and examine the patient to define the most appropriate broad class of movement disorder in which to place the problem. Abnormal movements must be considered a clinical sign for which there are many causes. Most types of movement disorder can be seen in pure form with no known or established cause. These "essential" or "idiopathic" disorders must be distinguished from the "symptomatic" or "secondary" varieties.

Movement disorders can be subdivided into those conditions resulting in the syndrome of parkinsonism or an akinetic rigid syndrome and those causing a variety of abnormal involuntary movements or "dyskinesias" ("hyperkinesias") including tremor, dystonia, athetosis, chorea, ballism, tics, myoclonus, and a small number of less common varieties. A principal source of disability in patients with *parkinsonism* is the reduction in speed and amplitude of movements, fatiguing, and later arrests in ongoing movement. These features are termed *akinesia* and *bradykinesia*. As part of the clinical picture of parkinsonism, there is a reduction in the normal repertoire of "associated movements," such as arm swing while walking. Increase in muscle tone, equally appreciated in flexors and extensors, is termed *rigidity* ("lead pipe"), which may have a ratchety or cogwheel consistency when tremor is superimposed. A flexed posture and impairment of postural stability is also a common feature of parkinsonism. The common association between the above features and tremor, as defined below, provides the acronym TRAP (T = Tremor, R = Rigidity, A = Akinesia, P = Postural Disturbances), which emphasizes the major components of the syndrome of parkinsonism. Tables 1 and 2 provide an outline of the causes of this disorder.

Tremor (Table 3) can be defined as a rhythmical oscillation of a body part, produced by either alternating or synchronous contractions of reciprocally innervated antagonistic muscles. Tremors usually have a relatively fixed periodicity although the rate may appear irregular clinically. Tremor is usually further categorized on the basis of the position, posture, or motor performance necessary to bring it out. A rest tremor is seen when the body part is in complete repose. Maintenance of a posture such as extending the arms parallel to the floor reveals a postural tremor, while moving the body part to and from a target brings out kinetic or intention tremor. One source of confusion is the fact that many postural tremors increase while approaching a target. The term *terminal tremor* is best used to describe this. Occasionally, a tremor is seen only with certain actions or limb positions. "Primary writing tremor" is an example of this. Orthostatic tremor is another uncommon but well-recognized form of tremor involving the proximal lower limbs and trunk when the

---

Table 1

Etiological Classification of Parkinsonism (Akinetic Rigid Syndrome)**

---

1. Idiopathic Parkinson's disease (? a single entity)
2. Secondary parkinsonism ("Parkinson's plus")
   A. Other primary "degenerative" CNS diseases (many inherited)
      a. Olivopontocerebellar atrophies ⎫
      b. Shy-Drager syndrome   ⎬ "Multiple System Atrophy"
      c. Striatonigral degeneration   ⎭
      d. Progressive supranuclear palsy
      e. Parkinson-dementia-ALS complex [a) Pacific b) non-Pacific]
      f. Alzheimer's disease
      g. Pick's disease
      h. Cortical-basal ganglionic degeneration (CBGD)
      i. Corticostriatospinal degeneration ("spastic pseudosclerosis")
      j. Azorean disease
      k. Huntington's disease*
      l. Familial basal ganglionic calcification*
      m. Pallidal degenerations*
      n. Neuroacanthocytosis
      o. Hallervorden-Spatz disease*
      p. L-dopa responsive dystonia-parkinsonism*
      q. Others* (e.g., familial depression, alveolar hypoventilation, and parkinsonism; X-linked Philippine dystonia-parkinsonism)
   B. "Secondary" parkinsonism due to other definable causes
      a. Drugs* (dopamine receptor blockers, dopamine depletors, lithium, alpha-methyldopa)
      b. Toxins* (manganese, MPTP, mercury, methanol, ethanol, carbon disulfide)
      c. Anoxic encephalopathy* (including carbon monoxide, cyanide)
      d. Vascular (atherosclerotic, hypertensive, amyloid angiopathy, Binswanger's, AVM)
      e. Postencephalitic* (encephalitis lethargica, other viral encephalitis, Creutzfeldt-Jakob, SSPE)
      f. Head Injury* (including "punch-drunk syndrome")
      g. Brain tumor*
      h. Hydrocephalus* (high pressure and NPH)
      i. Metabolic* (Wilson's disease, acquired hepatocerebral degeneration, hypoparathyroidism, GM1 gangliosidosis, Gaucher's disease, mitochondrial cytopathies, others).

---

* Disorders that may cause juvenile parkinsonism.
** Adapted from Lang.[7]

Table 2

Diseases Causing Dementia and Parkinsonism*

Idiopathic Parkinson's disease
  With: Concomitant Alzheimer's disease
         Cortical Lewy body disease
         No good explanation for dementia
Alzheimer's disease
Progressive supranuclear palsy
Multiple system atrophy
Huntington's disease
Cortical-basal ganglionic degeneration
Pick's disease
Parkinson-dementia-ALS complex: (a) Pacific; (b) non-Pacific
Creutzfeldt-Jakob disease
Multi-infarct state ("atherosclerotic pseudoparkinsonism")
Normal pressure hydrocephalus
Cerebral anoxia (including CO poisoning)
Dementia pugilistica
Wilson's disease
Hallervorden-Spatz disease
Calcification of basal ganglia (primary or secondary)
Others (e.g. Mn, neurosyphilis, Lafora body disease, ceriod lipofuscinosis,
  etc.)

---

* From Weiner and Lang.[1]

patient stands for any period of time. There are a variety of other rhythmical movements which can sometimes be confused with tremor (Table 3).

Chorea (Table 4) consists of irregular, unpredictable, brief, jerky movements that flit from one part of the body to another in a continuous random sequence. The movements are brisk and abrupt in some cases (e.g., Sydenham's chorea), while in others, they are somewhat slower and flowing (e.g., Huntington's disease). The term *choreoathetosis* has been used in this latter situation where chorea may be combined with features of dystonia and athetosis (see below). An important "choreatic" disorder discussed in Chapter 5 is tardive dyskinesia, a consequence of long-term treatment with dopamine receptor-blocking drugs. Although more typical or classic chorea can be seen in this condition, there are certain common features that often help to distinguish these movements from those seen in other choreas, for example, Huntington's disease. Table 5 lists some of these.

Table 3

Classification and Differential Diagnosis of Tremor*

1. Rest tremors
   a. Parkinson's disease
   b. Other parkinsonian syndromes (less commonly)
   c. Midbrain ("rubral") tremor: Rest < Postural < Kinetic
   d. Wilson's disease (also acquired hepatocerebral degeneration)
   e. Essential tremor—only if severe: Rest << Postural and Action

2. Postural and action ("terminal") tremors
   a. Physiological tremor
   b. Exaggerated physiological tremor (these factors can also aggravate other forms of tremor)
      (1) Stress, fatigue, anxiety, emotion
      (2) Endocrine: hypoglycemia, thyrotoxicosis, pheochromocytoma, adrenocorticosteroids
      (3) Drugs and toxins: Beta agonists, dopamine agonists, amphetamines, lithium, tricyclic antidepressants, neuroleptics, theophylline, caffeine, valproic acid, alcohol withdrawal, mercury ("Hatter's shakes"), lead, arsenic, others
   c. Essential tremor (familial or sporadic) ? Subtypes
   d. Primary writing tremor
   e. With other CNS disorders
      (1) Parkinson's disease
      (2) Other akinetic-rigid syndromes
      (3) Idiopathic dystonia, including focal dystonias
   f. With peripheral neuropathy
      (1) Charcot-Marie-Tooth (controversial as to whether to call this the Roussy-Levy syndrome)
      (2) Variety of other peripheral neuropathies
   g. Cerebellar tremor

3. Kinetic (intention) tremor
   Disease of cerebellar "outflow" (dentate nucleus and superior cerebellar peduncle): MS, trauma, tumor, vascular, Wilson's disease, acquired hepatocerebral degeneration, drugs, toxins (e.g., mercury), others

4. Miscellaneous rhythmical movement disorders
   a. Psychogenic tremor
   b. Orthostatic tremor
   c. Rhythmical movements in dystonia (dystonic tremor)
   d. Rhythmical myoclonus (segmental myoclonus, e.g., palatal or branchial myoclonus, spinal myoclonus, limb myorhythmia)
   e. Oscillatory myoclonus
   f. Asterixis
   g. Clonus
   h. Epilepsia partialis continua
   i. Hereditary chin quivering
   j. Spasmus nutans
   k. Head bobbing with third ventricular cysts
   l. Nystagmus

* From Weiner and Lang.[1]

Table 4

Etiological Classification of Chorea*

1. Developmental/aging choreas
   a. Physiological chorea of infancy
   b. Cerebral palsy—anoxic, kernicterus
   c. Minimal cerebral dysfunction
   d. Buccal-oral-lingual dyskinesia and edentulous orodyskinesia in elderly
   e. Senile chorea (probably several causes)

2. Hereditary choreas
   a. Huntington's disease
   b. Benign hereditary chorea
   c. Neuroacanthocytosis
   d. Other CNS "degenerations": OPCAs, Azorean disease, ataxia telangiectasia, tuberous sclerosis, Hallervorden-Spatz, familial calcification of basal ganglia, others
   e. Neurometabolic disorders: Wilson's disease, Lesch-Nyhan syndrome, lysosomal storage disorders, amino acid disorders, Leigh's disease, porphyria

3. Drug-induced: neuroleptics (tardive dyskinesia), antiparkinsonian drugs, amphetamines, tricyclics, oral contraceptives, anticonvulsants, anticholinergics, others

4. Toxins: alcohol intoxication and withdrawal, anoxia, carbon monoxide, Mn, Hg, thalium, toluene

5. Metabolic
   a. Hyperthyroidism
   b. Hypoparathyroidism (various types)
   c. Pregnancy (chorea gravidarum)
   d. Hyper- and hyponatremia, hypomagnesemia, hypocalcemia
   e. Hypo- and hyperglycemia (latter may cause hemichorea, hemiballism)
   f. Acquired hepatocerebral degeneration
   g. Nutritional: e.g., bereberi, pellegra, B_{12} deficiency in infants

6. Infectious
   a. Sydenham's chorea
   b. Encephalitis lethargica
   c. Various other infections and postinfectious encephalitides, including Creutzfeldt-Jakob disease

7. Immunological
   a. SLE (including ANF negative cases with lupus anticoagulant)
   b. Henoch-Schonlein disease
   c. Others rarely, sarcoid, MS, Behçet's, polyarteritis nodosa

(continued)

Table 4 (*continued*)

8. Vascular (often hemichorea)
   a. Infarction
   b. Hemorrhage
   c. AVM
   d. Polycythemia rubra vera
   e. Migraine
9. Tumors
10. Trauma, including subdural and epidural hematoma
11. Miscellaneous including paroxysmal choreoathetosis

---

* Altered from Shoulson.[2]

Table 5

Features Distinguishing Between Tardive Dyskinesia (TD) and Huntington's Disease (HD)*

	TD	HD
Repetitive stereotypic choreic-like movement	+	−
Flowing choreic movement	−	+
Forehead chorea	−	+
Lingual-facial-buccal dyskinesia	+	±
Oculomotor disturbances and head thrusts	−	+
Impersistence of tongue protrusion	−	+
Facial dyspraxia	−	+
Dysarthria	±	+
Respiratory dyskinesia	+	±
Milkmaid grip	−	+
Body rocking movements	+	±
Marching in place	+	−
Stuttering, bizarre ataxic gait	−	+
Dementia	±	+
Progressive course	−	+

+ = commonly present
± = occasionally present
− = absent
Altered from Fahn.[3]

Table 6

Causes of Ballism*

Infarction or ischemia including TIAs (usually lacunar disease, hypertensive, diabetic atherosclerosis, vasculitis, polycythemia, thrombocytosis, and other causes).
Hemorrhage
Tumor–Metastatic
        Primary
Hyperglycemia (nonketotic hyperosmolar state)
Other focal lesions (e.g., abscess, AVM, tuberculoma, MS plaque, encephalitis, subdural hematoma)
Drugs (e.g., phenytoin, dopamine agonists in Parkinson's disease)

---

* Taken from Lang.[7]

Ballism (Table 6) is comprised of wide amplitude flinging movements, usually involving the proximal limbs. This movement disorder most often involves only one side of the body (hemiballism[us]). Occasionally, bilateral movements occur (biballism or paraballism). Ballism is closely linked to chorea since many patients demonstrate additional distal choreic movements, and as recovery occurs, hemiballism often transforms into a milder hemichoreic state.

Dystonia (Table 7) can be defined as a disorder dominated by sustained muscle contractions which frequently cause twisting and repetitive movements or abnormal postures. Dystonic movements may be slow and twisting. When these are located distally, they are referred to as *athetosis*. Prolonged dystonic spasms result in characteristic posturing of various body parts. In addition, dystonic movements may be quite rapid, resembling the shock-like jerks of myoclonus. There may be additional rhythmical movements, especially when the patient attempts to resist the involuntary dystonic movement actively (sometimes referred to as "dystonic tremor"). Here, if the patient is asked to relax and allow the limb to move as it pleases, the abnormal dystonic posturing usually becomes evident and the rhythmical movements lessen. Failure to recognize the wide range of abnormal movement types that occur in dystonic syndromes often results in the misdiagnosis of dystonia as some other dyskinesia.

Dystonic movements and postures are often specific to selected actions ("action dystonia"), and many patients are able to use a variety of peculiar tricks to lessen the severity of the dystonia. These

---

Table 7

Etiological Classification of Dystonia*

---

1. Primary dystonia
   a. Generalized dystonia (dystonia musculorum deformans, idiopathic torsion dystonia)
      (1) Hereditary [dominant, ? recessive, X-linked recessive dystonia-parkinsonism (Philippines)]
      (2) Sporadic
   b. Focal, segmental, multifocal
      (1) Cranial dystonia (Meige's syndrome, blepharospasm-oromandibular dystonia)
      (2) Spasmodic torticollis
      (3) Writer's cramp (and other occupational dystonias)
      (4) Spasmodic dysphonia
      (5) Others
   c. Idiopathic paroxysmal dystonias
      (1) Kinesigenic
      (2) Nonkinesigenic
2. Secondary dystonia
   a. Diseases with known metabolic defect, e.g., Wilson's, GM_1 gangliosidosis, GM_2 gangliosidosis, metachromatic leukodystrophy, Lesch-Nyhan syndrome, glutaric acidemia, methylmalonic acidemia, homocystinuria, others
   b. Disease with presumed (but undefined) metabolic defect, e.g., Hallervorden-Spatz, calcification of basal ganglia, Leigh's disease, bilateral necrosis of basal ganglia ($\pm$ Leber's optic neuropathy), dystonic lipidosis (Niemann-Pick), ataxia telangiectasia, neuroacanthocytosis, ceriod lipofuscinosis, Hartnup
   c. "Degenerative" CNS diseases, e.g., Parkinson's, dopa-responsive dystonia, PSP, Huntington's, pallidal degenerations, OPCA, Azorean disease, CBGD
   d. (1) Perinatal anoxia/kernicterus (may be delayed)
      (2) Head trauma (often delayed)
      (3) Cerebral infarction/hemorrhage (often delayed)
      (4) AVM
      (5) Tumor
      (6) Encephalitis (various types)
      (7) Toxins (especially manganese)
      (8) Postoperative (thalamotomy)
      (9) MS (often paroxysmal)
      (10) Drugs (especially neuroleptics, dopamine agonists)
   e. Psychogenic dystonia
3. Disorders simulating dystonia
   a. Orthopedic disorders, e.g., rotational atlanto-axial subluxation
   b. Neurological, e.g., seizures, posterior fossa tumor causing torticollis, hemianopia, strabismus
   c. Miscellaneous, e.g., hiatus hernia in childhood (Sandifer's syndrome), congenital neck muscle lesions, abnormal posture in utero, others

---

* Altered from Lang.[7]

Table 8

Classification of Tics*

1. Simple motor tics
   e.g., eye blinking, eyebrow raising, nose flaring, grimacing, mouth opening, tongue protrusion, platysma contractions, head jerking, neck or trunk shuddering, shoulder shrugging or abduction, neck stretching, arm jerks, fist clenching, abdominal tensing, pelvic thrusting, buttock or sphincter tightening, hip flexion or abduction, kicking, knee extension, foot dorsiflexion, toe curling

2. Simple phonic tics
   e.g., sniffing, grunting, throat clearing, shrieking, yelping, barking, growling, squealing, snorting, coughing, clicking, hissing, humming, moaning

3. Complex motor tics
   e.g., head shaking, teeth gnashing, wrist shaking, finger cracking, touching, biting, jumping, skipping, stamping, squatting, kicking, smelling hands/objects, rubbing, finger twiddling, echopraxia, copropraxia, spitting, exaggerated startle

4. Complex vocal tics
   e.g., coprolalia (wide variety, including shortened words), unintelligible words, whistling, "Bronx cheer," panting, belching, hiccough, stuttering, stammering, echolalia, palilalia (also mental coprolalia and palilalia)

* From Weiner and Lang.[1]

features have frequently encouraged a misdiagnosis of hysteria (particularly in idiopathic dystonic syndromes but also in drug-induced states). The adult-onset idiopathic focal and segmental dystonias are much more common than previously recognized. These include cranial muscle involvement (blepharospasm, oromandibular/lingual dystonia, spasmodic dysphonia), spasmodic torticollis and other axial dystonias, and writer's cramp and other "occupational palsies."

Tics (Tables 8 and 9) are the most varied of all movements disorders. Patients may demonstrate a wide array of motor or vocal tics as well as a number of associated symptoms including hyperactivity, attention deficit disorder, and obsessive-compulsive disorder. Motor and vocal tics can be further subdivided as simple or complex. Tics are usually abrupt, transient, stereotypic, coordinated movements

Table 9

Etiological Classification of Tics*

Idiopathic
  a. Acute simple transient tic (<1 year)
  b. Persistent single or multiple tics of childhood (remits before adulthood)
  c. Chronic single or multiple motor tics (persists throughout life)
  d. Adult onset of senile tic
  e. Gilles de la Tourette syndrome

"Secondary" tics
  a. Postencephalitic (especially encephalitis lethargica: klazomania)
  b. Postrheumatic chorea
  c. Head injury
  d. Carbon monoxide poisoning
  e. Poststroke
  f. Neuroacanthocytosis
  g. Drugs: stimulants, levodopa, neuroleptics ("tardive Tourette"), carbamazepine, phenytoin, phenobarb
  h. Mental retardation syndromes, including chromosomal abnormalities
  i. Others

Related disorders
  a. Mannerisms
  b. Stereotypies
  c. Habitual manipulations of the body
  d. Hyperactivity syndrome
  e. Compulsions
  f. Excessive startle
  g. Jumping Frenchmen, latah, myriachit

* From Weiner and Lang.[1]

that vary in intensity and are repeated at irregular intervals. The movements are most often brief and jerky (clonic); however, slower, more prolonged movements (tonic or "dystonic" tics) also occur. Several other features are quite characteristic and helpful in distinguishing this movement disorder from other dyskinesias. Patients usually experience an inner urge to make the movement themselves, which is temporarily relieved by its performance. Tics are voluntarily suppressible for variable periods of time but this usually occurs at the expense of mounting inner tension and the need to perform the tic. Several other types of abnormal movements also may be voluntarily suppressible for short periods of time.

Myoclonus can be defined as sudden, brief, shock-like involuntary movements that may be caused by both active muscle contraction (positive myocolonus) or inhibition of ongoing muscle activity (negative myoclonus). Asterixis is the most common example of the latter phenomenon. The differential diagnosis of myoclonus is broader than any other movement disorder (Table 10). There is a wide range of clinical patterns of myoclonus. The frequency varies from single, rare jerks to constant, repetitive contractions. The amplitude may range from a small contraction that fails to move a joint, to a very large jerk that moves the entire body. The distribution ranges from focal involvement of one body part to segmental (involving two or more contiguous regions) to multifocal, to generalized. When the jerks occur bilaterally, they may be symmetrical or asymmetrical. When they occur in more than one region, they may be synchronous in two body parts (within milliseconds) or asynchronous. Myoclonus is usually arrhythmic and irregular, but in some patients it is very regular (rhythmical) and in others, there may be jerky oscillations that last for a few seconds and then fade away (oscillatory). Myoclonic jerks may occur spontaneously without a clear precipitant or as a response to a wide variety of stimuli. This stimulus sensitivity may occur in response to sudden noise, light, visual threat, pinprick, touch, or muscle stretch. Attempted movements (or even the intention to move) may initiate the muscle jerks (action or intention myoclonus).

Some dyskinesias occur intermittently rather than in a persistent fashion. This is typical of tics and certain forms of myoclonus. Dystonia often occurs only with specific actions, but this is usually a consistent response to the action rather than periodic or unpredictable. A small group of patients with chorea and/or dystonia have bouts of sudden-onset, short-lived involuntary movements known as *paroxysmal choreoathetosis* (Table 11).

There are a number of disorders in which abnormal or *excessive startle* occurs (Table 12). In some patients, one simply finds an exaggerated startle response that habituates poorly after repeated stimuli. In others, there is an abnormal response to the stimuli that normally evoked startle. Hyperexplexia, or hyperekplexia, also known as "startle disease," may be more akin to certain forms of myoclonus than to a normal startle response. A variety of other unusual disorders, first described in the 19th Century together with

Table 10

Etiological Classification of Myoclonus*

1. Physiological myoclonus (normal subjects)
   a. Sleep jerks (hypnic jerks)
   b. Anxiety-induced
   c. Exercise-induced
   d. Hiccough (singultus)
   e. Benign infantile myoclonus with feeding
2. Essential myoclonus (no known cause and no other gross neurological deficit)
   a. Hereditary
   b. Sporadic
3. Epileptic myoclonus (seizures dominate and no encephalopathy, at least initially)
   a. Fragments of epilepsy
      Isolated epileptic myoclonic jerks
      Epilepsia partialis continua
      Idiopathic stimulus-sensitive myoclonus
      Photosensitive myoclonus
      Myoclonic absences in petit mal
   b. Childhood myoclonic epilepsies
      Infantile spasms
      Myoclonic astatic epilepsy (Lennox-Gastaut)
      Cryptogenic myoclonus epilepsy (Aicardi)
      Awakening myoclonus epilepsy of Janz
   c. Benign familial myoclonic epilepsy (Rabot)
   d. Progressive myoclonus epilepsy: Baltic myoclonus (Unverricht-Lundborg)
4. Symptomatic myoclonus (progressive or static encephalopathy dominates)
   a. Storage disease:
      Lafora body disease
      Lipidoses, e.g., GM_2 gangliosidosis, Tay-Sachs, Krabbe's, Ceroid-lipofuscinosis (Batten/Kufs)
      Sialidosis ("cherry-red spot")
   b. Spinocerebellar degeneration:
      Ramsay-Hunt syndrome (several etiologies)
      Friedreich's ataxia
      Ataxia telangiectasia
   c. Basal ganglia degenerations:
      Wilson's disease
      Torsion dystonia
      Hallervorden-Spatz disease
      Cortical-basal ganglionic degeneration
      Progressive supranuclear palsy
      Huntington's disease
      Parkinson's disease
      Multiple system atrophy
      Dentato-rubro-luysian atrophy

Table 10 (*continued*)

  d. Mitochondrial encephalopathies
  e. Dementias:
     Creutzfeldt-Jakob disease
     Alzheimer's disease
  f. Viral encephalopathies:
     Subacute sclerosing panencephalitis
     Encephalitis lethargica
     Arbor virus encephalitis
     Herpes simplex encephalitis
     Postinfectious encephalitis
  g. Metabolic:
     Hepatic failure
     Renal failure
     Dialysis syndrome
     Hyponatremia
     Hypoglycemia
     Infantile myoclonic encephalopathy (polymyoclonus)
     ($\pm$ neuroblastoma)
     Nonketotic hyperglycemia
     Multiple carboxylase deficiency
  h. Toxic encephalopathies:
     Bismuth
     Heavy-metal poison
     Methyl bromide, DDT
     Drugs including levodopa, tricyclic antidepressants, others
  i. Physical encephalopathies:
     Posthypoxia (Lance-Adams)
     Posttraumatic
     Heat stroke
     Electric shock
     Decompression injury
  j. Focal CNS damage:
     Poststroke
     Postthalamotomy
     Tumor
     Trauma
     Dentato-olivary lesions (palatal myoclonus)
     Spinal cord lesions (segmental/spinal myoclonus)
  k. Rarely root, plexus or peripheral nerve disorders

* Altered from Fahn et al.[4]

Table 11

Differential Diagnosis of Paroxysmal Dyskinesias*

---

1. Idiopathic (familial or sporadic)
   a. Paroxysmal kinesigenic choreoathetosis
   b. Paroxysmal nonkinesigenic ("dystonic") choreoathetosis
   c. Paroxysmal hypnogenic dystonia
2. Symptomatic
   a. Seizures
   b. Multiple sclerosis
   c. Transient ischemic attacks
   d. Drugs
   e. Head trauma
   f. Cerebral palsy
   g. Metabolic disturbance, e.g., hypoparathyroidism, hyperthyroidism, Hartnup disease, pyruvate decarboxylase deficiency, D-glyceric acidemia
   h. Degenerative disorders (rarely)
   i. Psychogenic

---

* From Riley and Lang.[5]

Tourette's syndrome, manifest excessive startle. The jumping Frenchmen of Maine, latah, and myriachit also demonstrate sudden striking out, echo phenomena, automatic obedience, and several other less common features.

The term *akathisia* refers to a sense of restlessness and the feel-

---

Table 12

Startle and Related Syndromes*

---

1. Startle reflex
   a. Normal
   b. Exaggerated
2. Hyperexplexia
3. Reticular reflex myoclonus
4. Startle epilepsy
5. Startle reflex plus Moro reflex
6. Exaggerated startle in Tourette syndrome
7. Jumping Frenchmen of Maine, latah, myriachit

---

* Altered from Wilkins et al.[6]

ing of a need to move. This disorder may be accompanied by a variety of "akathitic" movements including repetitive rubbing, crossing and uncrossing the arms or legs, stroking the head and face with the hands, repeatedly picking at clothing, abducting and adducting, swinging or up and down pumping of the legs, shifting weight, rocking, marching in place, or pacing while sitting and standing. Occasionally patients demonstrate a variety of vocalizations such as moans, grunts, and shouts. Whether true akathitic movements can occur in the absence of the subjective sense of needing to move remains controversial. This disorder is more often a consequence of drug therapy than most other disorders defined in this chapter (except tardive dyskinesia, which by definition, is drug-induced). Chapters 4 and 6 discuss the types of akathisia in considerable detail.

Another disorder in which movements occur secondary to the subjective need to move is the *restless legs syndrome*. Here, unlike in akathisia, the patient typically complains of a variety of sensory disturbances in the legs, including pins and needles, creeping or crawling sensations, aching, itching, stabbing, heaviness, tension, burning, or coldness. Occasionally, similar symptoms are appreciated in the upper limbs. These complaints are usually experienced during recumbency in the evening and are often associated with insomnia. This condition is commonly associated with another movement disorder, *periodic movements of sleep* (sometimes inappropriately termed *nocturnal myoclonus*). These periodic, slow, sustained (1–2 seconds) movements range from synchronous to asynchronous dorsiflexion of the big toes and feet to triple flexion of one or both legs. More rapid myoclonic movements or slower, prolonged dystonic-like movements of the feet and legs also may be present in these patients while awake. Table 13 lists the movement disorders that usually persist in or occur primarily during sleep.

Another uncommon but well-defined movement disorder of the lower limbs has been termed *painful legs and moving toes*. Here, the patient typically complains of a deep pulling or searing pain in the lower limb and foot associated with continuous wriggling or writhing of the toes. Occasionally the ankle and less commonly more proximal muscles of the legs are involved. Rarely, a similar problem is seen in the upper limb as well. In some cases, there is a history of nerve insult or injury and the examination may demonstrate evidence of peripheral nerve dysfunction.

There are numerous "movement disorders" caused by dysfunction of the peripheral nerves (e.g., fasciculations, myokymia). These

---

Table 13

Abnormal Involuntary Movements in Sleep*

Hypnic jerks
Nocturnal myoclonus
Periodic leg movements in sleep
Seizures, including epilepsia partialis continua
Segmental myoclonus
Tics
Paroxysmal hypnogenic dystonia
Dystonic postures when contractures supervene or disorder that simulates
    dystonia (e.g., orthopedic)
Hemifacial spasm
Painful legs and moving toes ($\pm$)

---

* Other dyskinesias (e.g., tremor, chorea) may persist in the earlier stages and subside in deeper stages of sleep.
* Taken from Lang.[7]

are usually easily separated from the movement disorders described above. *Hemifacial spasm* is a common disorder in which irregular tonic and clonic movements involve the muscles innervated by one 7th cranial nerve. Eyelid twitching is usually the first symptom followed at variable intervals by lower facial muscle involvement. Rarely, both sides of the face are affected, in which case the spasms are asynchronous on the two sides in contrast to other pure facial dyskinesias such as cranial dystonia.

The nature and extent of the investigation of the patient presenting with a movement disorder will vary depending on the clinical circumstances (Table 14). When the historical and clinical features are typical of certain conditions (e.g., familial essential tremor, Tourette syndrome), further investigations may be unnecessary. This also applies to certain well recognized drug-induced movement disorders. In other situations, particularly when the association is poorly documented or previously unreported, all other possible causes for the same movements must be considered. As will be outlined throughout the remaining chapters, one must always consider a possible predisposing underlying disorder requiring further investigations even when the drug precipitant is obvious. The specifics related to investigations of movement disorder patients are beyond the scope of this brief introductory chapter and the reader is referred to several excellent references dealing with these conditions.[1-11] Fi-

Table 14

Investigation of Movement Disorders*

Investigation	Movement Disorder					
	A[a]	C[a]	B[a]	D[a]	T[a]	M[a]
Routine hematology (including sedimentation rate)	+ [b]	+	+	+	− [b]	+
Routine biochemistry (including Ca^{++}, uric acid, liver function tests)	+	+	+	+	± [b]	+
Serum Cu, ceruloplasmin (with or without 24-hour urine Cu, liver biopsy, radiolabeled Cu studies)	+ + [b]	+ +	−	+ +	±	+
Slit-lamp examination	+ +	+ +	−	+ +	±	+
Thyroid function	±	+ +	−	+	−	+
Antistreptolysin O test, antihyaluronidase	−	+	−	±	±	−
Antinuclear factor, LE cells, other immunological studies (also VDRL)	±	+ +	+	+	−	+
Blood acanthocytes	+	+	−	+	+	±
Lysosomal enzymes	+	+	−	+	±	+
Urine organic and amino acids	±	+	−	+	−	+
Urine oligosaccharides and mucopolysaccharides	±	+	−	+	−	+
Serum lactate and pyruvate	±	+	−	+	−	+
Bone marrow for storage cells (including electron microscopy [EM])	±	+	−	+	−	+
EM of leukocytes; biopsy of liver/skin/conjunctiva	±	+	−	+	−	+
Nerve/muscle biopsy	±	+	−	+	−	+
Oligoclonal bands	±	+	+	+	−	±
CT scan/MRI	+ +	+ +	+ +	+ +	±	+ +
Electroencephalography (EEG)	+	+	−	+	+	+ +
Electromyography (EMG) and nerve conduction studies	+	+	−	+	+	+
Evoked potentials	+	+	−	+	−	+ +
Electroretinogram	±	+	−	+	−	+

Note: The extent of investigation will depend on factors such as age of onset, nature of progression, and presence of historical or clinical atypical features suggesting a secondary cause of the movement disorder in question.
[a] A = akinetic rigid syndrome; C = chorea; B = hemiballism; D = dystonia; T = tics; M = myoclonus.
[b] + + very important or frequently useful; + sometimes helpful; ± questionably helpful; − rarely if ever helpful.
* Taken from Lang.[7]

nally, the importance of excluding Wilson's disease cannot be over-emphasized in view of its treatability and universally fatal outcome if left undiagnosed.

References

1. Weiner WJ, Lang AE. Movement Disorders: A Comprehensive Survey, Mount Kisco, NY, Futura Publishing Co., 1989.
2. Shoulson I. On chorea. Clin Neuropharmacol 1986; 9:S85-S99.
3. Fahn S. Tardive dyskinesia. In: Rowland LP (ed), Merritt's Textbook on Neurology, Philadelphia, Lea & Febiger, 1984, 7th edition, pp 539–541.
4. Fahn S, Marsden CD, Van Woert MH. Definition and classification of myoclonus. Adv Neurol 1986; 43:1–5.
5. Riley DE, Lang AE. Dystonia. In: Kennard C (ed), Recent Advances in Clinical Neurology, Edinburgh, Churchill Livingston, 1988, 5:175–200.
6. Wilkins DE, Hallett M, Weiss MM. Audiogenic startle reflex of man and its relationship to startle syndromes. Brain 1986; 109:561–573.
7. Lang AE. Movement disorder symptomatology. In: Bradley WG, Daroff RB, Fenichel GM, et al. (eds), Neurology in Clinical Practice, Boston, Butterworths, Heinemann, 1991, pp 315–336.
8. Fahn S, Marsden CD, Calne DB (eds). Dystonia 2, Raven Press, New York, 1988.
9. Fahn S, Marsden CD, Van Woert M (eds). Myoclonus, Raven Press, New York, 1986.
10. Jankovic J, Tolosa E (eds). Parkinson's Disease and Movement Disorders, Baltimore, Urban and Schwarzenberg, 1988.
11. Elble RJ, Koller W. Tremor, Baltimore, John's Hopkins University Press, 1992.

2

Neuroleptic-Induced Acute Dystonia

Daniel E. Casey, M.D.

History

The introduction of neuroleptic antipsychotic drugs in the early 1950s revolutionized the care of the severely mentally ill.[1] Soon thereafter, it became well recognized that in addition to the beneficial effects on disorders of thinking, these drugs also produced disorders of motor function. The types of syndromes associated with the initiation of these drugs are neuroleptic-induced dystonia (abnormal postures), akathisia (restlessness), and parkinsonism (tremor, rigidity, bradykinesia). Indeed, the term *neuroleptic*, meaning "to take the neuron," was coined to incorporate the two actions on psychoses and motor function.

It was once thought that adequate antipsychotic doses were obtained when motor disturbances were produced. However, it was eventually recognized that these effects were not inextricably linked. Currently it is believed that antipsychotic effects are mediated via mesolimbic or prefrontal cortex mechanisms, whereas the motor symptoms are localized to the basal ganglia. Though not linked, there is a narrow therapeutic index between desirable bene-

Lang AE, Weiner WJ (editors): *Drug-Induced Movement Disorders,* Mount Kisco, NY, © Futura Publishing Co., Inc., 1992.

21

fits and undesirable side effects as the majority of patients receiving these drugs experience both effects.[2]

The aim of this review is to focus on the specific syndrome of neuroleptic-induced acute dystonia. Literature will be reviewed to summarize clinical presentations, differential diagnosis, epidemiology, pathophysiology, treatment, and future research directions. While much is known about this clinically striking disorder, much remains to be learned.

Clinical Presentation

Neuroleptic-induced acute dystonia spans a wide range of symptom presentation and severity. Mild symptoms can lead to subjective distress with few physical findings, such as complaints of a thick tongue with little or no dysarthria. Moderate symptoms may produce briefly or temporarily sustained abnormal postures. Severe symptoms such as laryngopharyngeal spasms may greatly compromise airway function and lead to terrifying feelings of suffocation. This syndrome may be a rare cause of sudden death.

Common clinical presentations include opening or closing of the jaw, grimacing, tongue protrusion, difficulty in swallowing, tightness in the throat, turning the head to one side (torticollis), pulling the head straight back (retrocollis), or rolling the eyes upward, sometimes with deviation to the side (occulogyric crisis). Abnormal positions in the limbs with flexion or extension as well as torsion of the trunk can also lead to bizarre postures or complaints. Muscle tone is usually increased in the affected muscles. When acute dystonia occurs for the first time in a patient, it may be frightening, associated with painful muscle spasms, and can lead the patient to believe that something is controlling their body. Symptoms can also have a fluctuating course. When a patient is reporting a symptom, it may go away or the patient can demonstrate that they can voluntarily suppress it only to have it come back within a few minutes to hours later.

Differential Diagnosis

Exposure to neuroleptics is a required feature of the diagnosis of neuroleptic-induced acute dystonia. Since this information is not always available or accurate, other diagnoses should be considered. Symptoms of malingering or hysterical conversion reactions may mimic acute dystonia, though these are not common. More often, mild acute dystonic symptoms will come and go, leaving the observer to wonder if the patient is manipulating the situation for some unclear secondary gain (i.e., a misdiagnosis of malingering or "hysteria"). In most cases, this is not the correct interpretation as a waxing and waning course is a frequent feature of acute dystonia. If there is any reason to believe that the patient has taken neuroleptics within the last 4 to 5 days, it is better to give them the benefit of the doubt and consider complaints of muscular contractions or bizarre postures and movements as neuroleptic drug-induced.

In addition to the traditional neuroleptics used to treat schizophrenia and psychoses, other drugs can cause acute dystonia. Though some compounds are not marketed as neuroleptics, they share the same mechanism of action as neuroleptics—dopamine receptor blockade. Antiemetic compounds such as prochlorperazine (Compazine) have long been recognized as producing acute dystonia, particularly in children. Metoclopramide (Reglan), another antiemetic often used in oncology and a frequently prescribed agent for disorders of digestion such as diabetic gastroparesis or esophageal reflux, can cause acute dystonia. Prochlorperazine and metoclopramide can also cause the acute extrapyramidal syndromes of akathisia and parkinsonism, as well as the late-onset syndrome of tardive dyskinesia when these drugs are used chronically.[3]

Other drugs may cause acute dystonia though the mechanism of action is not known (see Chapters 10–12). For example, toxic levels of phenytoin can produce typical signs of acute dystonia that resolve when blood levels return to the therapeutic range.[4] Therapeutic doses of levodopa may produce dystonic syndromes in idiopathic parkinsonian patients.[5] The widely used quinine-based antimalarial drugs, such as chloroquine or amodioquine, are also known for their ability to produce dystonia and other dyskinesias.[6,7]

A variety of other causes of dystonia must be considered in a differential diagnosis.[8,9] Endocrinopathies (hyperthyroidism, hypoparathyroidism, hyperglycemia) are infrequently associated with dystonic syndromes. Neurological disorders such as temporal lobe seizures can produce bizarre behavior as well as peculiar postures. Central nervous system infections, both viral and bacterial, trauma, multiple sclerosis, or space-occupying lesions are other uncommon causes of dystonia. Several of the conditions listed may cause paroxysmal dystonia. Other cases are idiopathic, sometimes induced by movement (kinesigenic). Other idiopathic neurological syndromes with dystonic features as their hallmark include the focal or regional dystonic syndromes of torticollis, oromandibular dystonia with or without blepharospasm, writer's cramp, and other intention dystonias. The acute onset and the natural history of spontaneous resolution unless challenged with further causative medication (see below), usually serves to distinguish acute dystonic reactions from these more persistent and often progressive dystonic syndromes.

Epidemiology

Prevalence and Incidence

The prevalence (number of cases at a specific time) and incidence (number of new cases in a specific period, such as 1 year) are similar because neuroleptic-induced acute dystonia is a time-limited, short-duration event. This contrasts with other types of dystonia that may be chronic or progressive and have a higher prevalence than incidence.

Neuroleptic-induced acute dystonia prevalence/incidence has dramatically changed in the past 35 years. This is primarily due to changing patterns of neuroleptic use. The two main changes are a preference for more potent neuroleptics and a tendency toward using higher doses.[2] In the early to middle 1950s, low-potency agents, such as promazine and chlorpromazine, infrequently produced dystonia. In the late 1950s to early 1960s, when more potent phenothiazines were developed, neuroleptic-induced acute dystonia was noted in 2.3% of patients.[10] In the 1970s, more potent and long-acting depot neuroleptics were more often used and produced dystonia rates ranging from 15% to 25%.[11,12] A survey in 1980 reported a 39% dystonia rate[13] and a study of high-risk young male patients receiving high-potency neuroleptics identified acute dystonia in over 90% of the patients.[14] Recently, 21% of young healthy male volunteers were reported to develop acute dystonia in response to the catecholamine-depleting agent, alpha-methyl-para-tyrosine (AMPT).[14a]

Risk Factors

Vulnerability to acute dystonia is determined by several different risk factors. These can be categorized as patient characteristics, drug factors, and temporal aspects.

Patient Characteristics

Age is the most important characteristic in determining vulnerability to neuroleptic-induced acute dystonia. Children and young adults are highly vulnerable, whereas the elderly rarely develop acute dystonic reactions to neuroleptics (Fig. 1).[15] Though this has been attributed to the possibility that older patients receive lower doses of neuroleptics than young adult schizophrenics, children and teenagers also receive low doses of these drugs for either vomiting or behavioral problems and still develop high rates of dystonia. Gender plays an important role in dystonia. Males develop this syndrome twice as often as females. This contrasts with the increased vulnerability to tardive dyskinesia in females.[16] Prior vulnerability to acute dystonic reactions is also a good predictor of future vulnerability when patients are re-exposed to the same neuroleptic drug type and dose in a later treatment episode.[17]

Coexisting conditions such as hypocalcemia, hyperthyroidism, and hypoparathyroidism, as well as a family history of idiopathic

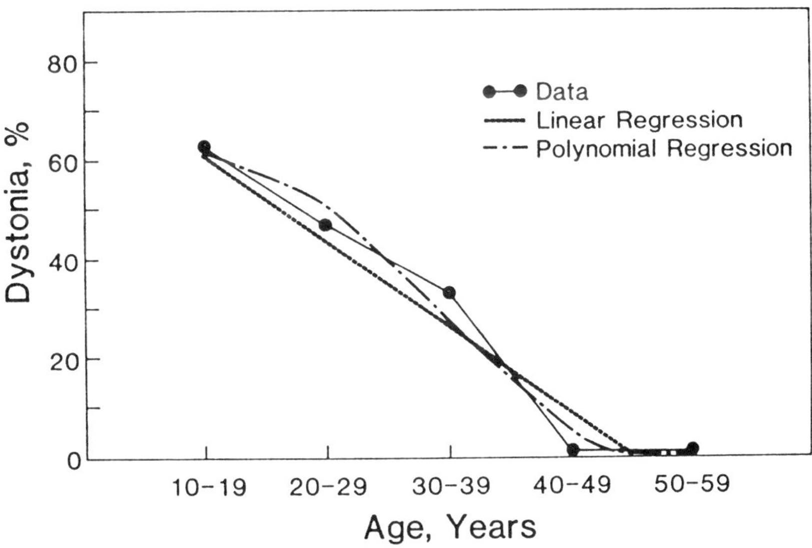

Figure 1: Age-related incidence of neuroleptic-induced acute dystonia. Linear (r^2 = 0.94) and polynomial (r^2 = 0.98) regression lines are shown with the actual data. Reprinted with permission.[17]

dystonia or recent cocaine abuse (see Chapter 11) have also been associated with increased vulnerability to drug-induced dystonia. However, these observations primarily derive from case reports and must be further substantiated before it can be concluded that they are true risk factors.

Drug Factors

Characteristics of neuroleptic drugs also substantially affect rates of dystonia. There is a complicated inverted U-shaped curve between the incidence of dystonia and neuroleptic dosage. Dystonia most commonly occurs in the middle to upper dose range of neuroleptics (400–1000 mg/day of chlorpromazine or its equivalents). When large and megadoses are used (over 1400 mg/day of chlorpromazine equivalents), the frequency of dystonia appears to decrease (Fig. 2).[15] Thus, at very low and very high doses, there is less dystonia than at moderate doses.[13,15,18]

Studies evaluating the correlation between neuroleptic blood

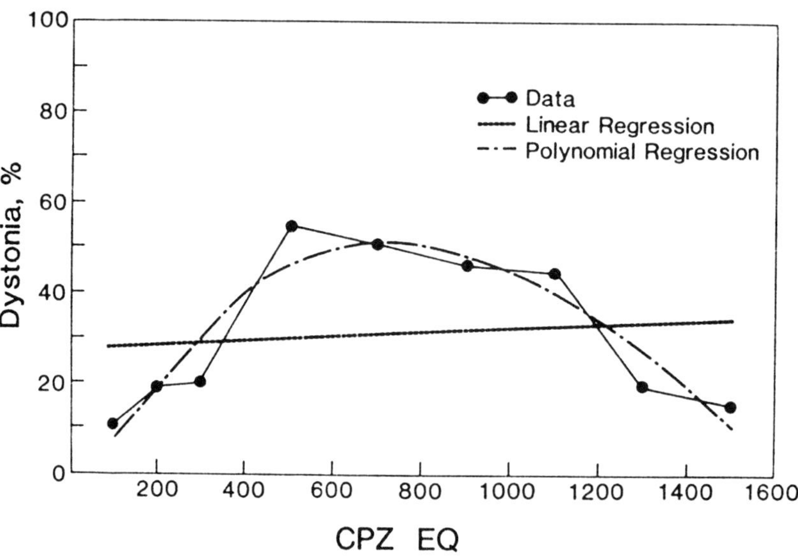

Figure 2: The relationship between neuroleptic dose and acute dystonia. Linear ($r^2 = 0.012$) and polynomial ($r^2 = 0.86$) regression lines are shown with the actual data. Reprinted with permission.[17]

levels and dystonia, as well as other extrapyramidal syndromes, have produced conflicting results. While one study found a significant positive correlation between these parameters,[19] other studies found no relation between blood level and extrapyramidal syndromes[20] or dystonia.[21] Though it seems obvious that there should be a relationship between dose or blood level and desirable or undesirable side effects, these associations are not easily demonstrated. For example, if a high side effect rate plateaus with low to moderate dosages, any further increase in the drug dose will not show a corresponding increase in the high plateau side effect rate. Thus, there will be a low correlation because one of the parameters does not change while the other parameter does. Also, if there is a nonlinear relationship, such as an inverted U-shaped curve, any evaluation with linear analyses will fail to find an association (Fig. 2).[15] In addition, wide interindividual differences in drug metabolism and blood levels are commonly found in neuroleptic studies. This problem is best solved by studying drugs in fixed-dose paradigms across a wide range of dosages and applying a variety of statistical assessments to evaluate the data.

Neuroleptic-induced acute dystonia is positively correlated with drug potency. Low-milligram, high-potency compounds (e.g., haloperidol, fluphenazine), produce high rates of dystonia, whereas high-milligram, low-potency compounds (e.g., thioridazine, chlorpromazine) produce low amounts of dystonia. Intermediate-potency neuroleptics (e.g., perphenazine) produce intermediate rates of dystonia. In corresponding fashion, low-milligram, high-potency drugs have minimal anticholinergic activity, whereas the high-milligram, low-potency drugs have high intrinsic anticholinergic aspects. This has been proposed as the mechanism for why one type of drug induces more dystonia than another type.[22] However, others have speculated that there is an additional, unknown component to this issue because adding an anticholinergic to low-milligram, high-potency compounds produces a side-effect profile that differs from the high-milligram, low-potency, high-intrinsic anticholinergic neuroleptic.[23]

It has also been proposed that some neuroleptics have a preferential binding affinity to the mesolimbic area of the brain and have a low affinity for the basal ganglia, but this hypothesis has yet to be verified.[2] Currently, the best working hypothesis to explain the differential rates of dystonia across the types of neuroleptics is that the receptor-blocking ratio between dopamine and acetylcholine adequately accounts for the data. Clozapine, which has the lowest dopamine/acetylcholine antagonist ratio of any neuroleptic, appears not to produce acute dystonia.[24]

Temporal Aspects

Time is also a critical component in determining the expression of acute dystonic reactions. Over 95% of these episodes occur within 96 hours of initiating neuroleptic therapy (Fig. 3) or within the same time period of a large dose increase.[13] Acute dystonia is only rarely seen after this time, but it may appear if anticholinergics are abruptly discontinued within the first few weeks of initiating neuroleptic treatment. If dystonic reactions occur after this period, one should suspect that the patient has either taken a larger neuroleptic dose than prescribed, combined the neuroleptic with other drugs, including alcohol, has not been taking the antiextrapyramidal syndrome medicines, or may have an underlying medical disorder.

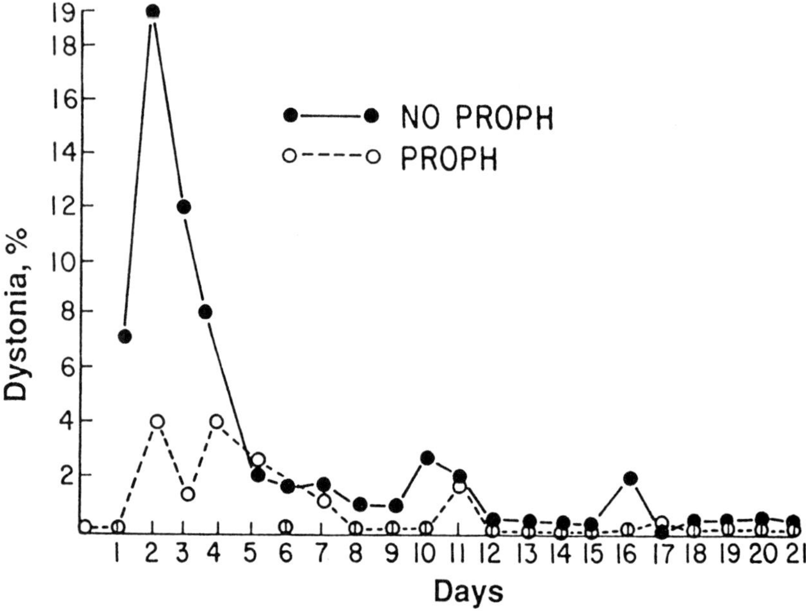

Figure 3: Time course of neuroleptic-induced acute dystonia with prophylaxis (PROPH) and no prophylaxis with anticholinergic drugs. Adapted with permission.[13]

In a single-dose neuroleptic blood level study, the majority of dystonic reactions occurred 20 to 26 hours after neuroleptic drug ingestion. At that time, blood levels were only 15% to 20% of their peaks. It was also found that the red cell-bound neuroleptic levels correlated somewhat better with dystonic reactions than the unbound neuroleptic levels.[25] This has led to the proposal that neuroleptic-induced acute dystonia occurs on falling blood levels and has been titled the "mismatch" hypothesis.[9] However, in a separate study where patients received continuing neuroleptic doses, as is the most common way these drugs are prescribed, acute dystonia occurred most often on the second day at approximately 10.6 hours after the last neuroleptic dose.[26] Though these dystonic reactions could be described as occurring during the falling phase of blood levels since it was more than 10 hours after the last dose, another interpretation is that the blood levels on the second day were higher than the blood levels on the first day and are certainly higher than they would be if the patient had only received a single dose of neuroleptic and was observed for the next 48 hours as described in the study above.[25] Thus, the data can be interpreted in two ways. If one chooses to emphasize the falling blood level concept, a patient's blood level is falling the vast majority of time after the rapid onset of peak blood levels in 1–2 hours following drug ingestion. Therefore, it is statistically likely that most events will occur when blood levels are falling. On the other hand, with each successive dose the overall blood level, or area under the curve, increases in each 24-hour period until it stabilizes at approximately 5 days of continued drug therapy, which is the timeframe in which most dystonic reactions occur.

Pathophysiology

Surprisingly little is known about the specific pathophysiological mechanisms underlying acute dystonia, though these drug reactions have been recognized for the past 35 years. It is commonly stated that acute dystonia is due to the onset of dopamine receptor blockade in the basal ganglia. However, most dystonic reactions occur in the 24- to 48-hour period after neuroleptics have been initiated. This is much later than the period of peak receptor occupancy, which occurs within 1 to 2 hours of administering neuroleptics.[27] While this may be used to argue the point that acute dystonia occurs on falling blood and brain levels, the counterpoint is made that the levels and receptor occupancy rates on day 2 are usually higher than blood and brain levels on day 1, when most dystonic reactions would be expected to occur if it were simply an issue of greatly falling levels after reaching peak levels in the first few hours of treatment (also see *Temporal Aspects* above).

Neuroleptic-induced acute dystonia has been most commonly attributed to blockade of the type 2 dopamine receptor (D_2), an effect that is found in all commercially available neuroleptics. The role of the type 1 dopamine receptor (D_1) has not been evaluated clinically because no pure D_1 antagonists have been available for clinical use. Nonhuman primate animal models can help clarify the specific roles of the D_1 and D_2 receptors. In monkeys receiving pure or nearly pure D_2 antagonists, such as raclopride or haloperidol, there is a clear dose-response relationship to the prevalence and severity of neuroleptic-induced dystonia.[28–34] Additionally, neuroleptics with mixed D_1/D_2 antagonist properties also produce dose-related acute dystonia in nonhuman primates.[28–30,35–37]

Recent studies with D_1 antagonists also show that these compounds can produce similar types of dystonic syndromes as those seen with the pure D_2 antagonists[31,33] when the compounds are given parenterally, though this was not seen when a D_1 antagonist was given orally.[38] This issue has been framed in the context of neuroleptic sensitized monkeys showing D_1 antagonist-induced dystonia[31,33] versus neuroleptic naive monkeys not developing this syndrome.[38] However, sensitization status is not the only parameter to be considered, as oral administration in sensitized monkeys did not always produce acute dystonia.[38] This negative finding may simply be due to a low bioavailability with oral administration, since parenteral administration of both D_1 and D_2 antagonists to neuroleptic naive monkeys can produce dystonic syndromes.[39] In those studies that have evaluated anticholinergic drugs in the nonhuman primate model, these compounds reversed both the D_1 and the D_2 acute dystonic symptoms.

Dopamine plays a central role in neuroleptic-induced acute dystonia. However, two conflicting hypotheses propose that this syndrome is due to either *increased* or *decreased* dopamine neurotransmission. The *increased* dopamine (or "mismatch") hypothesis argues that neuroleptic-induced dopamine receptor blockade produces increased release of dopamine due to a compensatory feedback system.[9,40] Evidence for this increased striatal dopamine hypothesis derives from reports that levodopa can cause dyskinesias resembling acute dystonia in idiopathic parkinsonian patients and in monkeys with central nervous system lesions that receive large parenteral doses of levodopa.[5,41] Dopamine directly applied intrastriatally can also cause acute dystonia in monkeys.[42]

These data are the main points used to support the "mismatch" hypothesis of neuroleptic-induced acute dystonia.[9,41] This theory proposes that the compensatory increase in dopamine release from neuroleptic drugs overrides the dopamine receptor blockade in the nigrastriatal dopamine receptors as neuroleptic blood and brain levels decline (see *Temporal Aspects* above). Indeed, at this time, dopamine receptors may be transiently supersensitive or up-regulated in response to their blockade by the neuroleptic. However, there are several points that are not consistent with this hypothesis. With continued drug treatment on a once a day or multiple times a day dosing regimen, the blood and brain levels in patients are actually going up in each 12- or 24-hour epoch so that the drug levels at the most common times of dystonia, during the second day of neuroleptic therapy, are higher when compared to the first day of treatment. Additionally, continuous oral levodopa therapy in nonhuman primates and in nonparkinsonian patients does not produce acute dystonia.[43] Furthermore, dopamine agonists such as amphetamine, apomorphine, and levodopa can have therapeutic benefits in acute dystonia in both man and monkeys.[28,44] If neuroleptic-induced acute dystonia were due to increase dopamine neurotransmission, then dopamine agonists should aggravate rather than improve this syndrome, which appears not to be the case in the large majority of investigations.

In contrast, the hypothesis of *decreased* striatal dopamine function as the underlying pathophysiology of neuroleptic-induced acute dystonia has much data to support it. First, neuroleptics block dopamine receptors in close correlation to their clinical potency and propensity to produce acute dystonia in humans and animals.[37,45] Pretreatment with dopamine synthesis inhibitors or depleters either caused or exacerbated neuroleptic-induced dystonia in most studies.[28,37,44,46,47] However, a separate study in baboons selected for sensitivity to dystonia found that a presynaptic depleter decreased rather than increased dystonia.[48] Further supportive evidence comes from a study observing that pargyline, a monoamine oxidase inhibitor, also reduced acute dystonia in monkeys.[49] Finally, the data cited above, noting that dopamine agonists can effectively treat acute dystonia, support the proposal that this syndrome is due to decreased dopamine neurotransmission.

Cholinergic mechanisms also play an important role in neuroleptic-induced acute dystonia. Several lines of evidence come together to support a consistent database on this issue. Anticholinergic drugs reverse or prevent acute dystonia in both man and monkey.[2,28] Neuroleptics with high intrinsic anticholinergic activities have low acute dystonia rates.[2,22] Also, clozapine, an atypical neuroleptic with very high anticholinergic activity does not produce dystonia in either man or monkeys.[24,30]

Cholinergic agonists produce acute dystonia in nonhuman primates when injected intrastriatally.[42] Cholinergic agonists will also produce or aggravate neuroleptic-induced acute dystonia in monkeys.[28,44] Finally, acutely administered neuroleptic drugs lead to increased acetylcholine in the striatum.[50] This leads to an absolute increase in cholinergic function with a corresponding relative decrease in dopaminergic neurotransmission.

The role of gamma-amino-butyric acid (GABA) in acute dystonia is much less well studied. Most of the data come from studies in nonhuman primates. GABA antagonists such as picrotoxin worsen acute dystonia in monkeys, but this may be due to the compound's toxic effects and very low seizure threshold.[28] GABA agonists such as muscimol increase acute dystonia in monkeys.[28] GABA agonists tested clinically in paradigms evaluating these compounds as potential treatments for tardive dyskinesia found that acute extrapyramidal syndromes were aggravated in some patients, but there were no cases of acute dystonia precipitated by these compounds.[51,52] Two compounds with unclear mechanisms of action on the GABA system, baclofen and diazepam, decreased acute dystonia in monkeys.[44] Diazepam is an effective treatment for acute neuroleptic-induced dystonia, but baclofen has not been evaluated for this purpose.[2]

Recently, it has been proposed that serotonin plays a critical role in the neuroleptic-induced acute extrapyramidal syndromes. The serotonin type 2 (S_2) antagonists decrease catalepsy in rodents (possibly a model of neuroleptic-induced acute dystonia), leading to the hypothesis that neuroleptics with intrinsic S_2 antagonist properties or S_2 antagonists by themselves may be effective antiextrapyramidal syndrome drugs.[53,54] However, studies in nonhuman primates have not been supportive of this proposal. In one investigation, serotonin antagonists only modestly reduced dystonia,[55] but similar agents had no significant effect on neuroleptic-induced acute dystonia in another investigation.[56] Extensive studies in monkeys have evaluated compounds across a wide range of dopamine D_2 and serotonin S_2 antagonist ratios. All these compounds produced acute dystonia.[29,30] The syndromes produced by each of these different drugs were clinically identical, the only difference was the threshold dose that was required to produce such symptoms. Therefore, it appears that S_2 antagonism does not have a central role in neuroleptic-induced acute dystonia.

Finally, there is considerable interest in the role of the sigma "opiate" receptor in psychoses and the action of antipsychotic drugs.[56a] Recent evidence supports a possible role of the haloperidol-sensitive sigma receptor in the induction of acute dystonia by neuroleptics.[56b]

Treatment

Treating neuroleptic-induced acute dystonic reactions is usually straightforward. Parenteral administration of anticholinergics [e.g., benzotropine (Cogentin), biperiden (Akineton), or the antihistaminic/anticholinergic diphenhydramine (Benadryl)] is impressively effective in reversing this drug-induced dystonia. The first injection is usually effective within 15 to 20 minutes or less, though a second treatment may be necessary after 30 minutes in particularly severe cases. Rarely, a third dose is necessary. If symptoms are not substantially improved or resolved after the third parenteral treatment, a search for other underlying medical illnesses as the cause of dystonia may be fruitful. In very rare circumstances, parenteral benzodiazepines may be effective when anticholinergics or antihistaminics have failed.

Once the acute dystonic reaction has resolved, oral anticholinergics should be continued for 24 to 48 hours in view of the possibility for early recurrence.

Opinion is divided about whether to automatically continue antiextrapyramidal syndrome medicines after the first dystonic reaction or whether to wait for a second episode to develop. Either strategy has its benefits and detriments which should be evaluated in each clinical situation.

Prophylaxis with antiextrapyramidal syndrome drugs (anticholinergics, antihistiminics, or amantadine) to prevent dystonia is far more controversial. Those in favor of prophylaxis argue that dys-

tonic episodes can be frightening, painful, and occasionally dangerous, such as the laryngopharyngeal dystonias. Those against prophylaxis argue that the antiextrapyramidal syndrome medicines have
their own side effects such as memory impairment, blurred vision,
and dry mouth, which may further complicate medical illnesses.
Both sides of this controversy contend that their approach leads to
the best therapeutic outcome with the maximum of benefits and a
minimum of side effects. By achieving this balance, it is most likely
that a patient will engage in a therapeutic alliance and continue to
take the prescribed medicine. No one treatment strategy appears to
be the best approach for all patients (Fig. 4).

Prophylaxis is highly appropriate and effective when specific
conditions occur (Fig. 4).[2] These include when a patient (1) is at high
risk of acute dystonia; (2) has a predisposition to acute dystonia; or
(3) may suffer detrimental sequelae from acute dystonia, such as
when paranoid patients already believe that external forces are controlling them. A review of studies evaluating the efficacy of prophylaxis in acute dystonia and other extrapyramidal syndromes indicates that prophylaxis is clearly beneficial.[2] Two prospective
investigations including 241 patients and three retrospective studies
including 336 patients, all consistently found a statistically significant benefit of this treatment approach.[13,14,57-59] However, when
there is a low likelihood of acute dystonia, treatment with only a
neuroleptic drug and no antiextrapyramidal syndrome prophylaxis
is the preferred strategy because the additional risks of an antiextrapyramidal syndrome drug outweigh the potential minimum benefit
from protection against a low-frequency event.

Rather than attempting to apply a single-treatment strategy of
prophylaxis or no prophylaxis for all patients, it is preferred to make
an informed treatment decision that includes patient characteristics
(age, gender, prior extrapyramidal syndromes), drug factors (dose,
milligram potency, intrinsic anticholinergic activity), and temporal
aspects (time since first dose). If the choice is to use prophylaxis, this
strategy is best employed for 7 to 14 days when neuroleptics are
first initiated. Then the antiextrapyramidal syndrome drug can be
tapered over a few days so as not to cause a rebound acute dystonic
reaction. However, it may be necessary to continue the antiextrapyramidal syndrome medicines in those patients who develop other
drug-induced motor side effects such as akathisia or parkinsonism
during their treatment course with neuroleptics.

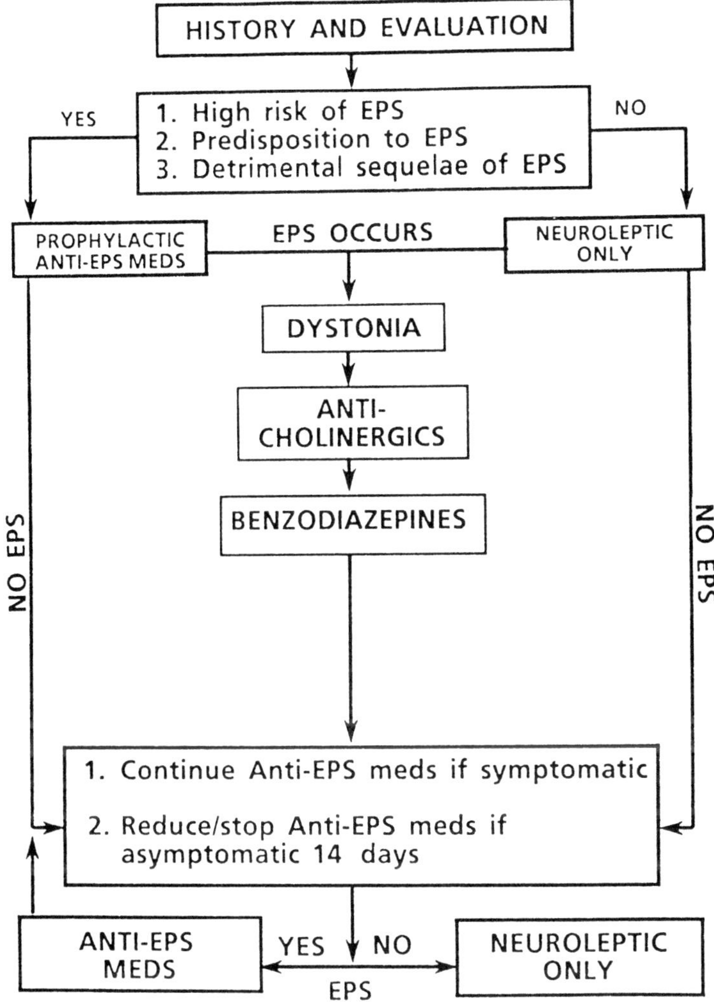

Figure 4: An algorithm for managing neuroleptic-induced acute dystonia. EPS = extrapyramidal syndrome. Adapted with permission.[2]

Future Research Trends

Unfortunately, only limited amounts of research are aimed at furthering our knowledge about neuroleptic-induced acute dystonia.

This is probably due to the perception that acute dystonia is not an important problem, particularly when its self-limited time course and very effective treatments are taken in the context of the far more troublesome extrapyramidal syndromes of akathisia and parkinsonism, as well as the long-term potentially irreversible tardive dyskinesia syndromes. The little research that is going on focuses on two areas. First is evaluating the increased versus decreased dopamine function hypotheses. The goal is to better understand the basic mechanism of action of neuroleptic drugs commonly used to treat psychosis in order to develop new agents that are free of the acute dystonia problem.

The second area of interest is to utilize the nonhuman primate model of neuroleptic-induced acute dystonia to test potential antipsychotic compounds. Compounds that do not produce this syndrome but fit other tests of antipsychotic efficacy are prime candidates for further development in the clinic. In contrast, compounds that do produce acute dystonia in monkeys are likely to do so in patients, unless the antipsychotic dose is several orders of magnitude below the acute dystonia-inducing threshold. To date, the best fit of this model is clozapine, a compound that does not produce acute dystonia in monkeys, has very little or no acute extrapyramidal syndrome liability in patients, appears not to produce TD in the clinic, and is antipsychotic.[24,30]

Summary

Neuroleptic-induced acute dystonia has had a steadily increasing prevalence/incidence due to the trend of utilizing more potent neuroleptics in higher doses over the past 35 years. Symptoms characteristically develop within the first 5 days of starting neuroleptics, with the highest frequency of symptom onset during day 2. The symptoms usually present as briefly sustained, abnormal muscular contractions of the face, head, and neck, though bizarre positions and postures of the limbs and trunk may also develop. Differential diagnosis includes the psychiatric syndromes of malingering and hysterical conversion as well as neurological syndromes of seizures, central nervous system infection, trauma, tumors, idiopathic focal or regional dystonic syndromes, and endocrinopathies. Other drug causes must also be considered in the differential diagnosis. Risk factors for developing neuroleptic-induced acute dystonia include patient characteristics (age, gender, prior symptoms), drug factors (dose, milligram potency), and temporal aspects.

The underlying pathophysiology of acute dystonia undoubtedly involves increased cholinergic mechanisms. Dopamine also plays a significant role in neuroleptic-induced acute dystonia, though it is unclear whether increased or decreased dopamine neurotransmission mediates this syndrome. Other neurotransmitters, such as GABA or serotonin, appear to play only secondary or tertiary roles. Treating acute dystonia is almost uniformly effective with anticholinergic or antihistaminic/anticholinergic agents. Benzodiazepines have been used in the uncommon situations where these other anti-extrapyramidal syndrome compounds are ineffective. Prophylaxis against neuroleptic-induced acute dystonia is controversial, although it is clearly efficacious and appropriate in selected patients. Future research efforts are aimed at understanding the basic mechanisms underlying acute dystonia and are attempting to identify compounds that are antipsychotic but do not have acute dystonia or other extrapyramidal syndromes associated with them. The ultimate goal is to develop new antipsychotic compounds with greater efficacy and little or no motor side effects.

Acknowledgments: Stefani Sackinger prepared the typescript. This work was supported in part by funds from the Veterans Administration Research Program and by NIMH Grant No. 36657.

References

1. Delay J, Deniker P, Hare JM. Utilisation en therapeutique psychiatrique d'une phenothiazine d'action centrale elective (4560 RP). Ann Medicopsychol 1952; 110:112–117.
2. Casey DE, Keepers GA. Neuroleptic side effects: acute extrapyramidal syndromes and tardive dyskinesia. In: Casey DE, Christensen AV (eds), Psychopharmacology: Current Trends, Berlin, Springer, 1988, pp 74–93.
3. Casey DE. Metoclopramide side effects. Ann Intern Med 1983; 98:673–674.
4. Chadwick D, Reynolds EH, Marsden CD. Anticonvulsant-induced dyskinesias: a comparison with dyskinesias induced by neuroleptics. J Neurol Neurosurg Psychiatry 1976; 39:1210–1218.
5. Parkes JD, Bedard P, Marsden CD. Chorea and torsion in parkinsonism. Lancet 1976; 1:155.

6. Akindele O, Odejide AO. Amodiaquine-induced involuntary movements. Br Med J 1976; 6029:214–215.

7. Umez-Eronini E, Eronini EA. Chloroquine-induced involuntary movements. Br Med J 1977; 6066:945–946.

8. Casey DE. The differential diagnosis of tardive dyskinesia. Acta Psychiat Scand 1981; 63(Suppl 291):71–87.

9. Marsden CD, Jenner P. The pathophysiology of extrapyramidal side effects of neuroleptic drugs. Psychol Med 1980; 10:55–72.

10. Ayd FJ. A survey of drug-induced extrapyramidal reactions. JAMA 1961; 175:1054–1060.

11. Groves JE, Mandel MR. The long-acting phenothiazines. Arch Gen Psychiatry 1975; 32:893–900.

12. Swett C. Drug-induced dystonia. Am J Psychiatry 1975; 132(5):532–533.

13. Keepers GA, Clappison VJ, Casey DE. Initial anticholinergic prophylaxis for neuroleptic-induced extrapyramidal syndromes. Arch Gen Psychiatry 1983; 40:1113–1117.

14. Boyer WF, Bakalar NH, Lake CR. Anticholinergic prophylaxis of acute haloperidol-induced acute dystonic reactions. J Clin Psychopharmacol 1987; 7(3):164–166.

14a. McCann UD, Penetar DM, Belenky G. Acute dystonic reaction in normal humans caused by catecholamine depletion. Clin Neuropharmacol 1990; 13:565–568.

15. Keepers G, Casey DE. Prediction of neuroleptic-induced dystonia. J Clin Psychopharmacol 1987; 7:342–344.

16. Casey DE. Tardive dyskinesia. In: Meltzer H (ed), Psychopharmacology: The Third Generation of Progress, New York, Raven Press, 1987, pp 1411–1419.

17. Keepers GA, Casey DE. Use of neuroleptic-induced extrapyramidal symptoms to predict future vulnerability to side effects. Am J Psychiatry 1991; 148(1):85–89.

18. Casey DE. Neuroleptic drug-induced extrapyramidal syndromes and tardive dyskinesia. Schizophr Res 1991; 4(2):109–120.

19. Hansen LB, Larsen NE, Vestergard P. Plasma levels of perphenazine (Trilafon) related to development of extrapyramidal side effects. Psychopharmacology 1981; 74:306–309.

20. Tune L, Coyle JT. Acute extrapyramidal side effects: serum levels of neuroleptics. Psychopharmacology 1981; 75:9–15.

21. Bateman DN, Craft AW, Nicholson E, Pearson ADJ. Dystonic reactions and the pharmacokinetics of metoclopramide in children. Br J Clin Pharmacol 1983; 15:557–559.

22. Snyder S, Greenberg D, Yamamura H. Antischizophrenic drugs and brain cholinergic receptors. Arch Gen Psychiatry 1974; 31:58–61.

23. Sayers AC, Burki HR, Ruch W, Asper H. Anticholinergic properties of antipsychotic drugs and their relation to extrapyramidal side effects. Psychopharmacology 1976; 51:15–22.

24. Casey DE. Clozapine: neuroleptic-induced EPS and tardive dyskinesia. Psychopharmacology 1989; 99:S47–S53.

25. Garver DL, Davis JM, Dekirmenjian H, Ericksen S, Gosengeld L, Hara-

szti J. Dystonic reactions following neuroleptics: time course and proposed mechanisms. Psychopharmacology 1976; 47:199–201.

26. Keepers GA, Brown WL, Casey DE. Timing of neuroleptic-induced dystonia and dystonia pathophysiology. Proc Soc Biol Psychiatry 1989; 334.

27. Farde L, Hall H, Ehrin E, Sedvall G. Quantitative analysis of D_2 dopamine receptor binding in the living human brain by PET. Science 1986; 231:258–261.

28. Casey DE, Gerlach J, Christensson E. Dopamine, acetylcholine, and GABA effects in acute dystonia in primates. Psychopharmacology 1980; 70:83–87.

29. Casey DE. Serotonergic aspects of acute extrapyramidal syndromes in nonhuman primates. Psychopharmacol Bull 1989; 25(3):457–459.

30. Casey DE. Extrapyramidal syndromes in nonhuman primates: typical and atypical neuroleptics. Psychopharmacol Bull 1991; 27(1):47–50.

31. Casey DE, Gerlach J. Is tardive dyskinesia due to dopamine hypersensitivity? Clin Neuropharmacol 1986; 9(Suppl 4):134–136.

32. Gunne LM, Barany S. Haloperidol-induced tardive dyskinesia in monkeys. Psychopharmacology 1976; 50:237–240.

33. Gerlach J, Casey DE, Kistrup K. D-1 and D-2 receptor manipulation in cebus monkeys: implication for extrapyramidal syndromes in humans. Clin Neuropharmacol 1986; 9(Suppl 4):131–133.

34. Rupniak NMJ, Jenner P, Marsden CD. Acute dystonia induced by neuroleptic drugs. Psychopharmacology 1986; 88:403–419.

35. Bedard P, Delean J, Lafleur J, Larochelle L. Haloperidol-induced dyskinesias in the monkey. Can J Neurol Sci 1977; 4:197–201.

36. Weiss B, Santelli S, Lusink G. Movement disorders induced in monkeys by chronic haloperidol treatment. Psychopharmacology 1977; 53:289–293.

37. Liebman J, Neale R. Neuroleptic-induced acute dyskinesias in squirrel monkeys: correlation with propensity to cause extrapyramidal side effects. Psychopharmacology 1980; 68:25–29.

38. Coffin VL, Latranyi MB, Chipkin RC. Acute extrapyramidal syndrome in Cebus monkeys: development mediated by dopamine D_2. J Pharmacol Exp Ther 1989; 249:769–774.

39. Casey DE. Neuroleptic drug-induced extrapyramidal syndromes: different sensitization by dopamine D_1 and D_2 antagonists. Proceedings of the 17th Congress of Collegium Internationale Neuropsychopharmacologium, 1990.

40. Kolbe H, Clow A, Jenner P, Marsden CD. Neuroleptic-induced acute dystonic reactions may be due to enhanced dopamine release on to supersensitive postsynaptic receptors. Neurology 1981; 31:434–439.

41. Sassin JF. Drug-induced dyskinesia in monkeys. In: Meldrum BS, Marsden CD (eds), Advances in Neurology: Primate Models of Neurological Disorders, vol. 10, New York, Raven Press, 1975, pp 47–54.

42. Cools AR, Hendricks G, Korten J. The acetylcholine-dopamine balance in the basal ganglia of rhesus monkeys and its role in dynamic, dystonic, dyskinetic, and epileptoid motor activities. J Neural Transm 1974; 36:91–105.

43. Paulson GW. Dyskinesias in monkeys. In: Huntington's Chorea, Advances in Neurology, vol. 1, Raven Press, New York, 1973, pp 647–650.

44. Neale R, Gerhardt S, Liebman JM. Effects of dopamine agonists, catecholamine depletors, and cholinergic and GABAergic drugs on acute dyskinesias in squirrel monkeys. Psychopharmacology 1984; 82:20–26.
45. Creese I, Burt DR, Snyder S. Dopamine receptor binding predicts clinical and pharmacological potencies of antischizophrenic drugs. Science 1976; 192:481–483.
46. Reches A, Burke RE, Kuhn CM, Hassan MN, Jackson VR, Fahn S. Tetrabenazine, an amine-depleting drug, also blocks dopamine receptors in rat brain. J Pharmacol Exp Ther 1983; 225(3):515–521.
47. Burke RE, Reches A, Traub M, Ilson J, Swash M, Fahn S. Tetrabenazine induces acute dystonic reactions. Ann Neurol 1985; 17:200–202.
48. Meldrum BS, Anlezark GM, Marsden CD. Acute dystonia as an idiosyncratic response to neuroleptics in baboons. Brain 1977; 100:313–326.
49. Heintz R, Casey DE. Pargyline reduces/prevents neuroleptic-induced acute dystonia in monkeys. Psychopharmacology 1987; 93:207–213.
50. Sethy VH, VanWoert MH. Modification of striatal acetylcholine concentration by dopamine receptor agonists and antagonists. Res Commun Chem Pathol Pharmacol 1974; 8(1):13–28.
51. Casey DE, Gerlach J, Magelund G, Rosted Christensen T. The effect of gamma-acetylenic GABA in tardive dyskinesia. Arch Gen Psychiatry 1980; 37:1376–1379.
52. Korsgaard S, Casey DE, Gerlach J. Effect of gamma-vinyl-GABA in tardive dyskinesia. Psychiatry Res 1983; 8(4):261–269.
53. Balsara JJ, Jadhav JH, Chandorkar AG. Effect of drugs influencing the central serotonergic mechanisms on haloperidol-induced catalepsy. Psychopharmacology 1979; 62:67–69.
54. Waldemier PC, Delini-Stula AA. Serotonin-dopamine interactions in the nigro-striatal system. Eur J Pharmacol 1979; 55:363–373.
55. Korsgaard S, Gerlach J, Christensson E. Behavioral aspects of serotonin-dopamine interaction in monkeys. Eur J Pharmacol 1985; 118:245–252.
56. Povlsen UJ, Noring U, Laursen AL, Korsgaard S, Gerlach J. Effects of serotonergic and anticholinergic drugs in haloperidol-induced dystonia in cebus monkeys. Clin Neuropharmacol 1986; 9(1):84–90.
56a. Deutsch SI, Weizman A, Goldman ME, Morihisa JM. The sigma receptor: a novel site implicated in psychosis and antipsychotic drug efficacy. Clin Neuropharmacol 1988; 11:105–119.
56b. Walker JM, Matsumoto MA, Bowen WD, Gans DL, Jones KD, Walker FO. Evidence for a role of haloperidol-sensitive σ-"opiate" receptors in the motor effects of antipsychotic drugs. Neurology 1988; 38:961–965.
57. Moleman P, Schmitz PJM, Ladee GA. Extrapyramidal side effects and oral haloperidol: an analysis of explanatory patient and treatment characteristics. J Clin Psychiatry 1982; 43:492–496.
58. Sramek JJ, Simpson GM, Morrison RL, Heiser JF. Anticholinergic agents for prophylaxis of neuroleptic-induced dystonic reactions: a prospective study. J Clin Psychiatry 1986; 47:305–309.
59. Winslow RS, Stillner V, Coons DJ, Robinson MW. Prevention of acute dystonic reactions in patients beginning with high-potency neuroleptics. Am J Psychiatry 1986; 143:706–710.

3

Drug-Induced Parkinsonism

Joseph H. Friedman, M.D.

The emergence of parkinsonism during chlorpromazine and reserpine therapy constitutes undoubtedly one of the most fascinating developments in psychiatric therapy.
Freyhan, 1957[1]

Introduction

Drug-induced parkinsonism (DIP) would appear to be the most straightforward of the drug-induced movement disorders.[2] In the most simplistic model, drugs that either block dopamine receptors[2,3] or deplete dopamine stores[3] cause a functional dopaminergic deficiency and thereby produce a condition that mimics idiopathic Parkinson's disease (IPD), a known dopamine deficiency state.[2] This model is heuristically valuable, but does not explain many of the observations made in this condition. This chapter will discuss what is known about DIP and the areas in which our understanding is incomplete.

History

Historically, the importance of drug-induced parkinsonism in understanding IPD cannot be overemphasized.[4] Although the neuro-

Lang AE, Weiner WJ (editors): *Drug-Induced Movement Disorders*, Mount Kisco, NY, © Futura Publishing Co., Inc., 1992.

pathology of IPD was relatively well understood by the 1920s, the biochemistry was not, until 1960.[5] Animal studies had demonstrated that reserpine acted by depleting catecholamine stores and that sufficiently high but nontoxic doses induced an akinetic syndrome in animals.[4] It was later noted in human studies that reserpine, when used for treating psychiatric disorders, often induced a syndrome identical to IPD.[3] This observation led to the momentous discovery that catecholamine stores were depleted in IPD and that dopamine, in particular, was drastically reduced.[5] Developments soon documented that this deficiency was in fact key to understanding IPD and led directly to the development of L-dopa and its use in treating IPD.[4,6]

For many years, it was debated whether DIP was required for an antipsychotic effect[3,7] or whether DIP was an untoward toxic effect of all known neuroleptic drugs. It has even been suggested that IDP protects against schizophrenia and vice versa. It has become clear in recent years that antipsychotic effects do not require the imposition of parkinsonism and that IPD and schizophrenia do not preclude each other.[8]

The importance of understanding neuroleptic side effects is not limited to psychiatrists and neurologists. The increasing population of elderly patients has resulted in a dramatically increased number of demented patients who have a wide spectrum of associated behavioral problems, often requiring treatment with antipsychotic drugs. Thus, virtually all physicians who see adult patients are confronted with those suffering from dementia and behavioral problems. As a result, antipsychotic medications are among the most commonly prescribed drugs in North America.

While DIP occurs mainly in patients treated for psychiatric disorders, increasing use of the antiemetics prochlorperazine (Compazine) and droperidol (Inapsine) and the gastric motility enhancer, metoclopramide (Reglan), has made recognition of DIP important in nonpsychiatric patients. Alpha-methyldopa, although rarely a cause of parkinsonism, is so commonly used as an antihypertensive that it too should be recognized as a potentially offending agent. New calcium channel blocking drugs, not yet approved in the United States, also are known to cause DIP (see chapter 12 for a discussion of movement disorders complicating alpha-methyldopa and calcium channel blocking drugs).

Clinical Aspects

The DIP Syndrome

Drug-induced parkinsonism cannot be clinically distinguished from IPD.[9] It can be defined as an akinetic rigid syndrome induced by pharmacological agents. The cardinal features are: rigidity, akinesia, bradykinesia, tremor at rest, and postural instability. Minor features that are helpful in the diagnosis include micrographia, seborrhea, and changes in speech. The *rigidity* is often described as cogwheeling in nature but is not always. The finding of cogwheeling rigidity is not pathognomonic of parkinsonism and may be difficult to distinguish from "gegenhalten" or paratonia, a resistance to passive movement caused by frontal lobe dysfunction. The rigidity can be appreciated by the examination of the elbows, wrists, and neck, but it may also affect other joints. It can often be brought out by reinforcement maneuvers such as opening and closing the nonexamined hand. The rigidity is not uniform and often affects one joint more than another in the same limb and one side more than the other.

Akinesia refers to a relative paucity of spontaneous, generally automatic and unconscious movements that are part of the normal resting repertoire. Akinetic patients blink less than normals, thus appearing to stare (the "reptilian stare"). They swallow less than normals, causing pooling of saliva and a tendency to drool. They exhibit fewer unconscious movements at rest such as crossing their legs while sitting or touching their hands to their face. The lack of such "natural" movements is often overlooked by inexperienced observers but is as obvious to trained observers as tremor and leads to an immediate diagnosis. The "masked facies" of parkinsonism, or facial hypomimia, is the result of akinesia and rigidity of the facial muscles.

Bradykinesia refers to slowness of movement. This can be demonstrated by observing how the patient performs various tasks. We often rate bradykinesia by asking the patient to tap fingers together or open and close a hand as fast as possible. More demanding tasks such as buttoning a shirt or putting on a coat reveal how severely compromised a patient may be in activities of daily living. In IPD, bradykinesia is one of the most debilitating features of the illness.

It is important to note that akinesia and bradykinesia, while often thought to be synonymous, are not. Frequently, patients will perform remarkably well on timed tasks, indicating only a mild degree of bradykinesia, while being profoundly akinetic. There are rare patients who exhibit "kinesia paradoxica," a condition in which severely akinetic subjects respond more quickly than expected when faced with startling or threatening stimuli. The tremor of DIP may be mild or severe. Typically it involves the fingers or the hands but may involve the jaw, feet, or tongue. It is uncommon to involve the head, although with a severe tremor that emanates from the elbow or shoulder, one often sees a reflection or conducted movement that involves the head passively. The tremor is present at rest and often with the arms held in a fixed posture, but usually resolves with movement. The "pill rolling" tremor of parkinsonism refers to a finger tremor, in which the thumb and opposing fingers appear to be rolling a pill back and forth in the hand. It is less common than hand tremor and is often absent. Because the tremor is often present in sustained postures, it can severely interfere with important functions of everyday living such as eating and writing. The *tremor,* present at rest, resolves as the patient picks up the utensil but recurs as the hand is positioned over the target, whether a pile of peas, a bowl of soup, or a writing pad. It resolves as the hand moves but then recurs as the fork or spoon stops to deliver its contents to the mouth. Patients also taking lithium may have a more prominent action tremor in addition to a resting and sustension tremor induced by a neuroleptic, complicating the clinical picture.

Postural instability refers to a diminished response to postural displacements resulting in loss of balance. In normal humans, the maintenance of the upright posture requires continuous muscle contractions. With perturbations induced by outside forces, the body reflexively attempts to maintain its center of balance to keep from falling. When a normal subject is pulled backwards, the arms go up in front and backward steps are taken. If a fall is imminent, the arms go up to break the fall if the subject is moving forward or to the side. The knees buckle to allow a cushioned landing on the buttocks if the fall is backwards. In parkinsonism, these responses are impaired. Subjects may take many steps, often increasing in frequency as they decrease in amplitude (festination) (retropulsion if pulled or falling backward) and they may fail to put out their arms entirely. Thus a parkinsonian may fall like a stiff board when knocked off balance and strike the occiput or the face, depending on the direction of the fall.

The *posture* of parkinsonism probably in part reflects truncal rigidity. Patients have stooped shoulders suggestive of accelerated aging, often referred to as a "simian posture" (ape-like). When advanced in the process, they are flexed at all joints. The gait has a normal narrow base but the stride is reduced from normal. Arm swing is also reduced and may be absent entirely. In severe cases, the arms are flexed at the elbows even while the patient is walking, producing an appearance much like the arm posture of hemiparetic patients after a stroke. Tremor in the hands and fingers is often evident during walking and may become more pronounced at this time. Shuffling is common in severe cases and some patients develop a tendency to run forward with increasingly small steps, the "festinating gait" of Parkinson's disease. Turning may be problematic, with patients turning "en bloc," that is, in one piece, requiring several steps rather than a pivot. Turning is a maneuver that is commonly associated with falls in subjects with advanced parkinsonism.

One generally conceives of toxic and metabolic derangements as causing symmetrical, nonfocal deficits. In DIP, as in IPD, asymmetry is common and should not be misconstrued as evidence against the correct diagnosis. Tremor, stiffness, akinesia, and bradykinesia may all be more prominent on one side, even to the extent that a parkinsonian sign is present only on one side. An occasional patient may have more facial hypomimia on one side and appear to have facial muscle weakness due to loss of wrinkling and an increased palpebral fissure on the affected side. The distribution of parkinsonian signs may be different in DIP and IPD, but a large study with age-matched groups would be necessary for comparison.

In a recent study[9] of 26 patients, median age 61, with DIP, the major sign of parkinsonism was rigidity in 18, bradykinesia in 14, tremor in 13, and gait abnormality in 5. The signs were asymmetrical in 14, and 11 had associated tardive dyskinesia (TD). In IPD, tremor is thought to be present in 80% of cases.

Some parkinsonian features may be intrinsic to the psychiatric illness and may not necessarily represent medication effect.[10] For example, depressed and catatonic patients may be akinetic and bradykinetic. This was noted in a large double-blind study[10] comparing neuroleptics and placebo for efficacy in treating psychosis. Signs of parkinsonism were identified as part of the general adverse effects screened. Since the age of the patients was very young (mean age

Table 1

Incidence in Percent of Parkinsonian Features in NIMH Study[10]

	Chlorpromazine	Fluphenazine	Thioridazine	Placebo
Facial rigidity	12.5	14.3	8.8	5.4
Tremors Loss of	5.7	12.1	13.2	5.4
associated movements	3.4	19.8	0.0	2.7

28.2), the incidence of parkinsonism was not great. Of particular note in this study was the incidence of parkinsonian features in placebo-treated subjects (Table 1), which could be explained either by poor assessment techniques or the natural occurrence of parkinsonian signs among psychotic patients. The youth of the subjects makes it unlikely that IPD was the explanation for the placebo-induced parkinsonism. Although patients may develop incapacitating parkinsonism that can mimic catatonia, patients are often unaware of their signs.[11,12] In general, patients with DIP are aware mainly of their tremor.[12] When tremor is absent, there are frequently no symptoms to correlate with the signs of rigidity and akinesia.

A rare form of DIP is the *rabbit syndrome*. It does not look like typical IPD. The "rabbit syndrome" is a peculiar-appearing disorder, aptly named,[13] that was only recognized in 1972. Patients exhibit "perioral muscular movements strikingly imitating the rapid chewing-like movements of a rabbit's mouth."[13] The tongue is said not to be involved. The syndrome is typically due to a tremor of the lips and perioral region. It is generally believed that this is a restricted form of DIP that responds to anticholinergic medications in the same fashion as the more typical resting limb tremor. Irregular lip movements and nasal flaring in some patients with TD may cause diagnostic confusion.

Differential Diagnosis

When all the features of parkinsonism are present and a history of drug exposure is obtained, the diagnosis is simple. Mild parkinsonism is more difficult to diagnose, and there is a large gray zone in which the transition from normal to abnormal occurs. This explains why DIP and IPD may have different clinical spectrums. The former has a high incidence in psychiatric patients where it is common to observe only asymptomatic facial hypomimia or a mildly stooped posture with diminished arm swing in screening surveys searching for DIP in at-risk populations. On the other hand, IPD patients generally seek help only when symptomatic or when some abnormality is noted by an observer.

When patients are evaluated for parkinsonism, a complete drug history is mandatory. The effects of neuroleptics can persist for surprisingly long periods, and sensitivity to the extrapyramidal effects of these drugs is surprisingly varied.

There are two clinical settings in which the differential diagnosis of DIP is important. Most commonly encountered is the older patient, on a stable dose of neuroleptic for many years without apparent adverse effects, who develops signs of parkinsonism. The question then arises as to whether the patient has IPD or DIP, with IPD being "unmasked" prematurely[14] by the dopamine receptor blockade. The alternative explanation is that the patient has simply become more sensitive to the neuroleptic[15] with aging. In either case, discontinuation of the neuroleptic, when possible, should ameliorate the syndrome, although the time course for this may be well over a year.[9,16] In the course of a year or more, if the neuroleptic is stopped, DIP should improve significantly and then resolve, whereas IPD always worsens after the improvement gained by stopping the neuroleptic recedes.

Less common, but more important is the clinical distinction between catatonia and severe DIP. Quite clearly the treatment is very different. While the obvious diagnostic differences include waxy flexibility versus cogwheeling rigidity, muteness versus dysarthria, absence of tremor in catatonia, and parkinsonian gait in DIP, these distinctions may prove difficult to elicit in practice. The catatonic may not keep his arms in a statuesque posture and probably won't attempt to walk. In addition, the catatonic patient is likely to have received neuroleptics, further complicating the picture. On the other hand, the patient with DIP may be psychotic and uncooperative and refuse to allow a full examination, leaving the examiner uncertain as to what degree of akinesia is drug-induced and how much is catatonia. Gait analysis may not be possible if the patient is uncooperative. Luckily, catatonia is rare and the history will hopefully help clear up the dilemma. When the history is unknown, the diagnosis may well be in doubt.

Other causes of parkinsonism aside from IPD must also be considered in the differential diagnosis. A long list of disorders including degenerative diseases, toxins, tumors, and hydrocephalus may cause parkinsonism. Certain of these may also cause psychiatric disorders early in the course. Progressive parkinsonism may then be mistakenly ascribed to the neuroleptics used for these psychiatric features rather than to a primary brain disorder causing both problems. Wilson's disease is probably the most important condition with potential to cause this scenario in view of its treatability and universally fatal outcome if the diagnosis is missed. In young people, Huntington's disease may occur in the "rigid form" which can be mistaken for Parkinson's disease.

Factitious parkinsonism is extremely rare. To make the diagnosis, the examiner must attempt to divert the patient or to observe the patient when the subject is unaware of the surveillance. A sodium amytal interview may also be considered. Depending on the underlying psychiatric problem, neuroleptics may even be helpful!

Clinical Course

Probably the most cited paper evaluating extrapyramidal drug side effects is that of Ayd.[15] It is the largest survey, looking at 3775 patients, and provides the broadest sweep of clinical overviews. Ayd reported that DIP generally occurs later than akathisia and dystonia, with 90% of cases developing within the first 72 days but that time of onset varied with the mode of drug administration (Fig. 1). He noted that patients complained of prodromal symptoms before the parkinsonism was evident. These consisted of weakness, paresthesias, and joint pains, mainly in limbs later affected by the DIP. Patients with the syndrome were "constantly aware of fatigue" in affected limbs. These descriptions are in contrast to other observations[11,12] and may reflect differences in the populations under study. Akinetic patients were apathetic and were less active.

The initial signs of DIP were rigidity and impaired arm swing in 65% of patients, with tremor heralding the syndrome onset in about 35%. The tremor usually began asymmetrically in an arm. Tremor eventually developed in 60% of patients. This is in contrast to IPD in which 80% of patients develop tremor.

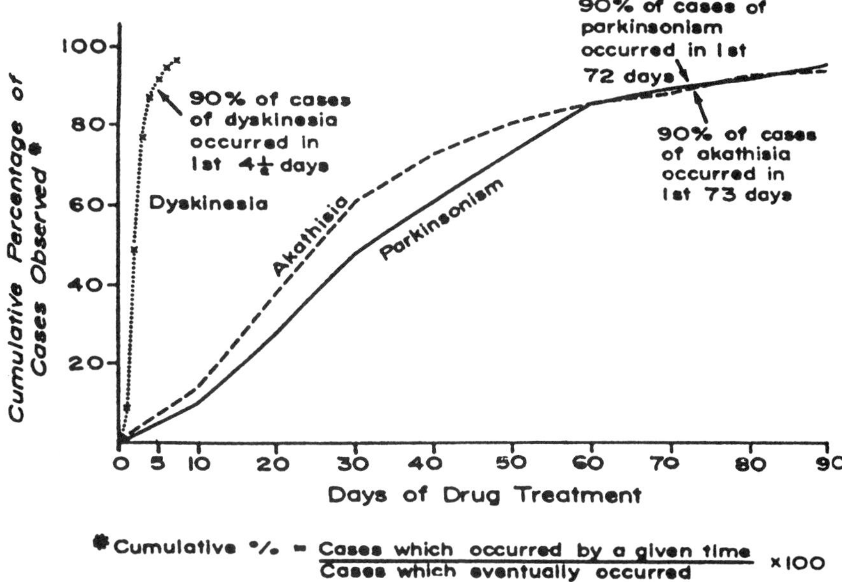

Figure 1: Drug-induced extrapyramidal reactions: time for onset.[15]

Freyhan[17] had reported earlier that the great majority of patients developed parkinsonism before the 20th day, whereas Medinar et al.[18] found that the majority of patients developed parkinsonism within the first week. A recent study[19] reported that with haloperidol, time of onset of parkinsonism was dose-related and that higher doses began producing akinesia within 2 weeks.

The natural course of DIP with continued drug exposure is unknown. Patients successfully treated with antiparkinson drugs for DIP can often have these drugs discontinued without a recurrence of DIP. This suggests that DIP is often a temporary phenomenon that ameliorates with time. Animal data[20,21] show that chronic exposure to dopamine receptor blocking agents causes an increase in dopamine turnover and alters the sensitivity of dopamine receptors. Thus, compensatory mechanisms occur in animals that, if present in humans, could explain a decline in parkinsonism in people chronically exposed to receptor-blocking drugs.

There are conflicting reports regarding the decline in DIP over time. One study[22] reports resolution within 2 months. In another study of patients who had taken trifluoperazine for over 3 years, 27 of 63 continued to have tremor and 24 had rigidity. This DIP prevalence of almost 50% was seen despite concurrent anticholinergic therapy in most cases.[23] Yet another report found that chronic antiparkinsonism therapy was rarely required, with only 9 out of 1000 chronic patients receiving it.[24] This of course only implies that severe, chronic DIP is uncommon but it does not help in assessing the actual incidence of the syndrome. Many reports document the tolerability of antiparkinson drug discontinuation.

Special Aspects

Drug-Induced Parkinsonism in the Elderly

The elderly may be at increased risk for DIP.[15,23] If true, this could relate to the increasing likelihood of IPD in this age group or it could simply be due to the diminished number of nigral dopaminergic neurons. Both of these changes would increase the sensitivity to dopamine agonists that occurs with normal aging. If DIP is more common in women,[15] as is reported in some studies (but not all[23]), then the increased incidence of DIP in the elderly would only be partly explained by subclinical IPD, as IPD is more common in men.[25]

In a prospective study, 9% of all new cases referred to a geriatrics unit had parkinsonism and of this total of 95 cases, 51% were drug-induced.[26] The most common offending agent was prochlorperazine (Compazine), an antiemetic, which the authors felt was not indicated in even a single case. The clinical features of DIP, difficulty turning in bed, rigidity, and tremor, were similar to those encountered in IPD. Twenty-five percent of the DIP patients couldn't walk, 60% gave a history of falls, and 45% required hospital admission. The DIP persisted for a mean of 7 weeks (range 1–36) before resolution in the two out of three who resolved during the study. Of special note was the later development of parkinsonism presumably due to IPD in five patients (11%) within 18 months, a higher number than anticipated in an age-matched control population. Interestingly, only 25% of referring physicians had recognized the parkinsonism.

The prognostic implications of recognizing DIP in the elderly are great since the disorder may not be benign.[27] Fifty-four percent of the elderly with DIP in one study died within 41 months of diagnosis, a far higher rate than expected for healthy, age-matched controls. Whether the mortality rate is higher for age in medically matched controls is unknown. This study found that 25% of DIP patients developed IPD within 41 months of drug discontinuation.

These studies emphasize the problems associated with parkinsonism in the elderly. The diagnosis of IPD cannot be made in a patient who has received dopamine antagonists within the past year or more unless the parkinsonism has slowly worsened off the drug. IPD develops in up to 25% of the elderly with DIP, presumably reflecting the extra sensitivity to dopamine blockade in pre- clinical IDP. And finally, the presence of DIP forewarns of a poor prognosis. It is associated with falling, gait dysfunction, prolonged hospitalization, and increased mortality. Of course, it is not simply the DIP that determines this prognosis. Undoubtedly, the indications for neuroleptic use also play a role.

DIP and Tardive Dyskinesia

The coexistence of DIP and tardive dyskinesia is a relatively common although not well-known fact. The heuristic concept of parkinsonism representing a dopamine deficiency state and tardive dyskinesia representing a dopamine excess state is clearly violated in its most simple formulation by the concurrence of these syndromes.

Richardson and Craig[28] surveyed 132 patients at a state psychiatric hospital of whom 91% were on neuroleptics and found that 28% had TD only, 19.7% had DIP only, while 17.4% had both. There were no significant differences in neuroleptic dose, duration of exposure, or antiparkinson drug use. Crane[29] had similar results in a population that was probably comparable (chronic state psychiatric in-patients). At the Institute of Mental Health,[30] the only state psychiatric hospital in Rhode Island, a survey of the entire in-patient population, acute and chronic patients, revealed a smaller percentage of patients with both syndromes, but the combination was not rare.

The coexistence of TD and DIP is analogous to the situation of the IPD patient with L-dopa-induced dyskinesias. In such a case, the patient may still be bradykinetic and rigid while showing obvious chorea. The explanation presumably lies in the differences in altered biochemistry occurring simultaneously in different regions of the brain. Thus in TD, the presumed receptor alterations have a predisposition, for unknown reasons, to affect neurons controlling the oral and facial regions (see Chapter 5). With an increase in dopamine blockade, the TD usually decreases (is masked) and parkinsonism develops. The relative balance between the receptor supersensitivity (hypothesized to account for TD) in certain brain regions involved in generating TD versus dopamine receptor blockade in those controlling other body segments may determine whether or not the TD is suppressed before DIP appears.

Withdrawal Emergent Parkinsonism

An unexplained and rarely reported[34,35] form of DIP is that caused by neuroleptic withdrawal ("withdrawal emergent parkinsonism"). In a single case study,[34] the first patient reported with this syndrome developed rigidity, drooling, and shuffling gait over a 2-week interval as thioridazine 100 mg, chlorpromazine 150 mg, and flurazepam 30 mg daily were tapered to a final schedule of chlorpromazine 50 mg daily. The syndrome rapidly responded to the addition of benztropine.

A second report[35] concerned a prospective study of abrupt neuroleptic withdrawal in 15 long-term hospitalized schizophrenics on chronic neuroleptics (mean dose 1081 chlorpromazine equivalents). Those taking anticholinergics had them withdrawn 5 to 7 days before the neuroleptic. Six patients developed new or worsened parkinsonism within 1 to 4 days of neuroleptic withdrawal. Three had not been on anticholinergics, and the other three had not worsened when the anticholinergics were stopped. All six had rest tremor, two were hypokinetic, two had excess salivation, and four had seborrhea. Two of these patients had choreoathetoid movements prior to the neuroleptic withdrawal. Of special note was the transient nature of the syndrome in one patient, lasting only for a few hours and the remarkable responsiveness to treatment of the DIP with either anticholinergics or neuroleptics. Two of these patients were taking only haloperidol, whereas three were taking a combination of low- and high-potency neuroleptics.

The authors of these reports provide no adequate explanation for their observations. This phenomenon certainly contradicts the simplistic theory that neuroleptics act primarily by blocking dopamine receptors and suggests a more complex set of actions for these drugs. It is troubling, however, that a syndrome that occurred in 40% of an unselected group of subjects is not recognized more often.

Abrupt discontinuation of neuroleptics is common among psychiatric patients, yet withdrawal emergent parkinsonism is almost unknown. Further corroborative reports will be required before the syndrome of withdrawal emergent parkinsonism can be generally accepted.

Epidemiology

Risk Factors

While a number of risk factors have been tentatively identified for the development of DIP, few have been confirmed by later studies and contradictory reports are common. Only one fact is unambiguous. All studies have demonstrated a rather remarkable individual variation in susceptibility to the extrapyramidal effects of dopamine-blocking drugs. This fact was noted as early 1957[1]: " . . . our observations reveal that neither drug quantity nor treatment duration can account for the severity of extrapyramidal symptoms." The author then went on to suggest that DIP subjects may have had an increased incidence of neurological disorders, brain injury, and subnormal intellect in family members, but he lacked sufficient data to compare this information on DIP subjects to non-DIP subjects.

The purported major risk factors for the development of DIP are: sex, age, drug potency, and drug dose.[36] These are potential risk factors only and individual patients with all of these predispositions may not develop any extrapyramidal syndromes (EPS).

Ayd conducted the first major study of the clinical epidemiology of DIP.[15] He identified three risk factors for DIP: female gender, old age, and the use of high-potency neuroleptics. Ayd surveyed 3775 phenothiazine-treated patients for all identifiable extrapyramidal reactions. All subjects had been taking high-potency medications for 3 months to 6 years. Since he used a classification system that allowed only one adverse effect per patient, his numbers may be artificially low. He observed (1) that women were almost twice as likely to suffer DIP than males in all age groups except for those below 10 and above 80 years old (both groups had small numbers of patients); (2) that DIP was related to drug potency with trifluoperazine causing a 42% higher incidence than chlorpromazine (chlorpromazine equivalent doses for the drugs were not given); and (3) that older patients

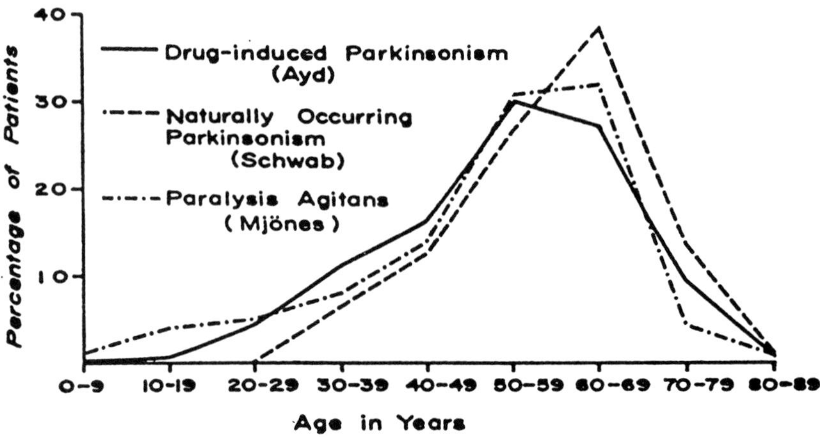

Figure 2: Parkinsonism: age distribution.[15]

were at greater risk than the younger in both sexes (Fig. 2). However, like Freyhan,[1] he noted that 61% of the patients had no extrapyramidal signs and that many of these were on larger doses of neuroleptics than those suffering from EPS. The NIMH study of 1964[10] also documented the relationship between DIP and potency of neuroleptic with thioridazine and chlorpromazine causing less DIP than fluphenazine. This study did not comment on age or sex factors.

These observations, although generally accepted,[36] are not universally supported. Other studies have found no sex differences[23] and even age as a risk factor has been contested.[37] In IPD, there is a clear male predilection,[25] so that the reversal of sex predominance in DIP, if true, is perhaps surprising.

Many other potential risk factors have been explored. Myrianthopoulos et al.,[38] noting that many cases of IPD appeared to be inherited in an autosomal dominant fashion, evaluated family history of parkinsonism as a potential risk factor. Detailed family histories on psychiatric patients taking neuroleptics were obtained, 59 of whom had moderate to severe DIP and 67 of whom were without any signs of parkinsonism (controls), despite being on neuroleptics. They found a history of parkinsonism in 15 relatives of patients in the first group but in only three relatives of the controls, concluding that there may be a familial susceptibility to DIP. Unfortunately, although the patients and controls were matched for age, gender, and drug exposure, the identification of affected family members was based solely on history. The authors repeated their study[39] and again found similar results but only for American Caucasian patients, not for Afro-Americans. This racial discrepancy may be real since there is some evidence that Afro-Americans are less prone to IPD than American Caucasians,[25] although no data exist on the relative risks of race on DIP.

Pursuing the possibility of an hereditary predisposition to DIP, one group of investigators[40] performed HLA typing in 52 chronically hospitalized schizophrenic white men on neuroleptics. They found a single antigen, B44, significantly more common in the group with DIP than in the group without. This antigen had not been associated with IPD in previous HLA studies. The authors speculated on a variety of potential mechanisms to explain this association, although the possibility of a chance association in one of 80 antigens tested must be entertained. Thus, a comparable study from a different center will be required to confirm these results.

A puzzling risk factor cited for DIP is taste sensitivity for quinine. One study found that more sensitive tasters had a greater sensitivity to DIP at low doses of trifluoperazine yet less sensitivity at high doses.[41]

Brain damage has been implicated as a risk factor for DIP in some other studies. For example, 11 of 18 lobotomized schizophrenics[43] suffered DIP whereas only 3 of 11 nonlobotomized had DIP despite their use of lower doses of anticholinergics. This result, however, was not found in another group of leukotomized patients.[43] In a separate study looking at the effects of structural brain damage, the lateral ventricular size as measured by the ventricular to brain ratio (VBR) was found to correlate with DIP in patients taking the same doses of chlorpromazine.[44] However, DIP was defined as the ward physicians' use of antiparkinson medication. In addition, there was not a one-to-one correlation between VBR and DIP. Some normal controls and non-DIP neuroleptic-treated patients had larger VBR than some patients with DIP.

Serum levels of neuroleptic have been shown to correlate only variably with DIP.[40,45–47] However, the question of a relationship between DIP and serum levels of neuroleptic is somewhat misleading since DIP may persist for months after a drug is discontinued.[16] In such cases, the serum drug level may be zero but the dopamine receptors in the brain may remain strongly blocked.

The question of a correlation between DIP and psychiatric response has been debated. Alpert et al.[48] found that DIP, as measured by tremor in a single finger, was dose-related and negatively correlated with psychiatric response. This has not been confirmed with repeat studies, and such studies are complicated by the dissociation between the temporal motor and psychiatric responses to neuroleptics.

Neuroleptic potency and neuroleptic dose are unequivocal risk factors for DIP. Increasing age and brain damage are possible predisposing factors. However, the development of DIP is notoriously unpredictable. In one study, a patient receiving 480 mg trifluoperazine had no DIP,[49] and I have seen a patient on long-term haloperidol 200 mg/d without parkinsonism.

Pathophysiology

Pharmacology

The term "neuroleptic" was coined by Delay and Deniker and is used in a somewhat arbitrary fashion.[21] Delay and Deniker used the term, literally meaning "that which grips the nerve," to refer to all antipsychotic drugs.[21] Some authorities include dopamine depleting drugs such as reserpine and tetrabenazine,[20] whereas others only include antipsychotic drugs that block dopamine receptors.[21] In common neurological parlance, the term "neuroleptic" is used to mean a dopamine receptor-blocking drug, including the antipsychotics, the antiemetics, and metoclopramide. The latter drugs, if used in high doses, also possess some antipsychotic efficacy. Dopamine-depleting drugs are usually considered separately.

The Five General Categories of Neuroleptic Drugs

Phenothiazines

This class of drug has the general structure shown in Figure 3, which is tricyclic. Replacements at R_1 and R_2 determine the nature of the drug. The presence of a halogen at R_1 is evidently essential for neuroleptic activity since other substitutions will impart many phenothiazine actions without significant antipsychotic properties. Phenothiazines are classified into three groups depending on

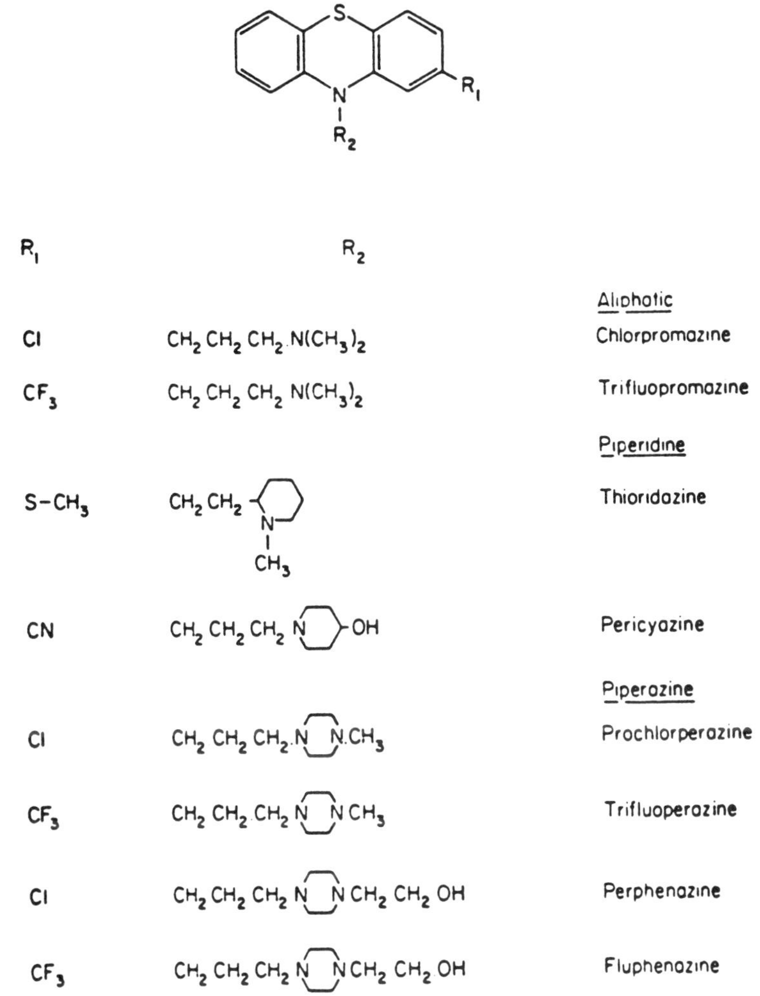

Figure 3: The chemical structures of some phenothiazine neuroleptics.[20]

R_1	R_2	
		Aliphatic
Cl	$CH_2 CH_2 CH_2 N(CH_3)_2$	Chlorpromazine
CF_3	$CH_2 CH_2 CH_2 N(CH_3)_2$	Trifluopromazine
		Piperidine
$S-CH_3$	$CH_2 CH_2$ (piperidine, N–CH_3)	Thioridazine
CN	$CH_2 CH_2 CH_2 N$ (ring)–OH	Pericyazine
		Piperazine
Cl	$CH_2 CH_2 CH_2 N$—$N \cdot CH_3$	Prochlorperazine
CF_3	$CH_2 CH_2 CH_2 N$—$N CH_3$	Trifluoperazine
Cl	$CH_2 CH_2 CH_2 N$—$N CH_2 CH_2 OH$	Perphenazine
CF_3	$CH_2 CH_2 CH_2 N$—$N CH_2 CH_2 OH$	Fluphenazine

whether the R_2 side chain is an aliphatic, a piperidine, or a pipera-zine. The piperidine drugs tend to be more sedating, while the piper-azines are generally less sedating, with more potent antipsychotic efficacy and with a greater tendency to induce extrapyramidal ad-verse effects. These drugs in general tend to have additional pro-nounced antihistaminic and anticholinergic properties.

Butyrophenones

These drugs evolved from studies aimed at finding analgesics related to meperidine (Demerol). In animal models, they shared properties with chlorpromazine rather than narcotics. The butyrophenones in common use are haloperidol and droperidol. The latter is primarily used for induction in anesthesia and as an antiemetic. They tend to be nonsedating and lack the antihistaminic and anticholinergic properties of the phenothiazines.

Thioxanthenes

The structure of these drugs is similar to that of the phenothiazines with the substitution of a carbon for a nitrogen atom where the R_2 chain attaches. The compounds resulting from substitution of identical R_2 side chains in the phenothiazine and thioxanthene rings result in compounds with similar pharmacology.

Dibenzazepines

These are also tricyclic compounds but with a structure different from the phenothiazines and thioxanthenes. Loxapine and clozapine are two commercially available antipsychotics from this group with very different properties. While loxapine is similar to other standard neuroleptics, clozapine is classified as an "atypical" neuroleptic because of its failure to induce extrapyramidal syndromes, yet its antipsychotic efficacy is as good or better than other neuroleptics.

Substituted benzamides

These drugs derive from studies of procainamide. Only metoclopramide (Reglan) is used in this country, but not as an antipsychotic. Sulpiride and tiapride have been used elsewhere for their antidyskinetic properties. Remoxipride is another of the "atypical" neuroleptic class of drugs.

Catecholamine-Depleting Agents

Reserpine is a naturally occurring substance derived from the rauwolfia shrub. It acts to deplete intraneuronal catecholamines by blocking their reuptake. Tetrabenazine also acts to deplete intraneuronal catecholamine stores but is less potent than reserpine. The action of tetrabenazine is considerably shorter than reserpine, so that adverse effects reverse more readily and the onset of action is quicker. However, tetrabenazine, in addition to depleting catecholamines, also may block dopamine receptors.[50] Alphamethyltyrosine (metyrosine) is a competitive inhibitor of tyrosine hydroxylase, the rate-limiting enzyme that converts tyrosine to diorthophenylalanine (levodopa) in the synthesis of dopamine, norepinephrine, and epinephrine. It depletes catecholamine stores by reducing synthesis.

Mechanisms of Action

All neuroleptics (if one excludes the catecholamine depletors) block dopamine receptors.[51] With the exception of clozapine and remoxipride, they induce similar biochemical, physiological, and behavioral changes in animals and presumably in man. In animals, they induce catalepsy (the prolonged maintenance of abnormal postures), reduce aggressive and hostile behavior, and decrease normal exploratory and locomotor behavior. In humans, they lessen emotions and interest in the environment in normal controls, and they reduce psychotic symptoms in psychiatric patients. They inhibit the actions of dopamine agonists in animals such as apomorphine-induced motor and stereotypic behaviors, vomiting, and climbing. The neuroleptics have diverse profiles with respect to which dopamine agonist actions they antagonize best. For example, some are better or worse than others in inducing catalepsy or in reducing vomiting.

There are several dopaminergic systems within the brain but the one that is particularly important in understanding parkinsonism is the nigrostriatal pathway. Within this and the other dopamine systems there have been at least three classes of dopamine receptors identified, each of which has a high and low affinity state.[52] The D_1 receptor is linked to adenylate cyclase and the D_2 receptor is not. The D_2 receptor has been most closely linked to both the parkinsonian side effects of neuroleptics and to the antipsychotic properties of these drugs. Neuroleptics vary considerably in their affinity for the D_2 receptor. This has been most extensively studied in the striatum (Table 2, Fig. 4). The importance of the D_1 receptor has still not been elucidated and has been described as "a receptor in search of a function."[53] This search constitutes an active area of

Table 2

Affinities of Neuroleptics for the Dopamine (D-2) Receptor of Human Brain Caudate Nucleus[103]

Neuroleptics	Affinity*
Spiperone**	625
cis-Thiothixene	222
Fluphenazine	125
d-Butaclamol**	116
Perphenazine	71
Trifluoperazine	38
Triflupromazine	36
Haloperidol	25
Prochlorperazine	14
Chlorprothixene	13
Mesoridazine	5.3
Chlorpromazine	53
Thioridazine	3.8
Loxapine	1.4
Molindone	0.83
Promazine	0.62
Clozapine**	0.56

* $10^{-7} \times 1/K_D$, where K_D = equilibrium dissociation constant in molarity.
** Not available for clinical use in the US.

neuropharmacology research.[54] The recent successful cloning of this receptor should encourage rapid advances in our understanding of its function. The existence of a D_3 receptor has only recently been demonstrated[55] with properties significantly different than the D_1 and D_2. Like D_2 receptors, D_3 receptors are not linked to adenyl cyclase. Unlike D_2 receptors, D_3 receptors are not located in the posterior pituitary gland. Neuroleptic binding profiles are different for each of the three receptor types.

Different regions of the brain have different ratios of D_1 and D_2 receptors,[56] and some drugs appear to have differential dopamine receptor binding affinities in different brain loci[57] despite the apparent uniformity of the dopamine receptors in these different regions. These facts, along with differing dopamine receptor binding affinities and anticholinergic potencies (Table 3) may help explain the variable extrapyramidal profiles of the neuroleptic drugs.

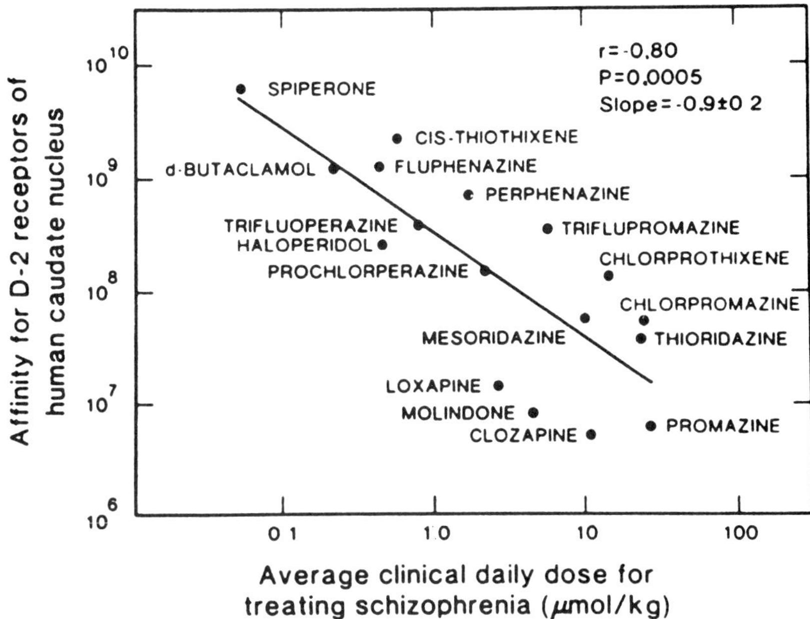

* **The equation for this regression is y = 8.5 + 0.92 × (r = − 0.80; p = .0005).**

Figure 4: Relationship between neuroleptics for the dopamine (D_2) receptor of human brian caudate nucleus and average daily dose for treating schizophrenia.[103]

The blockade of dopamine receptors by neuroleptics results in two further effects over time: an increase in dopamine synthesis and an increase in the number of dopamine receptors[21] (denervation supersensitivity). The drugs also affect nondopaminergic systems.[51] Most have a certain degree of antimuscarinic (anticholinergic) activity, with butyrophenones having the least and the atypical drugs such as clozapine having the most (Table 3).

The phenothiazines were initially developed as antihistamines and have considerable activity as H-1 antagonists. The butyrophenones are considerably less effective. Many neuroleptics antagonize serotonin (5-hydroxytryptamine) binding in the brain and inhibit the generation of serotonin-sensitive cAMP.[57] Some drugs also displace clonidine from its alpha-2 binding side, but this effect is mark-

Table 3

Affinities of Neuroleptics for the Muscarinic Acetylcholine Receptor of Human Brain Caudate Nucleus[103]

Drug	Affinity*
Neuroleptics	
Clozapine**	8.3
Thioridazine	5.6
Mesoridazine	1.4
Chlorpromazine	1.4
Promazine	0.67
Loxapine	0.22
Prochlorperazine	0.18
Trifluoperazine	0.15
Perphenazine	0.067
Fluphenazine	0.053
Spiperone**	0.037
cis-Thiothixene	0.034
d-Butaclamol**	0.0083
Haloperidol	0.0042
Molindone	0.00026
Antimuscarinics***	
Quinuclidinyl benzilate	2270
Atropine	42

* $10^{-7} \times 1/K_D$; where K_D = equilibrium dissociation constant in molarity.
** Not available for clinical use in US.
*** These are not neuroleptics but are shown here for comparison.

edly weaker than the alpha-1 binding affinity. There is virtually no effect on beta receptors by neuroleptics.[20] The alpha blockade provided by neuroleptics causes increased norepinephrine synthesis and turnover without affecting norepinephrine re-uptake.[20]

Neuroleptics have strong affinities for sigma receptors[58] and have complex effects on neuropeptides themselves, affecting levels of at least four neuropeptides (neurotensin, somatostatin, substance P, and met-enkephalin) in animals.[59] Exploration of neuroleptic effects on peptides in humans is still in its infancy. Of note, however, is the association between neuroleptic effects on sigma receptors and dystonia.[58] An association between sigma or other peptide receptors and DIP is not yet known.

Although neuroleptics do not appear to have direct effects on GABA, they undoubtedly do have indirect effects.[20]

The extrapyramidal profile of a neuroleptic has generally been interpreted as a balance between dopamine receptor blocking and anticholinergic activities.[60] This hypothesis appears to be useful for all typical neuroleptics but fails for clozapine, an atypical neuroleptic that blocks dopamine receptors but does not induce EPS. In addition, the combination of anticholinergics with high-potency neuroleptics does not always preclude the development of DIP.

Miscellaneous

Chlorpromazine Equivalents

A common and very useful standardization regimen has been developed to enable clinicians and researchers to compare one neuroleptic with another. Since there is a large number of antipsychotics commercially available, it is obviously important to be able to compare drugs both for efficacy and adverse effects. Using an "empirically based" method, Davis[61] published a table of the relative potencies of 19 neuroleptics (Table 4). For this analysis, he assessed clinical results of only double-blind studies which compared one antipsychotic to another, usually chlorpromazine. The averaged results were then compared with the average of seven individual experts' opinions concerning drug equivalence. There was an impressive degree of agreement between the two methods.

These results are comparisons of clinical efficacy only and are not comparisons of the potential for extrapyramidal side effects, although, for the standard neuroleptics, there is probably a very strong correlation in this clinical area as well. That is, drugs that treat psychosis at low milligram doses (i.e., high-potency medications) are most likely to produce DIP.

Treatment of DIP

Introduction

Problems in the Treatment Literature

DIP is usually treated with anticholinergics or amantadine. Diphenhydramine is another possible option. However, the data to sup-

Table 4
Chlorpromazine Equivalent Doses for Antipsychotic Efficacy[61]

Generic Name	Trademark	Defined Dosage, mg	Dose Equivalent, mg
Chlorpromazine	Thorazine	100	100
Thioridazine	Mellaril	97 ± 7	100
Mesoridazine	Serentil	56 ± 6	51
Chlorprothixine	Taractan	44 ± 8	100
Triflupromazine hydrochloride	Vesprin	28 ± 2	28
Carphenazine maleate	Proketazine	25 ± 2	28
Acetophenazine maleate	Tindal	23 ± 1	19
Prochlorperazine	Compazine	14 ± 2	15
Piperacetazine	Quide	11	14
Butaperazine maleate	Repoise maleate	9 ± 1	13
Perphenazine	Trilafon	9 ± .6	
Molindone hydrochloride	Moban	6 ± .9	
Thiothixene	Navane	4.4 ± 1	10
Trifluoperazine hydrochloride	Stelazine	2.8 ± .4	10
Haloperidol	Haldol	1.6 ± .5	3
Fluphenazine hydrochloride	Prolixin, 5 mg	1.2 ± .1	5
Fluphenazine hydrochloride	Permitil, 10 mg	1.2 ± .1	2
Fluphenazine enanthate	Prolixin enanthate	.67	2
Fluphenazine decanoate	Prolixin decanoate	.61	2

port these choices are scanty. Few double-blind trials have been performed to prove efficacy and even fewer have compared active drug to placebo. Most have compared one drug with another. The problems inherent in this area have been well reviewed by Mindham,[62] including problems with rating instruments, the natural tendency of untreated DIP to improve over time, the reporting of results that strain credibility, the occasional failure to obtain baseline measurements, the use of nonblinded raters, the use of untrained raters, and the use of different populations. Treatment studies for DIP fall into three categories: treatment of symptomatic DIP, prophylaxis against DIP, and chronic treatment/prophylaxis of DIP while on neuroleptics. The last category refers to the questionable need for continued long-term antiparkinsonian medication in view of the fact that for many patients DIP resolves spontaneously even though the patient remains on a neuroleptic.

Rating Scales

Although it was evident quite early that DIP and IPD appeared to be the same clinically, the Parkinson syndromes were evaluated differently. As has been the case with investigations of IPD, psychiatric papers have used a variety of rating instruments to score parkinsonian severity. In neurological trials in IPD, there has been an increasing trend to use the Unified Parkinson's Disease Rating Scale (UPDRS),[63] whereas a similar trend toward a single scale has not been evident in the studies of DIP. This problematic lack of standardization compromises any attempt to compare severity from one study to the other. The various scales clearly measure DIP, although some, such as the Rating Scale for Extrapyramidal Symptoms (REPS),[64] blur distinction between dystonia, akathisia, and DIP by providing a summed score for all extrapyramidal syndromes without distinguishing the various subsets.

1. The Simpson-Angus scale[65] uses a five-point scale to rate each of nine different items. It is readily apparent that scoring is heavily weighted towards rigidity. Seven of nine items are measures of rigidity. Glabellar tapping to measure akinesia and gait analysis for posture and arm swing are the only other items analyzed. Aside from overly stressing rigidity, tremor, bradykinesia, and postural instability are notably absent from the scale. Furthermore, many of the tests advocated for rigidity are extremely difficult to perform because of limited patient compliance.

2. The Rating Scale for Extrapyramidal Symptoms (REPS)[64] consists of four ratings of parkinsonism, plus two on akathisia and dystonia. The parkinson section rates tremor, akinesia, rigidity, and facial expression equally on a 0 (not present) to 3 (severe) scale. The akinesia scale actually measures gait and thus assumes that gait dysfunction and akinesia are synonymous, which is not true. In addition, the scale fails to include bradykinesia, and rates a mask-like face as being as important as a slow and rigid gait. For assessing treatment outcome, it is useful for subjects whose parkinsonism is not severe. It is easy to use, reproducible, and fast. Subjective symptoms are not assessed.

3. The Extrapyramidal Symptom Rating Scale (ESRS)[67] assesses nine subjective symptoms on a 0 to 3 scale and five signs of DIP on a 0 to 6 scale. The signs of DIP are scored by the results from each limb so that measures of tremor or rigidity acquire extra weight by being multiplied by the number of limbs involved. The problem with the scale is illustrated by noting that a severely disabled person "barely able to walk" scores the same as a patient with occasional low-amplitude tremors of multiple limbs. While this is true of the UPDRS as well, the ESRS has a much briefer objective component than the UPDRS and is therefore more subject to bias by a single aspect of the DIP. Having patients rate their own symptoms of parkinsonism is extremely difficult in the psychiatric hospital. It may be neither reliable nor accurate.

4. The clinical assessment of parkinsonism by Mindham[62] does not score akinesia and bradykinesia but includes the useful concept of a global assessment of parkinsonism. An advantage of this scoring system is that the scale is not meant to be summed, so that total severity is the observer's global score and not simply the sums of rigidity and tremor in each limb.

5. Some methods for rating parkinsonism employ objective tasks, which are usually timed. One method has the subject maximally squeeze a sphygmomanometer cuff blown up to 60 mm Hg.[68] A grooved pegboard[69] test requires patients to insert pegs into grooved holes in a fixed period of time. Speed of walking can be assessed by having a subject walk a fixed distance, including a turn, or, in a variation, measure the time for the patient to stand up from a chair, walk a fixed distance, and return to sit in the chair.[63] The number of completed movements such as hand taps performed in a certain period can be measured.[70] Timed writing for standardized items and even size of handwriting can be assessed.[69]

While objective measures provide clearly defined and easy to compare results, they require consistent cooperation from the subject. This is readily achievable with some subjects but can be virtually impossible in severely affected psychiatric patients. Diminished attention for any reason impairs reliability of the results and since individual patients act as their own controls, the tests must be reliable.

Treatment of Symptomatic DIP

Anticholinergics

Negative reports

Simpson[71] treated patients with advanced phenothiazine-induced parkinsonism with single boluses of intravenous anticholinergics and found no difference compared to placebo. He then treated six patients with oral biperiden in standard doses for 5 weeks. Only one patient improved. The surprising conclusion of the study was that it is exceedingly difficult to measure DIP. "As benztropine and biperiden are widely used for the treatment of Parkinsonism, we may be justified in rejecting" the conclusion that there is no difference between active drug and placebo. This study exemplifies the problems of clinical trials in this area.

In looking at individual variations in response to neuroleptics, Simpson et al.[49] treated those who developed DIP with benztropine and reported benefit "in a small number of cases" only.

In one of the only double-blind, placebo-controlled studies, amantadine and orphenadrine were compared in a crossover fashion[67] and no differences from placebo were found.

Positive reports

In an open study[18] of phenothiazine-induced DIP, biperiden in doses up to 18 mg daily was used. The majority responded well to 6 mg/d. In another double-blind controlled trial[67] comparing procyclidine, piribedil, and placebo, procyclidine was found to be more effective than placebo on clinical evaluations, yet timed tasks (which are presumably more objective or measure different functions than the clinical assessment) showed no differences. Kelly et al.,[72] using young male patients as their own controls, found in a double-blind controlled study of DIP that benztropine 2–4 mg/d was able to induce virtually total clinical remission. However, here too, objective scores using timed tasks showed no changes. Amantadine, though helpful, was less effective. DiMascio et al.[64] also reported benefit from anticholinergics in a blind study without placebo.

Amantadine

The mechanism of action of amantadine is thought to be dopamine enhancement. One hypothesis is that amantadine increases dopamine release. Another hypothesis is that amantadine blocks dopamine re-uptake. Although it lacks anticholinergic effects on the brain, it occasionally has anticholinergic side effects such as urinary retention and visual disturbances.[73]

In an open study, amantadine produced moderate to marked benefit in 9 of 10 cases.[74] In a double-blind comparison of benztropine and amantadine,[64] both were found to be equally effective in DIP but amantadine was better tolerated. Greenblatt and DiMascio[75] reported in a separate study that amantadine was beneficial and that, in general, improvement paralleled serum levels of amantadine. They also found that improvement continued at each assessment, which is not the case for amantadine in IPD. Presumably this reflects diminishing severity of DIP rather than improving efficacy of amantadine over time. Stenson et al.[76] reported benefit in 100% of patients on amantadine and found that it was as effective as benztropine, with a similar incidence of adverse effects. Pacifici et al.[77] found that amantadine led to a rapid and marked improvement within 4 to 6 days in rigidity and tremor in 15 patients whose DIP had been unresponsive to anticholinergics. There was no relationship found between individual responses and serum amantadine levels. Only the placebo-controlled study of Mindham et al.[67] has reported negative results using amantadine. Thus, the results for amantadine are somewhat less conflicting than for anticholinergics.

Treatment with Levodopa

Treating DIP with levodopa initially seems somewhat counter-intuitive. While DIP clinically is identical to IDP, the fundamental pathophysiology is quite different. On the one hand, since dopamine receptors are blocked, increasing dopamine should not have any effect. On the other hand, it is known that dopamine receptor blockade in animals produces a reactive increase in dopamine turnover and an increase in dopamine receptors. Thus, one could argue that DIP occurs when there are too few available receptors or the reactive dopamine increase has been insufficient. This might justify a trial of levodopa in order to increase dopamine production. Whether levodopa actually increases available dopamine in neuroleptic-treated patients is unknown. In reserpinized rodents,[78] it does not reverse locomotor changes that are due to catecholamine depletion.

Several reports have been published concerning both the mental and the motoric effects of levodopa in neuroleptic-treated psychiatric patients. As with other treatment aspects of DIP, the published results are contradictory both for the psychiatric and for the parkinsonian aspects.

In a nonblinded study[79] comparing single intravenous boluses of levodopa given at 2 mg/kg over 5 minutes to placebo in treating DIP, all 40 patients were improved in terms of akinesia and rigidity, with tremor being the least responsive. The least severely affected cases of DIP responded best. Men and women responded equally, but the patients taking chlorpromazine benefitted more than those taking haloperidol. Improvement began within 5 to 20 minutes. Psychiatrically, there was a "trend towards euphoria." Maximum effect occurred between 1 and 2 hours and the benefit was mostly lost by 3 hours. There was no response to the placebo. Angrist et al.[80] reported behavioral worsening in 10 of 10 schizophrenics treated with 3–6 gm of levodopa, possibly because they had discontinued ongoing neuroleptic therapy.

Twenty patients taking neuroleptics and "standard" antiparkinson medication for observed extrapyramidal syndromes were taken off their antiparkinson drugs and then placed on increasing doses of levodopa.[81] Sixteen subjects failed to tolerate removal of their antiparkinson medications and the four who received levodopa (maximum daily doses 1400–2600 mg for 8–23 days) all worsened psychiatrically without motor improvement. Resumption of the previous medications resulted in improvement. Given the small numbers of patients and the relatively small doses of levodopa used, one could only conclude that levodopa was not promising rather than that it simply didn't work.

A study[82] involving 84 chronic schizophrenics given levodopa up to 1200 mg daily reported a moderate to marked improvement in the "negative" symptoms of the disease such as rapport, emotional blunting, and autism. Howevere, no comments were made on the response of DIP.

From a referred population of patients with disabling DIP, Hardie and Lees[9] treated 15 (5 maintained on neuroleptics and 10 withdrawn from them) with levodopa plus benserazide in doses of 300–1000mg of levodopa. Seven had a moderate (41–75%) and 2 had a complete response to levodopa while the rest had no (<20%) or slight (20–40%) benefit. However, theirs was a highly selected population referred to a movement disorders clinic. These patients had been on anticholinergics and therefore may have been referred precisely because they were unresponsive to typical antiparkinson medications. Thus, they may have constituted a refractory population.

Other levodopa studies in small populations have also produced conflicting results. Thus, it would seem that there is a limited role for levodopa in the routine treatment of DIP. It appears to be ineffective in most cases where anticholinergics fail and possibly less effective than anticholinergics in cases where the latter work. The reports of levodopa's beneficial effects on psychiatric symptoms are counterbalanced by negative reports. It is, therefore, not recommended for treatment of typical DIP. On the other hand, some investigators have found it extremely effective in the management of young patients with severe, disabling DIP persisting after neuroleptic withdrawal (A. Lang, personal communication).

Electroconvulsive Therapy (ECT)

ECT has been helpful in Parkinson's disease for treating depression and paranoid psychosis and has been reported to ameliorate the motoric features as well. In two studies, ECT[83,84] was used to treat "on-off" clinical fluctuations in subjects who had no psychiatric problems and was found to improve parkinsonism for periods of time lasting from hours to several weeks. Isolated case reports have documented similar effects in DIP but few prospective studies have been performed. One study[85] found that bilateral ECT given at the rate of three shocks weekly progressively improved parkinsonism beginning within the first week and continuing until therapy was concluded after which the DIP began to worsen again. By the end of the second week post ECT, the DIP was still improved compared to baseline but anticholinergics had been increased, making interpretation difficult. However, this one prospective study does, in fact, support the antiparkinson properties of ECT. This may influence a decision on whether or not to use ECT. For example, depressed patients with DIP unresponsive to anticholinergics might benefit from ECT for treatment of both problems.

Negative aspects of ECT also need to be kept in mind since they can offset the benefits. In the elderly especially, transient delirium and memory dysfunction may occur. The duration of the antiparkinson effect is measured in days to weeks, so this potential benefit should be considered only secondarily.

How ECT works in ameliorating parkinsonism is unknown but appears to be independent of improvement in mood and thinking ability. In animal models, ECT has been shown to enhance dopaminergic transmission and the sensitivity of dopamine receptors but its biochemical effects are so manifold that a definitive explanation for its antiparkinson action is lacking.

Management of Coexistent DIP and TD

Management of these coexistent conditions is extremely difficult and is usually quite unsatisfactory. In a double placebo-controlled study,[31] both amantadine and trihexiphenidyl worsened TD as they improved DIP. DeFraites et al.[32] demonstrated in a single patient that benztropine improved DIP and worsened TD, while physostigmine, a centrally acting muscarinic agent, did the opposite. Aggravation of dyskinesias was dose-limiting in two patients whose DIP was treated with 1000 mg of levodopa and benserazide, while there was no mention of change in TD in another six patients treated with 300–1000 mg.[9]

Fahn and Mayeux[33] have argued that dopamine-depleting drugs such as reserpine and alpha-methyltyrosine ameliorate TD without worsening parkinsonism. Jankovic and Casabona[86] reported a beneficial response of the combined syndromes to catecholamine-depleting agents and levodopa. Their patients had all been off neuroleptics for at least 6 months. Treatment of these patients depends on a careful analysis of the contribution to disability of the DIP, the various features of the TD, and the underlying psychiatric illness. One is then faced with attempting to balance potential benefit with complications of drug intervention. Ideally, prolonged neuroleptic withdrawal may allow both DIP and TD to resolve, but this may not be feasible. There may be a role for ECT in the management of difficult or refractory cases.

Prophylaxis

The issue of whether patients started on a neuroleptic should be treated simultaneously with an antiparkinsonian drug is controversial. On the one hand, these drugs do reduce the risk of extrapyramidal adverse reactions but the tradeoff is the potential for other adverse effects.

Positive Studies

In a prospective study[87] comparing perphenazine to perphenazine plus benztropine in acutely disturbed female psychotic patients, the benztropine-treated patients had less parkinsonism and were more likely to be discharged from the hospital. Fourteen of 41 (34%) perphenazine-treated patients had DIP in contrast to only 3 of 33 (7%) prophylaxis patients, but the dropout rate from the study was almost 40% in each group before results could be obtained.

A retrospective[37] chart review of 215 schizophrenic patients who had not been taking neuroleptics prior to hospital admission found that 16% of patients receiving prophylaxis suffered DIP versus 32% of those who did not. Men benefitted more than women and the young did better than the old. Although the treated and untreated patients appeared to be comparable, one cannot completely eliminate physician treatment bias in this study, primarily with respect to how some patients were chosen for prophylaxis while others were not.

Chien et al.[88] prospectively looked at benztropine 2 mg b.i.d. prophylaxis for depot injections of fluphenazine enanthate and found that tremor, akinesia, and rigidity were reduced but that more than one-third of prophylactically treated patients still had clear parkinsonian features.

Negative Studies

Few negative studies exist. In a retrospective review, DiMascio and Demirgian[24] found a greater prevalence of both EPS and other adverse effects in patients receiving prophylaxis. The population was possibly biased by the selection for prophylactic intervention. For example, patients with a prior history of problems may have been more likely to be treated, and those on higher potency medications, presumably also at greater risk, might have been singled out for prophylaxis.

Chronic Use of Antiparkinson (AP) Medication

The issue of whether and when to stop AP medications has been addressed many times. Conclusions have again been strikingly different despite the fact that many studies used similar populations. One confounding feature was whether the AP drug was initially used to treat established signs of parkinsonism or used prophylactically. In addition, mild evidence of DIP might be considered irrelevant clinically and not reported, whereas a study specifically looking for DIP might find the same degree of parkinsonism important. As the following review indicates, there is no resolution to the issue of chronic prophylaxis. Much of the data concerns extrapyramidal syndromes in general without focusing on DIP.

Studies Recommending Chronic Prophylaxis

In a double-blind study[90] of patients on neuroleptics for more than 6 months (mean duration 8 years) and AP drugs more than 3 months (mean 5 years), Manos et al. replaced the AP drug with either placebo or trihexyphenidyl. Fifty-one placebo-treated patient versus one trihexyphenidyl-treated patients had severe worsening and 21 placebo versus two actively treated subjects had mild worsening. Grove and Cramer,[91] in a single-blind study, reported a doubling in parkinson severity when placebo was substituted for benzhexol. Mandel et al.[92] found that chronic neuroleptic-treated patients using AP medications for more than 3 months required this therapy. One hundred percent of the males and 60% of the females suffered recurrent DIP when placebo was substituted for the AP medication.

St. Jean et al.[93] replaced trihexyphenidyl with placebo or another anticholinergic in 30 chronically treated patients and found anticholinergics more helpful than placebo. Rifkin et al.[94] found that half of the placebo-treated patients developed akinesia when their procyclidine was stopped, whereas those maintained on procyclidine had no akinesia.

Chronic Prophylaxis Negative Studies

Although AP drugs may ameliorate the signs of DIP, they certainly do not eliminate the problem. Hershon et al.[95] found a very high incidence of DIP despite AP therapy, with 68% demonstrating increased tone or akinesia and about 70% coarse static tremor. This raises the question of whether chronic AP prophylaxtic therapy is necessary and how effective it is in ameliorating DIP. In one study, of 80 patients[96] receiving AP medications while on neuroleptics or reserpine, only eight suffered a recurrence of any EPS when the AP drug was withdrawn. Similarly, in another study,[81] only 4 of 20 chronically AP treated patients required treatment for recurrence of DIP on stopping the prophylactic therapy. Stratos et al.[97] reported that 88 patients, one-fourth of their female ward population, were on chronic AP prophylaxis at the beginning of their study and that only 27% developed DIP when this treatment was stopped. Of those who developed DIP, the majority experienced a remission with a decreased dose of neuroleptic and most of the remainder improved when thioridazine was substituted as the principle neuroleptic. The authors concluded that chronic AP was rarely needed.

Cahan and Parrish[98] found that only 21% of patients developed DIP when AP drugs were withdrawn. Orlow et al.[99] examined 78 patients who lacked DIP after taking AP medication for over 3 months. Only two developed DIP after being free of their AP drug for 3 weeks.

In one institution[24] of 1000 chronically hospitalized psychiatric patients, only nine were thought to require AP medications despite the fact that most were on neuroleptics.

Recommendations on Chronic Prophylaxis

The argument over whether or not to chronically use AP medications has not been definitively resolved. The data are conflicting yet a reasonable approach is evident. Antiparkinson medications should be tapered after about 3 months. Quite clearly, many patients do not need AP medications at all and fewer need them long term. The acute dystonic and acute akathitic reactions are less likely at this time and DIP should develop relatively slowly, unlike the other syndromes, and thus should not precipitate sudden emotional stress. The various studies quoted do indicate that if DIP recurs on stopping an AP drug, restarting it should control the DIP. In discontinuing the AP medication, it is wise to slowly taper the drug rather than stop it abruptly, which could induce a more precipitous onset of the parkinsonism.

Adverse Effects of Treatment Medications

All anticholinergics may produce prominent adverse effects.[18,66] Dry mouth and constipation are very common. Blurred vision, urinary retention, organic mental syndromes, and memory impairment are other potential side effects. The elderly are considerably more prone to all of these side effects, especially the latter group of mental disturbances. It should be noted that adverse effects are not always dose-related.[18]

Amantadine is generally well tolerated in younger patients, although there are reports of recurrent psychosis induced by this drug in previously stable schizophrenics.[100] Organic mental syndromes are generally more common in the elderly. Amantadine appears to be better tolerated than the anticholinergic drugs.[101]

Conclusion on Treatment of DIP

The data on treatment of DIP are confusing. Part of the problem stems from the evolution of medical practice with certain drugs having entered into common use by habit or consent rather than via strict clinical trials. This has kept investigators from performing the many placebo-controlled trials that are necessary. The focus has been on comparing one agent to a "standard" drug, the latter accepted as effective on the basis of previous habit rather than on trials establishing efficacy. The type of patient treated is also crucial. Not all patients with DIP are the same. It is clear that for many individuals DIP is a transitory phenomenon that will resolve with or without intervention. It is also clear that some individuals with DIP are refractory to all antiparkinson therapy. Chronic neuroleptic-treated patients who remain parkinsonian are more likely to be refractory to antiparkinsonian therapy. Neuroleptic differences probably have an effect on outcome, too, as parkinsonism induced by a neuroleptic with pronounced anticholinergic activity may prove more refractory to anticholinergic intervention than DIP caused by drugs with only a minor degree of anticholinergic action. The severity of DIP is likely to be another significant factor in determining drug response in that severe disability is less likely to respond to treatment than mild parkinsonism. Another potential explanation for different results could be the variable pharmacokinetics of the anticholinergics. Tune and Coyle[45] found no relationship between benztropine dose and anticholinergic activity in the blood but did find an inverse relationship between serum anticholinergic activity and extrapyramidal syndromes. In addition, a threshold for anticholinergic activity was found, above which extrapyramidal problems were unlikely to occur. Thus, some patients may require higher doses of anticholinergics than are generally given.

This author recommends treating DIP *only* when the patient is truly symptomatic, using either anticholinergic medications or amantadine, monitoring both for adverse and beneficial effects. Patients who fail to respond to a trial of one drug should have a second added (anticholinergic plus amantadine). If no benefit ensues, the AP medication should be stopped. It must be stressed that AP medications for DIP should be used only when symptomatic benefit is required and continued use should be justified by a documented response and a continuing symptomatic need. Continued use of these drugs despite lack of improvement or need only places the patient at risk of accruing unnecessary adverse effects.

It is recommended that a trial off all AP medications be attempted after 3 months and periodically thereafter whether the patient is parkinsonian or not. Should existing parkinsonism worsen or symptomatic DIP ensue, the medications should be restarted.

Prophylactic use of antiparkinson drugs for the prevention of acute dystonia and akathisia are discussed in Chapters 2 and 4, respectively.

Future Trends

The development of safe antipsychotic medications that do not induce prominent side effects is clearly the next step in psychopharmacology. The development of clozapine reveals that antipsychotics do not need to induce extrapyramidal side effects.[102] This drug, documented as being at least as or more efficacious[103] than the "typical" antipsychotic agents, has been classified as an "atypical neuroleptic" because of its failure to induce catalepsy and to antagonize amphetamine- and apomorphine-induced stereotypy in rodents. In humans, it not only fails to induce parkinsonism, dystonia, akathisia, or tardive dyskinesia[104] at antipsychotic doses, but it even ameliorates tremor in IPD[105,106] without worsening rigidity, bradykinesia, or other parkinsonian features. Unfortunately, it induces potentially life-threatening but reversible granulocytopenia in approximately 1% of the population.[107] Thus, close monitoring of blood counts is essential.

The explanation for clozapine's special properties is unknown. Although it has potent anticholinergic properties,[108] this alone is clearly insufficient to explain its lack of EPS. The two-drug combination of an anticholinergic and a typical neuroleptic does not mimic clozapine's lack of extrapyramidal adverse effects, and low-potency neuroleptics such as thioridazine have relatively similar antimuscarinic properties[109] yet do not have clozapine's extrapyramidal profile.

Clozapine does block dopaminergic receptors in the brain[110] but it exerts potent influences on other neurotransmitter systems.[110] It is possible that the combination of clozapine's effects on various neurotransmitter systems or perhaps its seeming ability to bind preferentially to dopamine receptors outside of the basal ganglia[57] renders it free of extrapyramidal adverse effects.

The development of this novel drug clearly points the way to a future class of drugs that do not induce EPS. Hopefully these drugs will be less toxic than clozapine.

When speculating about the future of antipsychotic medication, one must keep in mind the major limitations of all currently available drugs. Aside from their adverse effect profiles, all antipsychotics have limited efficacy.[19] For example, in schizophrenia, the most common psychosis, the utility of neuroleptics in treating the "positive" symptoms such as thought blocking and psychotic speech is greater than in treating the negative symptoms.[111] The adverse effect profile of drugs that will better ameliorate the "negative" symptoms such as anhedonia, lack of affect, and autism is unknown. Unfortunately, a significant number of psychotic patients do not respond to any of the available antipsychotics drugs.

Many research questions of interest remain. For example, an obvious question, not yet answered, is whether DIP from one drug predicts DIP on another, either of the same class or of another class. Does the presence of an active nonbasal ganglia brain disease such as Alzheimer's or another dementing illness predispose one to DIP? Is the development of DIP at low doses predictive of the later development of IPD? Do different ethnic groups have a different sensitivity to neuroleptics? Is the presence or absence of DIP predictive of the likelihood of later development of tardive dyskinesia?

References

1. Freyhan FA. Comments on the biological and psychopathological basis of individual variation in chlorpromazine therapy. Encephale 1957; 45:913–919.
2. Hornykiewicz O. Parkinsonism induced by dopaminergic antagonists. Adv Neurol 1975; 9:155–164.
3. Freyhan FA. Psychomotility and parkinsonism in treatment with neuroleptic drugs. Arch Neurol Psychiatry 1957; 78:465–472.
4. Carlsson A. The occurrence, distribution and physiological role of catecholamines in the nervous system. Pharmacol Rev 1959; 11:490–493.
5. Ehringer H, Hornykiewicz O. Verteilung von noradrenalen und dopamine (3-hydroxytyramine) im gehirn des menschen und ihr berhatten bei erkrankingen des extrapyramidalen systems. Klin Wochenschr 1960; 24:1236–1239.
6. Cotzias GC, Van Woert MH, Schiffer LM. Aromatic amino acids and modification of parkinsonism. N Engl J Med 1967; 276:374–379.
7. Haase HJ. Extrapyramidal modification of fine movements: a "conditio sine qua non" of the fundamental therapeutic action of neuroleptic drugs. Rev Can Biol 1961; 20:425–449.
8. Friedman JH, Max J, Swift R. Idiopathic parkinson's disease in a chronic schizophrenic patient: long-term treatment with clozapine and levodopa. Clin Neuropharmacol 1987; 10:470–475.
9. Hardie RJ, Lees AJ. Neuroleptic-induced Parkinson's syndrome: clinical features and results of treatment with levodopa. J Neurol Neurosurg Psychiatry 1988; 51:850–854.
10. National Institute of Mental Health Psychopharmacology Service Center Collaborative Study Group. Phenothiazine treatment in acute schizophrenia. Arch Gen Psychiatry 1964; 10:246–261.
11. Lohr JB, Lohr MA, Wasli E, et al. Self perception of tardive dyskinesia and neuroleptic induced parkinsonism: a study of clinical correlates. Psychopharmacol Bull 1987; 23:211–214.
12. Friedman JH. Personal observation.
13. Villeneuve A. The rabbit syndrome: a peculiar extrapyramidal reaction. Can Psychiatric Assoc J 1972; Suppl 2:SS69–72.
14. Duvoisin RC. Problems in the treatment of parkinsonism. Adv Exp Med Biol 1977; 99:131–155.
15. Ayd F. A survey of drug-induced extrapyramidal reactions. JAMA 1961; 175:1054–1060.
16. Klawans HL, Bergen D, Bruyn GW. Prolonged drug-induced parkinsonism. Confin Neurol 1973; 35:368–377.
17. Freyhan FA. Therapeutic implications of differential effects of new phenothiazine compounds. Am J Psychiatry 1959; 115:577–585.

18. Medinar C, Kramer MD, Kurland AA. Biperiden in the treatment of phenothiazine-induced extra-pyramidal reactions. JAMA 1962; 182:1127–1128.
19. Levinson DF, Simpson GM, Singh H, et al. Fluphenazine dose, clinical response and extrapyramidal symptoms during acute treatment. Am J Psychiatry 1990; 47:761–769.
20. Bradley PB. Pharmacology of antipsychotic drugs. In: Bradley PB (ed), Psychopharmacology and Treatment of Schizophrenia, Oxford, Oxford Univ Press, 1986, pp 27–70.
21. Jenner P, Marsden CDE. Neuroleptic agents: acute and chronic receptor actions. In: DC Howell (ed), Drugs in Central Nervous System Disorders, New York, Marcel Dekker, Inc, 1985, pp 149–262.
22. Azima H, Ogle W. Effects of largactil in mental syndromes. Can Med Assoc J 1954; 71:116–121.
23. Kennedy PF, Hershon HI, McGuire RJ. Extrapyramidal disorders after prolonged phenothiazine therapy. Br J Psychiatry 1971; 118:509–518.
24. DiMascio A, Demirgian E. Antiparkinson drug overuse. Psychosomatics 1970; 11:596–601.
25. Kessler II. Parkinson's disease in epidemiologic perspective. Adv Neurol 1978; 19:355–384.
26. Stephen PJ, Williamson J. Drug-induced parkinsonism in the elderly. Lancet 1984; 2:1082–1083.
27. Wilson JA, MacLennan WJ. Drug-induced parkinsonism in the elderly. Age Ageing 1989; 18:208–210.
28. Richardson MA, Craig TJ. The coexistence of parkinsonism-like symptoms and tardive dyskinesia. Am J Psychiatry 1982; 139:341- 343.
29. Crane GE. Pseudoparkinsonism and tardive dyskinesia. Arch Neurol 1972; 27:426–430.
30. Kucharski LT, Friedman JH, Wagner RW. An investigation of the co-existence of abnormal involuntary movements, parkinsonism and akathisia in chronic psychiatric patients. Psychopharmacol Bull 1987; 23:215–217.
31. Fann WE, Lake CR. On the coexistence of parkinsonism and tardive dyskinesia. Dis Nerv Syst 1974; 35:324–326.
32. DeFraites EG, Davis KL, Berger PA. Coexisting tardive dyskinesia and parkinsonism: a case report. Biol Psychiatry 1977; 12:267–272.
33. Fahn S, Mayeux R. Unilateral parkinson's disease and contralateral tardive dyskinesia: a unique case with successful therapy that may explain the pathophysiology of these two disorders. J Neural Transm 1980; Suppl 16:179–185.
34. Inoue F, Vanikowski AM. Withdrawal akinesia. J Neurol Neurosurg Psychiatry 1981; 44:958.
35. Nelli AC, Yarden PE, Feinberg I. Parkinsonism following neuroleptic withdrawal. Arch Gen Psychiatry 1989; 46:383–384.
36. Marsden CD, Mindham RHS, Mackay AVP. Extrapyramidal movement disorders produced by antipsychotic drugs. In: Bradley PB (ed), Psychopharmacology and Treatment of Schizophrenia, Oxford, Oxford Univ Press, 1986, pp 340–402.

37. Keepers GA, Clappison VJ, Casey DE. Initial anticholinergic prophylaxis for neuroleptic induced extrapyramidal syndromes. Arch Gen Psychiatry 1983; 40:1113–1117.
38. Myrianthopoulos NC, Kurland AA, Kurland LT. Hereditary predisposition in drug-induced parkinsonism. Arch Neurol 1962; 6:19–23.
39. Myrianthopoulos NC, Waldrop FN, Vincent BL. A repeat study of hereditary predisposition to drug-induced parkinsonism. Prog Neurogene 1967; 175:486–491.
40. Metzen WS, Newton JEO, Steele RW, et al. HLA antigens in drug-induced parkinsonism. Mov Disord 1989; 4:121–128.
41. Knopp W, Fischer R, Kech J, Teitelbaum A. Clinical implications of the relation between taste sensitivty and the appearance of extrapyramidal side effects. Dis Nerv Syst 1966; 27:729–735.
42. Holden JMC, Itil TM, Keshiner A. The treatment of lobotomized schizophrenic patients with butaperazine. Curr Ther Res 1969; 11:418–428.
43. Demars JPCA. Neuromuscular effects of long-term phenothiazine medications, electroconvulsive therapy and parkinsonism. J Nerv Mental Dis 1966; 143:73–79.
44. Luckins DJ, Jackman H, Meltzer HS. Lateral ventricular size and drug-induced parkinsonism. Psychiatr Res 1983; 9:9–16.
45. Tune L, Coyle JT. Acute extrapyramidal side effects: serum levels of neuroleptics and anticholinergics. Psychopharmacology 1981; 75:9–15.
46. Hansen LB, Larsen NE, Vestergard P: Plasma levels of perphenazine related to development of extrapyramidal effects. Psychopharmacology 1981; 74:306–309.
47. Hansen LB, Larsen NE. Plasma concentrations of perphenazine and its sulphoxide metabolite during continous oral treatment. Psychoparmacology 1977; 53:127–130.
48. Alpert M, Diamond F, Kesselman M. Correlation between extrapyramidal and therapeutic effects of neuroleptics. Comp Psychiatry 1977; 18:333–336.
49. Simpson GM, Kunz-Bartholini E. Relationship of individual tolerance and behavior in phenothiazine produced extrapyramidal system disturbance. Dis Nerv Syst 1968; 29:269–274.
50. Reches A, Burke RE, Kuker CM, et al. Tetrabenazine, an amine-depleting drug, also blocks dopamine receptors. J Pharmacol Exp Ther 1983; 225:515–521.
51. Snyder SH, Banerjee SP, Yamaura HI, Greenberg D. Drugs, neurotransmitters and schizophrenia. Science 1974; 184:1243–1253.
52. Clark D, White FJ. Review: D_1 dopamine receptor. The search for a function: a critical evaluation of the D_1/D_2 dopamine receptor classification and its functional implications. Synapse 1987; 1:347–388.
53. Stoof JC, Kebabian JW. Opposing roles for D_1 and D_2 dopamine receptors in efflux of cAMP from rat neostriatum. Nature 181; 294:366–368.
54. Boyce S, Rupnick NMJ, Steventon MS, Iversen SD. Differential affects of D_1 and D_2 agonists in MPTP treated primates: functional implications for Parkinson's disease. Neurology 1990; 40:927–933.

55. Sokoloff P, Giros B, Martres MP, Bouthenet ML, Schwartz JC. Molecular cloning and characterization of a novel dopamine receptor (D_3) as a target for neuroleptics. Nature 1990; 347:146–151.
56. Wolf ME, Roth RH. Heterogeneity of midbrain dopamine neurons: implications for psychiatry. Psychiatry Lett 1988; 6:24–32.
57. Borison RL, Fields JZ, Diamond BI. Site-specific blockade of dopamine receptors by neuroleptic agents in human brain. Neuropharmacology 1981; 20:1321–1322.
58. Walker JM, Matsumatoa RR, Bowen WB,Gans D, Walker FO. Evidence for a role of haloperidol-sensitive sigma-"opiate" receptors in the motor effects of antipsychotic drugs. Neurology 1988; 38:961–965.
59. Nemeroff CB, Bissette G. The role of neuropeptides. In: Henn FA, Delisi LE (eds), Handbook of Schizophrenia, Vol II: Neurochemistry and Neuropharmacology of Schizophrenia, New York, Elsevier, 1987, pp 297–318.
60. Miller RJ, Hiley CR. Antimuscarinic properties of neuroleptics and drug-induced parkinsonism. Nature 1974; 248:596–597.
61. Davis JF. Comparative doses and costs of antipsychotic medical. Arch Gen Psychiatry 1976; 33:858–861.
62. Mindham RHS. Assessment of drug-induced extrapyramidal reactions and of drugs given for their control. Br J Clin Pharmacol 1976; (Suppl)3:395–400.
63. Parkinson's Study Group. DATATOP: A multicenter controlled clinical trial in early Parkinson's disease. Arch Neurol 1989; 46:1052–1060.
64. DiMascio A, Bernardo DL, Greenblatt D, Marder JE. A controlled trial of amantadine in drug-induced extrapyramidal disorders. Arch Gen Psychiatry 1976; 33:599–602.
65. Simpson GM, Amuso D, Blair JH, Farhas T. Phenothiazine produced extrapyramidal disturbance. Arch Gen Psychiatry 1964; 10:127–136.
66. Chouinard G, Annable L, Ross-Chouinard A, Kropsky ML. Ethopropazine and benztropine in neuroleptic-induced parkinsonism. J Clin Psychiatry 1979; 40:147–152.
67. Mindham RHS, Gaind R, Anstee BH, Rimmer L. Comparison of amantadine, orphenadrine and placebo in drug-induced parkinsonism. Psychol Med 1972; 2:406–443.
68. Onuaguluchi G. Parkinsonism. London, Butterworths, 1964.
69. Meier MJ, Martin WE. Measurement of behavioral changes in patients on levodopa. Lancet 1979; 1:352–353.
70. Nutt J, Woodward WR, Hammerstad JP, et al. "On/off" phenomenon in Parkinson's disease: relationship to levodopa absorption and transport. N Engl J Med 1984; 310:483–488.
71. Simpson GM. Controlled studies of antiparkinsonism agents in the treatment of extrapyramidal syndromes. Acta Psychiatr Scand 1970; 212:44–51.
72. Kelly JT, Zimmerman RL, Abuzzahab FS, Schiele BC. A double blind study of amantadine HCl versus benztropene mesylate in drug-induced parkinsonism. Pharmacology 1974; 12:65–73.
73. Huzulakova I, Dukes MNG. Drugs affecting autonomic functions or

the extrapyramidal system. In: Dukes MNG (ed), Meyler's Side Effects of Drugs, 10th edition, New York, Elsevier, 1984.

74. Kelly JT, Abuzzahab FS. Antiparkinsonian properties of amantadine in drug-induced parkinsonism. J Clin Pharmacol New Drugs 1971; 11:211–214.

75. Greenblatt DJ, DiMascio A, Harmatz JS, et al. Pharmacokinetics and clinical effects of amantadine in drug-induced extrapyramidal syndromes. J Clin Pharmacol 1977; 17:704- 708.

76. Stenson RL, Donlon PT, Mayer JE. Comparison of benztropine and amantadine in neuroleptic-induced extrapyramidal syndromes. Comp Psychiatry 1976; 17:762–768.

77. Pacifici GM, Nardini M, Ferrani P, et al. Effect of amantadine on drug-induced Parkinsonism: relationship between plasma levels and effect. Br J Clin Pharmacol 1976; 3:883–889.

78. Carlson A. The occurrence, distribution and physiologic role of catecholamines in the nervous system. Pharmacol Res 1959; 11:490–493.

79. Bruno A, Bruno SC. Effects of levodopa on pharmacological parkinsonism. Acta Psychiatr Scand 1966; 42:264–271.

80. Angrist B, Sathanathan G, Gershon S. Behavioral effects of levodopa in schizophrenic patients. Psychopharmacologica (Berl) 1973; 31:1–12.

81. Yaryura-Tobias, Wolpert A, Dana L, Malis S. Action of L-dopa on drug-induced extrapyramidal syndromes. Dis Nerv Syst 1973; 31:60–63.

82. Inanga K, Inouye K, Tachibana H, et al. Effect of levodopa in Schizophrenia. Folia Psychiatr Neurol Japn 1972; 26:145–157.

83. Balldin J, Eden S, Granerus AK, et al. Electroconvulsive therapy in Parkinson's syndrome with "on-off" phenomenon. J Neural Transm 1980; 47:11–21.

84. Andersen K, Balldin J, Gottfries CG, et al. Double blind evaluation of electroconvulsive therapy in Parkinson's disease with "on-off" phenomena. Acta Neurol Scand 1987; 76:191–199.

85. Goswami U, Dutta S, Jurivilla K, et al. Electroconvulsive therapy in neuroleptic-induced parkinsonism. Biol Psychiatry 1989; 26:234–238.

86. Jankovic J, Casabona J. Dyskinesia and parkinsonism. Clin Neuropharmacol 1987; 10:511–521.

87. Honlon TE, Shoenrich, C, Freinek W, et al. Perphenazine- benztropine mesylate treatment of newly admitted psychiatric patients. Psychopharmacologica (Berl) 1966; 9:328–329.

88. Chien CP, DiMascio A, Cole JO. Antiparkinson agents and depot phenothiazine. Am J Psychiatry 1974; 131:86–90.

90. Manos N, Ghiouzepas J, Logothetis J. The need for continuous anti-parkinsonian medication with chronic schizophrenic patients receiving long-term neuroleptic therapy. Am J Psychiatry 1981; 138:184–188.

91. Grove L, Cramer JL. Benzhexol and side effects with long lasting fluphenazine therapy. Br Med J 1972; 1:276–279.

92. Mandel W, Claffey B, Margolis LH. Recurrent thioperazine induced extrapyramidal reaction following placebo substititions for maintenance antiparkinsonian drugs. Am J Psychiatry 1962; 118:351–352.

93. St. Jean A, Donald M, Ban T. Interchangeability of antiparkinsonian medication. Am J Psychiatry 1964; 120:1189–1190.

94. Rifkin A, Quitkin F, Kane J, et al. Are prophylactic antiparkinson drugs necessary? Arch Gen Psychiatry 1978; 35:483- 489.
95. Hershon HI, Kennedy PF, McGuire RJ. Persistence of extrapyramidal disorders and psychiatric relapse after withdrawal of long-term phenothiazine therapy. Br J Psychiatry 1972; 120:41- 50.
96. McGeer PL, Bouling JE, Gibson WC, Foulkes RG. Drug-induced extrapyramidal treatment with diphenhydramine hydrochloride and dihydroxyphenylalanine reactions. JAMA 1961; 177:166–170.
97. Stratos NE, Phillips RD, Walker PA, Sandifer MG. A study of drug-induced parkinsonism. Dis Nerv Syst 1963; 24:180–181.
98. Cahan RB, Parrish DD. Reversibility of drug-induced parkinsonism. Am J Psychiatry 1960; 116:1022–1023.
99. Orlow P, Kasparian G, Dimascio A, Cole JO. Withdrawal of antiparkinson drugs. Arch Gen Psychiatry 1971; 25:410–412.
100. Nastelbaum Z, Siris SG, Rifkin A, et al. Exacerbation of schizophrenia associated with amantadine. Am J Psychiatry 1986; 143:1170–1171.
101. Borison RL. Amantadine in the management of extrapyramidal side effects. Clin Neuropharmacol 1983; 6(Supp 1):S57-S63.
102. Povison UJ, Noring U, Fog R, et al: Tolerability and therapeutic effect of clozapine. Acta Neurol Scand 1985; 71:176- 185.
103. Kane J, Honigfeld G, Singer J, Meltzer H. Clozapine for the treatment-resistant schizophrenic, a double-blind comparison with chlorpromazine. Arch Gen Psychiatry 1988; 45:789–796.
104. Honigfeld G: Personal communication, 1989.
105. Friedman JH, Lannon MC: Clozapine treatment of tremor in Parkinson's disease. Mov Disord 1990; 5:225–229.
106. Pakkenberg H, Pakkenberg B. Clozapine in the treatment of tremor. Acta Neurol Scand 1986; 73:295–297.
107. Lieberman JA, Johns CA, Kane JM, et al. Clozapine-induced agranulocytosis: non-crossreactivity with other psychotropic drugs. J Clin Psychiatry 1988; 49:271–277.
108. Fjalland B, Christensen AV, Hyttel J: Peripheral and central muscarinic receptor affinity of psychotropic drugs. Naunyn-Schmiedebergs' Arch Pharmacol 1977; 301:5–12.
109. Richelson E. Neuroleptic affinities for human brain receptors and their use in predicting adverse effects. J Clin Psychiatry 1984; 45:331–336.
110. Wolters ECH, Hurwitz TA, Peppard RF, Calne DB. Clozapine: an antipsychoactive agents in Parkinson's disease? Clin Neuropharmacol 1989; 12:83–90.
111. Andreasen NC. Negative symptoms in schizophrenia: definition and reliability. Arch Gen Psychiatry 1982; 39:784–788.

4

Acute Neuroleptic-Induced Akathisia

Lenard A. Adler, M.D., Burt Angrist, M.D.,
John Rotrosen, M.D.

Introduction

Akathisia, a frequent and disturbing side-effect of neuroleptic treatment, literally means an inability to remain seated. Patients with acute neuroleptic-induced akathisia (NIA) have complaints of restlessness, most often referable to the legs, and often have objective motor movements including "leg waggling," inability to remain seated, and rocking from foot to foot. This discussion will focus on acute akathisia, the most typical form encountered. Other akathisia variants, such as chronic akathisia and pseudoakathisia, are covered more extensively in Chapter 6. This chapter will review: (1) the history of spontaneously occurring syndromes of restlessness and acute NIA, (2) the clinical significance of acute NIA, (3) epidemiology of NIA, (4) pathophysiology of NIA, (5) treatment of NIA, and (6) conclusions and trends for future directions.

History

Syndromes of spontaneously occurring restlessness were indentified long prior to the introduction of neuroleptic medications.

Lang AE, Weiner WJ (editors): *Drug-Induced Movement Disorders,* Mount Kisco, NY, © Futura Publishing Co., Inc., 1992.

These syndromes were felt to be secondary to psychological causes, rather than a motor disorder. The earliest descriptions were in the 1600s,[1] with reports in the 1800s attributing the restlessness to neurasthenia or hysteria.[2]

The term akathisia, from Greek derivation (*kathisia*—"the act of sitting" and *a*—"negative prefix"), was first used by Haskovec,[3] who also felt that the syndrome derived from psychological causes. Two reports in 1923 were the first to attribute akathisia to extrapyramidal disease. Bing[4] noted the condition in patients with encephalitis lethargica (Von Economo's disease) and recognized that Haskovec's "akathisia" was a symptom of extrapyramidal dysfunction; moreover, he speculated that Haskovec's patients may also have been victims of a prior encephalitis epidemic known as the "Nona."[5] In 1923, Sicard also described akathisia in patients with idiopathic and postencephalitic Parkinson's disease.[6]

Ekbom decribed an idiopathic disorder, restless leg syndrome (RLS), which was similar to akathisia with subjective complaints of restlessness in the legs and associated motor movements.[7,8] He stressed the disturbing nature of the symptoms with vivid descriptions given by patients, such as "it is something crawling, irritating, unpleasant, deep in the tissues," or "it feels as if ants were running up and down in my bones." RLS, although qualitatively quite similar to akathisia, differs in that patients with RLS have symptoms predominantly in the evening and when at rest.[9,10]

With the introduction of neuroleptics, there were an increasing number of reports of syndromes of restlessness associated with these agents, which the investigators also termed akathisia.[11-13] The first report of drug-induced akathisia was by Sigwald, who reported this syndrome prior to the introduction of neuroleptics in patients treated with promethazine.[11]

Clinical Significance of Acute NIA

Signs and Symptoms

The akathisia syndrome is composed of both subjective complaints of restlessness and objective motor movements. Subjective complaints include a sense of inner restlessness, most often referable to the legs, a compulsion to move one's legs, dysphoria, and anxiety.[9,14,15]

The subjective distress of akathisia is significant in that it can lead to decreased compliance with treatment or a worsening of psychosis. Van Putten,[16] in a study of 85 patients on neuroleptics, found that akathisia was significantly more prevalent in patients who refused medication versus those who were compliant with neuroleptics. Van Putten et al.[17] coined the term *phenothiazine-induced decompensation* to refer to an increase in psychosis associated with akathisia. They found that such decompensations were similar to the original psychosis and that "thought processes became disorganized, secondary symptoms recurred, quality of contact deteriorated, and many complained of an abject fear or terror that was difficult to articulate." Additionally, the syndrome can be so dysphoric that it has been associated with aggressive behavior and violence[18-20] or suicide attempts.[20-24]

The diagnosis of akathisia may be difficult in patients with the mild form of the syndrome, who exhibit only subjective complaints, without showing objective movements.[14,25,26] Objective motor movements almost always accompany subjective restlessness in moderate and severe akathisia. These motor movements include: rocking from foot to foot, "walking on the spot," swinging of the legs (leg waggling), leg shuffling, pacing, or in its most severe form, tasikinesia, an inability to maintain any position.[9,14,26,27,28] The restlessness and accompanying movements are typically bilateral and relatively symmetrical. Recently, cases of unilateral NIA have also been reported.[28a]

Differential Diagnosis

Disorders that can be confused with NIA occur both in patients who are and who are not receiving neuroleptics. As noted above, akathisia was originally felt to be secondary to psychological causes and a variety of psychological diagnoses should be considered in the differential diagnosis of NIA. Restless leg syndrome and other movement disorders (such as chronic akathisia, pseudoakathisia, and tardive dyskinesia) can also be difficult to distinguish from NIA.

Agitation Seen With Other Psychiatric Disorders

The agitation in a major depression, mania, or psychosis may result in significant restlessness or motor movements similar to that seen with akathisia. If these patients are receiving neuroleptics, it may not be possible to distinguish these symptoms from akathisia. A pattern of worsening of agitation with increasing neuroleptics may particularly alert the clinician to Van Putten's "phenothiazine-induced decompensation." In such cases, treatment of suspected akathisia is usually warranted.

Patients with generalized anxiety disorder may be restless and can pace. Akathisia may be differentiated from generalized anxiety in that in akathisia there is a compulsion to move and the feelings are described as "driven" or "unnatural";[15,29] however, not all patients can articulate such "fine" distinctions. Treatment response may again help differentiate these conditions. Adler et al.[30] found that in patients with akathisia the benzodiazepine lorazepam improved subjective complaints of restlessness, but not objective motor movements, while both elements of the syndrome were improved by propranolol. Conversely, one study found that propranolol improved both the subjective restlesssness and objective movements of akathisia without significantly affecting Hamilton Anxiety Scale ratings.[31]

Drug Withdrawal States

Restlessness, painful sensations in the legs, and leg movements are common symptoms of opiate withdrawal. Similarities between opiate withdrawal and akathisia also extend to agents used to treat these conditions. The alpha$_2$ agonist clonidine has been found to improve both opiate withdrawal[32] and akathisia.[33,34] Additionally, low doses of the β-blocker propranolol have been reported to improve the restlessness of both opiate withdrawal[35] and akathisia.[30,31,36–39]

Other Movement Disorders

Restless Leg Syndrome (RLS)

As mentioned above, patients with RLS complain of uncomfortable sensory phenomena in the legs, especially in the evening or at night when attempting to fall asleep. On the other hand, akathisia does not occur more frequently at any particular time of the day. It is not necessarily worsened by lying down and, indeed, many patients find this to be their most comfortable or preferred position.

Chronic Akathisia

Chronic akathisia occurs late in the course of treatment; this differs from acute akathisia, which is an early effect. Both forms of the syndrome have subjective complaints of restlessness along with objective motor movements. Barnes and Braude[40] defined chronic akathisia as occurring more than 6 months after initiation of, or increase in the dose of, neuroleptic.

Chronic akathisia may be more difficult to treat than acute akathisia.[41] The chronic form may also behave like tardive dyskinesia. Jeste and Wyatt[42] noted that in some patients chronic akathisia "has pharmacological characteristics similar to those of other manifestations of tardive dyskinesia." Braude and Barnes[43] reported two patients with chronic akathisia. The akathisia was more pharmacologically similar to tardive dyskinesia than acute akathisia, in that it was (1) improved by increasing the dose of neuroleptic, (2) worsened by reduction of the available dose of neuroleptic, and (3) unresponsive to anticholinergics.

Pseudoakathisia and Tardive Dyskinesia

Patients with pseudoakathisia have objective motor movements of akathisia, without subjective complaints of restlessness. The importance in establishing a differential between acute akathisia and pseudoakathisia is that it has been hypothesized that acute akathisia, chronic akathisia, pseudoakathisia and tardive dyskinesia may be points in a continuum.[43-47] This supposition is based upon several studies finding a relationship between pseudoakathisia and dyskinetic movements. Munetz and Cornes[45] studied 45 patients with tardive dyskinesia; they found that 21 patients had an acute akathisia at some prior time and that 11 of these 21 had a pseudoakathisia at the time of the examination. Barnes and Braude[40] studied 39 patients receiving depot neuroleptics who also had akathisia. They divided the patients as to whether they had acute akathisia, chronic akathisia, or pseudoakathisia. None of the patients with acute akathisia had tardive dyskinesia, while over one-half of the patients with chronic akathisia or pseudoakathisia also had dyskinesias.

Munetz[47] suggested "in distinguishing akathisia from tardive dyskinesia, one tries to determine whether the patient is restless and is therefore moving (akathisia) or moving and therefore restless (tardive dyskinesia)." However, in practice the differentiation of acute akathisia from some of the movements seen in patients with tardive dyskinesia and akathisia variants is often difficult, if not at times impossible, especially when the conditions coexist.

Epidemiology of Acute NIA

Timing of Onset of Effect

Akathisia can develop very rapidly after initiating or increasing the dose of neuroleptics or dopamine antagonists. Barnes et al.[48] have reported akathisia developing within an hour of receiving preoperative medication with droperidol and metoclopramide. The development of akathisia also appears to be dose-dependent. Ayd[49] surveyed 3775 patients receiving neuroleptics and found that patients started on higher doses of neuroleptics were more likely to develop akathisia than patients started on lower doses. Braude et al.[27] prospectively studied the development of akathisia in 109 inpatients followed over 23 days and also found a dose-dependent relationship. Frequently, it can take several weeks for akathisia to develop.[14] Acute akathisia tends to persist, although fluctuate in intensity, over time.[9] Although infrequent, akathisia has been reported to persist after discontinuation of neuroleptics.[50,51]

Prevalence of Acute Akathisia

The reported prevalence of akathisia in patients receiving neuroleptics varies widely. Lower estimates of prevalence, ranging from 3% to 13%,[52–54] were found in earlier studies.[14] More recent investigations have found higher prevalences. Gibb and Lees[14] and Van Putten[15] found figures in the 40% to 45% range. Most recently, Van Putten et al.[55] studied 32 schizophrenics, who were off neuroleptics and then treated with haloporidol 10 mg/day for 7 days and found a 75% incidence of akathisia. The most common estimate of prevalence is 20%.[27,49,56] Several factors may account for this wide variability in prevalence.[38] These include: (1) a lack of recognition of akathisia,[57] (2) the fact that some investigators exclude patients with only subjective complaints of restlessness, without objective motor movements (as may exist in mild forms of akathisia), and (3) the degree to which high- versus low-potency neuroleptics are used. Although all neuroleptics can cause akathisia, the syndrome occurs more frequently with higher potency agents).[49,58]

Evaluation/Quantification of Akathisia

There are six main scales that have been used to evaluate akathisia. Lipinski et al.[36,37] have used the akathisia item from the Chouinard Extrapyramidal Symptom Rating Scale (ESRS).[59] Subjective complaints are rated 0 to 3 ("none" to "severe"). Objective movements are rated 0 to 6 (0 = "none"; 1 = "looks restless, nervous, impatient, uncomfortable"; 2 = "needs to move at least one extremity"; 3 = "often needs to move one extremity or to change position"; 4 = "moves one extremity almost constantly if sitting or stamps feet while standing"; 5 = "unable to sit down for more than a short period of time"; 6 = "moves or walks constantly").

Adler et al.[30,31,38] have measured objective movements with the akathisia item from the Hillside/Long Island Jewish modification of the Simpson/Angus Extrapyramidal Symptom (EPS) Scale. Movements of akathisia are rated 0 to 4 (0 = "absent"; 1 = "mild; occasional restlessness observed during exam"; 2 = "moderate; continuous restlessness observed"; 3 = "marked; subject in and out of chair during exam; unable to maintain concentration"; and 4 = "extreme; heightened activity; panic".)

These authors have assessed subjective complaints of restlessness by having the patient mark a 100-mm line with anchor points, relating to the frequency of restlessness and degree of distress (0 = "none"; 20 = "sometimes a little"; 40 = "most of the time, a little"; 60 = "all of the time, sometimes annoying"; 80 = "all of the time, always very annoying"; and 100 = "can't stand it anymore").

Braude et al.[27] developed a 23-item rating scale. Subjective complaints were assessed by four items (limb sensations, inner restlessness, inability to remain still, and inability to keep legs still). Objective movements were rated 0 (absent) to 3 (continuous movement) with the patient in three positions (seated, standing, and lying). These authors found that this scale was able to distinguish akathisia from "illness-related movements" (secondary to psychopathology).

These authors have subsequently condensed the critical items from this 23-item scale into a four-item scale.[28] Patients are observed for at least 2 minutes in three situations: (1) when they do not know they are being observed and (2) during formal interview, both seated and standing. Objective movements are rated 0 to 3 based upon their frequency (e.g., more or less than one-half the time) and severity. Subjective complaints are divided into awareness and distress subsets, each rated 0 to 3. A global assessment of akathisia is scored 0 ("absent") to 5 ("severe"); the global rating includes assessments of the awareness of, and distress from, subjective complaints and the severity and frequency of objective movements.

The final scale is the Hillside akathisia scale.[60] As in the Braude et al.[27] 23-item scale, patients are rated sitting, standing, and lying down. Subjective complaints are divided into two subsets, the sensation of inner restlessness and the urge to move, each rated 0 ("absent") to 4 ("present and not controllable"). Objective movements are assessed separately in the head and trunk, hands and arms, and feet and legs; they are rated 0 to 4 (0 = "no akathisia"; 1 = "questionable"; 2 = "small amplitude movements, part of the time"; 3 = "small amplitude movements, all of the time or large amplitude movements, part of the time"; 4 = "large amplitude movements, all of the time"). There is also a clinical global impression item, which asks the rater to score the severity of akathisia, based on their experience with patients with akathisia, on a 1 ("normal, not at all akathisic") to 7 ("among the most akathisic of patients") scale.

The Hillside scale's inclusion of ratings of movements in the head/trunk and hands/arms in addition to those in the lower extremity constitutes a double-edged sword. Two systematic studies of patients with akathisia have found that movements of the lower extremities (e.g., rocking from foot to foot, pacing, leg waggling, etc.) are more specific for the syndrome of akathisia and help differentiate it from other syndromes.[14,27] Although akathisia may cause movements of other body areas, by including ratings of movements in the head/trunk and upper extremity, the Hillside scale might be more sensitive (by missing fewer cases since it includes movements of these other areas), but less specific than the other scales.

Pathophysiology of Acute Akathisia

The pathophysiology of acute akathisia is far from established, but appears to involve dopaminergic, noradrenergic, and other neurotransmitter systems. Dopaminergic dysfunction is implicated as akathisia: (1) occurs in both idiopathic Parkinson's disease (up to one in four patients)[61] and postencephalitic Parkinson's disease, and (2) is associated with the administration of dopamine-blocking agents. Marsden and Jenner[56] hypothesize that blockade of post-synaptic dopamine receptors in mesocortical tracts may be involved in the pathophysiology of akathisia. They base this concept on a variety of preclinical studies that indicate that these mesocortical tracts inhibit spontaneous locomotion and that dopamine blockade may remove this inhibition.

Dopaminergic hypofunction, while critical to the pathophysiology of akathisia, is likely to be an oversimplification. Agents affecting other neurotransmitters affect akathisia in a variety of ways. These include: (1) GABAergic agents: benzodiazepines have been shown to improve akathisia,[62-64] (2) adrenergic agents: an extensive body of literature exists that documents the efficacy of β-blockers in akathisia.[30,31,36,37,39] The α_2 agonist clonidine has also been found to improve the syndrome,[33,34] and (3) serotonergic agents: agents that increase or decrease serotonergic function have been shown to both improve and worsen akathisia.[65-73] Obviously, this does not disprove a primary role for dopamine since these other neurotransmitter systems have been shown to modulate dopaminergic function.[74-79]

Treatment of Akathisia

Adjusting the Dose of Neuroleptic Medication

The simplest treatment of acute akathisia is to lower the dose of neuroleptics. Braude et al.[27] treated 39 patients with akathisia and found that all 10 patients whose neuroleptic dose was decreased had improvement in akathisia. Obviously, however, dose reduction is not always a viable strategy in floridly psychotic patients. Switching the patient to a lower potency neuroleptic is another potential strategy.[49]

Pharmacological Treatment of NIA

The agents that have been used to treat NIA include[38]: (1) anti-parkinsonian agents, including anticholinergics and amantadine,

(2) benzodiazepines, and (3) agents that affect noradrenergic function, such as β-blockers and clonidine.

Antiparkinsonian Agents

Antiparkinsonian medications are commonly used to treat akathisia. However, there are few formal prospective studies of these agents in NIA. Many clinicians feel that antiparkinsonian agents are only partially effective; their use is limited by side effects to anticholinergics[49,58] or tolerance to the therapeutic effect of amantadine.[80]

Anticholinergics

There are many open studies of anticholinergic medications in drug-induced parkinsonism, few of which specifically examine affects on akathisia. Kruse[81] treated 112 patients with extrapyramidal symptoms for 3 months each with the anticholinergics benztropine and procyclidine; nearly equal numbers of patients predominantly had akathisia versus rigidity/tremors as their major symptoms. He found that patients who had akathisia responded less well to the anticholinergics than those who had rigidity/tremor. (Response rates: (1) benztropine/akathisia group – 21%; (2) rigidity and tremor group – 86%; (3) procyclidine/akathisia group – 57%; (4) rigidity and tremor group – 81%.)

Neu et al.[82] compared the efficacy of single versus multiple dose schedules of benztropine (4–6 mg/day) in 71 patients with drug-induced parkinsonism under double-blind conditions. They found that all of the patients with akathisia had substantial improvement after benztropine treatment (regardless of dose schedule).

Van Putten et al.[17] administered double-blind test doses of the anticholinergic agent biperiden (5 mg IM) and placebo to patients in whom the diagnosis of akathisia was uncertain. Patients were considered to have akathisia if their restlessness improved with biperiden, but not with placebo.

Van Putten and co-workers[55] examined the response of akathisia to open treatment with anticholinergic medications (benztropine or trihexyphenidyl) in patients receiving 1 week of treatment with 10 mg/day of thiothixene (n = 37) or haloperidol (n = 32). In the thiothixene group, four patients had a dysphoric reaction to anticholinergics and were excluded, and 30 of the remaining patients had a complete response of their NIA to anticholinergics. In the haloperidol cohort, 14 had a complete remission after anticholinergics. In this study, the investigators were screening for the development of akathisia and therefore rapidly instituted treatment for NIA. Thus, it is not clear what percentage of the patients would have also developed concomitant parkinsonian EPS if anticholinergic treatment had not been initiated.

Friis et al.[83] performed a double-blind, crossover study of 4 weeks of treatment each with biperiden (6–18 mg/day), the anticonvulsant sodium valproate, and placebo in 15 patients with NIA. Akathisia was rated on a 0 to 3 scale. Seventy-three percent of the patients responded to biperiden (mean akathisia score decreased from 1.4 after placebo to 0.6 after biperiden); no significant effects of sodium valproate or placebo were seen. It is of interest that 11 of the 15 patients had concurrent parkinsonian EPS.

Braude et al.[27] found that only 6 of 20 patients had improvement in NIA after open treatment with anticholinergics. Those patients who improved also had significant parkinsonian EPS. They suggest that there may be two distinct types of akathisia, distinguished by associated parkinsonian EPS and response to anticholinergics in one form, but not the other. This may explain the findings by: (1) Kruse[81] of a low response rate to anticholinergics in patients who had akathisia alone (versus those who had parkinsonian EPS alone) and (2) Friis et al.[83] of a high response rate to biperiden in patients with NIA, many of whom had concomitant parkinsonian EPS.

Amantadine

Merrick and Schmitt[84] treated 11 patients with drug-induced parkinsonism in a double-blind, crossover design study of 3 weeks of treatment with amantadine (200 mg/day) versus benztropine (2–4 mg/day). Substantial and fairly equal improvements in NIA were seen with both medications.

DiMascio et al.[85] compared amantadine (n = 13) and benztropine (n = 11) under double-blind conditions in patients with drug-induced EPS and NIA. Comparable improvement in NIA occured over 4 weeks of treatment with both agents.

Stenson et al.[86] treated 11 patients with NIA (under parallel group, double-blind conditions) with matching benztropine (4–6 mg/

day) (n = 6) or amantadine (200–300 mg/day) (n = 5) for up to 7 days. All of patients treated with amantadine improved; in the cohort receiving benztropine, four patients improved, one was unchanged, and one had a worsening of akathisia.

Zubenko et al.[80] treated four patients with NIA with amantadine. All four patients initially showed substantial benefit; however, within 1 week, tolerance developed to amantadine. Transient improvement occurred after raising the dose of amantadine again. One of these four patients had concomitant EPS that responded to amantadine, without the developement of tolerance.

Benzodiazepines

Donlon[87] noted improvement in akathisia in 10 of 13 patients who received open treatment with diazepam (15 mg/day). All patients had not improved with prior treatment with diphenhydramine (antihistaminic/anticholinergic) 75 mg/day.

Gagrat et al.[88] performed a double-blind, parallel-group trial of single intravenous (IV) doses of diazepam (5 mg) (n = 9) versus diphenhydramine (50 mg) (n = 11). NIA was rated at baseline and four times up to 2 hours after infusion. Mean postinfusion ratings (at all four times) were significantly lower than baseline for both diazepam- and diphenhydramine-treated groups.

Kutcher et al.[63] reported the results of an open 1-week trial of clonazepam (0.5 mg/day) in 10 adolescents with NIA. Mean akathisia scores (on the ESRS) decreased significantly from 4.1 at baseline to 1.6 at the end of clonazepam. They noted that possible advantages of clonazepam over other benzodiazepines were: (1) the low doses required and (2) the long half-life, making once-a-day treatment possible.

These authors then conducted a double-blind, parallel-group study of treatment with clonazepam 1 mg (n = 7) versus placebo (n = 7).[64] Substantial improvement was seen in all patients receiving clonazepam; five of the patients receiving placebo were unchanged, while two patients had mild improvement (of one point on the akathisia subscale of the ESRS). Also, all four of the patients in the placebo cohort who received a subsequent open trial of clonazepam responded to this agent.

Bartels et al.[62] studied the effects of 2 weeks of open treatment with lorazepam (1.5–5 mg/day) in 16 schizophrenic patients with

NIA. Fourteen patients improved with lorazepam (nine had marked response, and five had moderate response), while two patients were unchanged. Improvement occurred after the first week of treatment, with minimal additional amelioration after the second week of treatment.

Beta-Blockers

β-blockers are currently considered to be the most promising treatments for akathisia. These medications can be classified according to four properties: (1) selectivity, (2) lipophilicity, (3) intrinsic sympathomimetic activity (ISA), and (4) nonspecific properties, such as membrane stabilizing effects (MSE). Those that solely block β_1 receptors (the predominant beta-receptor in cardiac tissue) or β_2 receptors (e.g., lung, pancreas) are referred to as "selective" beta-blockers. Those that block both β_1 and β_2 receptors are refered to as "nonselective" beta-blockers. The more lipophilic beta-blockers cross the blood-brain barrier (BBB) during acute administration, while the less lipophilic (relatively hydrophilic) agents have a lower rate of penetrance of the BBB.[89] Beta-blockers with ISA have some partial agonist activity and therefore do not lower the heart rate as much as those agents without this property. Membrane stabilization is a term used to refer to decreased conductivity in isloated preparations of cardiac tissue, which correlates with local anesthetic effects of β-blockers.[90,91]

Table 1 classifies beta-blockers according to these four properties.[91] This table also shows the β_1 blockade potency ratios for each agent[38,91-93] so that dose comparisons can be made in the treatment studies. Table 2 summarizes studies with propranolol; Table 3 summarizes studies with other beta-blocking agents.

We will divide and discuss the studies of beta-blockers in NIA according to these properties. In general, centrally active beta-blockers (i.e., relatively lipophilic agents) have proven more efficacious than relatively hydrophilic ones. The data are less clear regarding the relative contributions of β_1 and β_2 receptors as agents selective for either receptor subset are effective. Membrane stabilizing effects do not seem to contribute significantly to the therapeutic effects.

Studies of Propranolol (Lipophilic, Nonselective) (Table 2)

Strang[94] originally described the beneficial effects of propranolol (5–30 mg/day) in parkinsonian patients who had restless leg syn-

Table 1

Characteristics of β-Blockers

Drug	Blockade of β-1 Receptors	Blockade of β-2 Receptors	MSE	Lipophilicity	β-1 Blockade Potency Ratio (D/L-Propranolol = 1)
d/l-Propranolol	+ +	+ +	+ +	+ + +	1.0
d-Propranolol	0	0	+ +	+ + +	—
Metoprolol*	+ +	0– +	0– +	+ +	1.0
Nadolol	+ +	+ +	0	0– +	1.0
Atenolol	+ +	0– +	0	0	1.0
Pindolol	+ +	+ +	+	+ +	6.0
ICI 118,551	0	+ +	+ +	+ + +	—
Betaxolol**	+ +	0– +	0	+ +	3.0–10.0
Sotalol	+ +	+ +	0	0	0.3

MSE = Membrane stabilizing effects.
* Metoprolol is selective for β-1 receptors at doses ≤ 100 mg/day.
** Betaxolol is selective for β-1 receptors at doses ≤ 10 mg/day.

drome. This led Lipinski et al.[36] to undertake the first trial of propranolol in NIA. Twelve patients with NIA were treated with propranolol (mean dose = 30 mg/day) in an open design. All patients improved, with nine having a complete response. This improvement was rapid with "a considerable clinical response typically [occurring] within an hour of the first dose and the maximum clinical response . . . in 24–48 hours." No significant changes in blood pressure or pulse were observed. Concomitant EPS were also unaffected. The rapidity of the response to propranolol and the absence of effects on blood pressure/pulse and parkinsonian symptoms have also been noted consistently in subsequent studies of low-dose propranolol in NIA. In the same year, another case of NIA successfully treated with propranolol was reported by Kulik and Wilbur.[95]

There have been several other reports, which are detailed below, of the efficacy of propranolol in NIA. Although the results of these studies have been uniformly positive, these investigations have each studied a relatively small number of patients.

Lipinski et al.[37] also reported an extension of their original open study which further documented the efficacy of propranolol in NIA.

Adler et al.[30] compared propranolol 20–30 mg/day, lorazepam 2 mg/day, and periods of no treatment in six patients with NIA; this

Table 2

Studies of Propranolol in Acute Neuroleptic-Induced Akathisia

Author	# of Subjects/ Design	Drug (Mean mg/ day)	Response
I. Open Studies			
Lipinski et al.[36]	12 patients	propranolol: 30	9 patients: complete response
			1 patient: 50% response; 2 patients 70% response
Kulik and Wilbur[95]	1 patient	propranolol: 160	response upon initial treatment and rechallenge
Lipinski et al.[37]	14 patients	propranolol: 42	all improved; 9 patients with complete response
Adler et al.[96]	17 patients; parallel group	propranolol: 56	9 patients: significant reductions in subjective and objective NIA
		benztropine: 2.9	8 patients: little change in subjective and objective NIA
II. Controlled Studies			
Adler et al.[30]	6 patients	propranolol: 25	significant reduction in subjective and objective NIA
	single-blind	lorazepam: 2	significant reduction only in subjective NIA
	crossover	no treatment	no significant difference from baseline
Adler et al.[31]	12 patients; double-blind; crossover	propranolol: 51	significant reduction in subjective and objective NIA
		placebo	no significant change from baseline
Kramer et al.[39]	20 patients; double-blind; crossover	propranolol: 60 placebo	significant improvement in NIA after 5 days of propranolol
Lipinski et al.[97]	20 patients; double-blind; parallel group	propranolol placebo	improvement in NIA greater on propranolol
Adler et al.[98]	11 patients; double-blind; crossover and parallel group	d-propranolol: 80 placebo d/L propranolol: 80	no difference in subjective and objective NIA after d-propranolol or placebo; significant improvement in 8 patients after open d/l propranolol

Table 3

Studies of Other β-Blockers in Acute Neuroleptic-Induced Akathisia

Study	Agent	Characteristics	Results
I. Hydrophilic Agents			
Lipinski et al.[37]	nadolol	hydrophilic nonselective	nadolol less effective than propranolol
Ratey et al.[104]	nadolol	hydrophilic nonselective	3 patients; good response after 2 weeks
Adler et al.[105]	nadolol	hydrophilic nonselective	6 patients; good response with at least 9–11 days of treatment 1 patient with CNS syphilis; rapid response in 1 day
Dupuis et al.[115]	sotalol	hydrophilic nonselective	6 patients with prior response to propranolol were unresponsive to sotalol
II. Selective Agents			
Derom et al.[106]	atenolol	hydrophilic β-1 selective	1 patient; no response to atenolol; good response to propranolol
Reiter et al.[107]	atenolol	hydrophilic β-1 selective	7 patients; no improvement on atenolol, while propranolol was effective
Zubenko et al.[111]	metoprolol	β-1 selective $\leq$ 100 mg/day	5 patients; metoprolol as effective as propanolol only at doses $\geq$ 200 mg/day
Kim et al.[113]	metoprolol	β-1 selective $\leq$ 100 mg/day	9 patients; metoprolol effective only doses < 100 mg/day; no additional benefit with subsequent propranolol treatment
Adler et al.[114]	metoprolol	β-1 selective $\leq$ 100 mg/day	8 patients; equal effects of 1 day treatment with metoprolol (75 mg/day) vs. propranolol
Dupuis et al.[115]	betaxolol	β-1 selective	4 patients with prior response to propranolol had good response to betaxolol
Adler et al.[117]	betaxolol	β-1 selective	6 patients; equal response to betaxolol and propranolol
Adler et al.[118]	ICI 118,551	β-2 selective	improvement with both ICI 118,551 and propranolol (n = 6); no significant effect of placebo (n = 4)

was a crossover study, in which the rater was blind. Propranolol significantly decreased subjective and objective measures of NIA, while lorazepam diminished subjective, but not objective akathisia scores. Scores at the end of no treatment periods did not differ from baseline.

These authors also performed a randomized, double-blind, crossover design study of the efficacy of propranolol (20–60 mg/day, mean dose = 51 mg/day) and matching placebo in treating NIA.[31] Propranolol caused significant overall improvement in both subjective and objective measures of akathisia compared to ratings done both at baseline and on placebo. Placebo caused no significant change of akathisia ratings from baseline. No significant effect of either propranolol or placebo was seen on Hamilton Anxiety scores. Parkinsonian EPS (cogwheeling, rigidity, tremor, akinesia), as measured by the Simpson/Angus EPS Scale were not significantly affected by treatment with propranolol.

Adler et al.[96] treated 17 patients with akathisia with propranolol (n = 9) 40–80 mg/day or benztropine (n = 8) 1.5–4.0 mg/day. This was a parallel-group design in which nonblind akathisia ratings were obtained at baseline and at the end of either treatment. Assessments of memory, performed by a rater blind to treatment assignment, were also obtained to examine for possible effects on cognition. As in prior studies, we found approximately 50% decreases in both subjective and objective NIA after treatment with propranolol. No change in objective NIA and a small decrease in subjective NIA occurred after treatment with benztropine. The relative lack of efficacy of benztropine in this study was hypothesized to be possibly due to: (1) atypical responses in the small sample and (2) only one of the patients having significant concomitant parkinsonian EPS. Braude et al.[27] also found that patients who had NIA, but not parkinsonian EPS, responded poorly to anticholinergics. Three measures of recent memory (Buschke recall, Buschke consistent retrieval, and superspan digits subtests) and one measure of immediate memory (WAIS digits forward) were impaired in those patients who received benztropine, but not in those who were treated with propranolol.

Kramer et al.[39] also completed a double-blind, crossover study of propranolol (60 mg/day) and placebo in 20 patients. Patients were divided into two cohorts, those who received (1) 2 days of placebo, followed by 5 days of propranolol, or (2) 2 days of propranolol followed by 5 days of placebo. There was an overall trend of decrease in subjective and objective akathisia after propranolol. Furthermore, ratings on two akathisia subscales were significantly lower after 5 days of treatment with propranolol than after 5 days of placebo. Interpretation of the data from this study is compromised by (1) unequal length of treatment in the two groups (i.e., 2 versus 5 days), and (2) possible carryover effects of 5 days of propranolol into the 2-day treatment period on placebo.

Lipinski and co-workers[97] have completed a randomized, parallel-group study of propranolol in 20 patients with NIA. Changes in akathisia scores from baseline were significantly greater with propranolol than with placebo.

We have recently completed a study[98] in collaboration with Lipinski and co-workers at McLean Hospital of d-propranolol in akathisia. Eleven patients (8 at the New York VAMC and 3 at McLean) completed this double-blind, crossover design study of d-propranolol 80 mg/day versus placebo. The clinical formulation of propranolol is a racemate. The d-isomer has a variety of pharmacological actions in common with the racemate, including membrane stabilization; however, the d-isomer does not have clinically significant β-blocking properties (only 1.7% to 6.7% of the racemate, based on clinical and preclinical studies of antagonism of isoproterenol-induced tachycardia).[99–101] In this study of d-propranolol in NIA, there were no differences in ratings at baseline versus after placebo versus after d-propranolol. Significant reductions in akathisia were seen in the eight patients who received racemic propranolol (80 mg/day) after the study was completed. This indicates that antagonism of β-receptors and not nonspecific properties, such as MSE, mediates the therapeutic effect of propranolol in NIA.

In all of these studies of racemic propranolol maximal improvement was noted within 3 days of initiation of treatment (except for Kramer et al.,[39] who found significant improvement after 5 days, but not 2 days, of treatment with propranolol).

Studies of Other β-Blockers in NIA (Table 3)

Other Nonselective β-Blockers

Pindolol (Lipophilic, Nonselective, with ISA): We have studied pindolol, another nonselective, lipophilic β-blocker, which additionally has the partial agonist property of intrinsic sympathomimetic activity (ISA), at first in one patient with sinus bradycardia and

NIA[102] and then in an additional eight patients[103] with akathisia. Of these nine patients, four had substantial or complete remissions in their akathisia after pindolol 5 mg/day. The five patients who did not respond were then treated with propranolol (mean = 72.0 mg/day) for 2–8 days; four of these five subjects had further improvement with propranolol. We suggested that the differential response may have been due to pindolol: (1) being less lipophilic than propranolol and (2) having partial agonist activity (ISA).

Nadolol (Nonlipophilic, Nonselective): Lipinski et al.[37] made the first attempt to treat NIA with other β-blockers besides propranolol, in order to evaluate central versus peripheral and β_1 versus β_2 mechanisms in the therapeutic effect. They found that nadolol (a nonselective, relatively hydrophilic agent) was less effective after acute treatment than propranolol (nonselective, lipophilic) in the treatment of NIA.

In contrast, Ratey et al.[104] described three cases of NIA that improved with nadolol (hydrophilic, nonselective). Interpretation of these data is difficult because (1) the improvement was also co-incident with the starting of benzodiazepines, and (2) the clinical effects required approximately 2 weeks with nadolol versus hours to days with propranolol.

Adler et al.[105] recently treated six patients with NIA with nadolol 60 mg/day for 12 to 14 days. Akathisia ratings were subdivided into the following epochs: day 0 (baseline), day 1, day 3–4, day 6–7, day 9–11, and day 12–14. Significant improvement in akathisia was not seen until 9–11 days (subjective ratings) and 12–14 days (objective and global ratings) of nadolol treatment. These findings verify both Lipinski's and Ratey's findings of a subacute, but not an acute, onset of action of nadolol, in that the effect was not seen until at least 9–11 days of treatment. During this study, a seventh patient with NIA, a chronic schizophrenic who also had neurosyphilis was treated. He had a complete cessation of akathisia after 1 day of nadolol therapy. The rapid response of this patient suggests a central site of action, as the active CNS syphilis infection presumably led to a more permeable blood-brain barrier and more rapid penetration of nadolol.

Studies of Selective β-Blockers

Atenolol (Nonlipophilic, β_1-Selective): Derom et al.[106] have reported a patient whose akathisia was improved with propranolol 120 mg/day, but not with atenolol (a nonlipophilic, selective β_1 antagonist) 100 mg/day. Reiter et al.[107] treated seven patients in a parallel-group design with atenolol (mean maximum dose = 60.7 mg/day) and propranolol (mean maximum dose = 60.0 mg/day). Propranolol significantly improved both subjective and objective akathisia versus baseline ratings; atenolol did not improve objective akathisia, and in fact worsened subjective complaints of restlessness in several patients. The authors note the following possible reasons for worsening:

1. Differences in these agents in lipophilicity and selectivity (atenolol: hydrophilic, β_1-selective; propranolol: lipophilic, nonselective).

2. An indirect effect of selective peripheral β_1 blockade (with atenolol, but not propranolol) leading to a compensatory increase in central noradrenergic activity. Patterson's[108] report of a syndrome similar to akathisia in a hypertensive patient treated with atenolol (but not receiving neuroleptics) supports this possibility.

3. Pharmacokinetic effects of beta-blockers on neuroleptic plasma levels: Two studies have shown increased plasma neuroleptic levels in patients treated with propranolol for aggressive behavior. Silver et al.[109] found that high-dose propranolol (up to 800 mg/day) increased thioridazine levels in two patients. Greendyke and Kanter[110] studied 12 patients with organic brain disease who were receiving high doses of propranolol; they found that propranolol increased plasma thioridazine levels, but not haloperidol levels. If atenolol also increases neuroleptic levels, these higher levels plus lack of acute central effects of atenolol could lead to a worsening of akathisia.

Metoprolol (Lipophilic, β_1-Selective): Zubenko et al.[111] found that metoprolol, which is a lipophilic/β_1-selective (in low doses) blocker, was effective in treating akathisia only in doses (>200 mg/day) where both β_1 and β_2 receptors are blocked.[112]

Kim and co-workers[113] examined the effect on NIA of increasing doses of metoprolol in nine patients (in the first six, ratings were nonblind; in the last three, the rater was blind to initiation of treatment). All patients were started at 25–50 mg/day of metoprolol, with the dose of metoprolol increased by 25 mg every several days up to a maximum of 100 mg/day or where maximal clinical improvement occurred. Ratings were obtained prior to each dosage increase. All patients were subsequently treated with open propranolol 60 mg/ day. The mean dose of metoprolol where maximal improvement occurred was 66.7 mg/day, a dose where selectivity for the β_1 receptor is putatively maintained. Seven patients had substantial improvements in akathisia after metoprolol. No significant further improvement was seen with subsequent propranolol treatment.

We conducted a second study[114] of the effects of metoprolol at β_1-selective doses: (1) because of the conflicting results of studies of this agent at β_1-selective doses and (2) to control for possible carryover effects that may have been present in our first metoprolol study (as patients were treated with propranolol immediately after their metoprolol trial). This study was a single-blind crossover design study of 1 day trials of metoprolol (75 mg/day) and propranolol (60 mg/day), with an intervening washout period. Eight patients with NIA participated. Both propranolol and metoprolol produced significant decreases in NIA, which were of equal magnitude.

Betaxolol (Lipophilic, β_1-Selective): Dupuis et al.[115] studied three different β-blockers, propranolol (20–40 mg/day), sotalol (nonlipophilic, nonselective) (40–80 mg/day), and betaxolol (lipophilic, β_1-selective) (10–20 mg/day), with an intervening washout period between each trial. Eight of 16 patients had complete remission of akathisia after propranolol. Six of these eight had recurrences of akathisia after discontinuation of propranolol. These patients were then unsuccessfully treated with sotalolol. Four of these remaining, initally propranolol-responsive patients were then treated with betaxolol, with each having a complete response of their akathisia.

Until recently, oral betaxolol was not available in the United States market. Betaxolol appears to maintain its β_1 selectivity over a larger dose range than metoprolol.[116] We have treated eight patients with NIA with betaxolol 5 mg/day, a dose where β_1 selectivity is quite likely to be maintained.[117] All eight patients improved and there was no further improvement with subsequent treatment with propranolol.

ICI 118,551 (Lipophilic, β_2-Selective): We have also examined the effects of ICI 118,551 (the only lipophilic β_2-selective agent developed to date) in a double-blind, parallel group study versus placebo in 10 patients (ICI 118,551 = 6; placebo = 4) with NIA.[118] Mean measures of akathisia were lower in the patients who received ICI

118,551 than in those who received placebo. Five of the six patients treated with ICI 118,551 had improvement in akathisia, while only one of the placebo-treated patients improved (chi-square, $x^2 = 6.53$, df = 2, p≤0.05). This study, however, was terminated prematurely when ICI 118,551 was withdrawn from clinical evaluation.

Clonidine

Clonidine is an alpha$_2$ agonist that decreases central noradrenergic activity.[119] Zubenko et al.[33] conducted an open trial of clonidine (0.2–0.8 mg/day) in six patients with NIA. All six patients improved, with four having complete remission. Treatment was limited by hypotension in two cases. These two patients also developed sedation and had only partial responses to clonidine. This lesser response in the patients who developed hypotension/sedation led Zubenko and co-workers to conclude that the therapeutic efficacy of clonidine was not related to its sedative properties.

Adler et al.[34] treated six patients with clonidine (0.15–0.40 mg/day) in a single-blind (rater-blind) design. Both subjective and objective akathisia were significantly decreased after treatment versus ratings at baseline. Akathisia ratings were substantially improved in all patients. Hamilton Anxiety Scale scores were also significantly lowered. The use of clonidine was limited by hypotension in five cases and clinically apparent sedation in four patients. Thus the possibility exists that in this study, the efficacy of the clonidine was due to a nonspecific sedative effect rather than a specific pharmacological effect on noradrenergic transmission. Both Adler et al. and Zubenko et al. noted that the sedation encountered with clonidine was not observed with beta-blockers. Clonidine also differed from propranolol in that clonidine decreased Hamilton Anxiety scores, while propranolol did not.

Conclusions and Future Directions

Quantification of Akathisia

The Barnes four-item akathisia scale seems to be the best available rating instrument (Table 4). Both the Barnes and the Hillside akathisia scales were developed to specifically rate akathisia (and

Table 4

Barnes Akathisia Scale

Patients should be observed while engaged in neutral conversation while seated, and then standing (for a minimum of 2 minutes in each position). Symptoms observed in other situations, e.g., engaged in activity on the ward, may also be rated. Subsequently, the subjective phenomena should be elicited by direct questioning.

OBJECTIVE   SCORE

0 = Normal occasional fidgety movements of the limbs.

1 = Presence of characteristic restless movements of the legs/feet, or swinging one leg, while sitting, AND/OR rocking from foot to foot or "walking-on-the-spot" when standing, BUT movements present for less than half the time.

2 = Observed phenomena, as described in (1) above, which are present for at least half the observation period.   _____

3 = The patient is constantly engaged in characteristic restless movements, AND/OR has the inability to remain seated or standing without walking or pacing, during the time observed.

SUBJECTIVE

Awareness of Restlessness

0 = Absence of inner restlessness.

1 = Nonspecific sense of inner restlessness.

2 = The patient is aware of an inability to keep the legs still, AND/OR complains of inner restlessness aggravated specifically by being required to stand still.   _____

3 = Awareness of an intense compulsion to move most of the time AND/OR reports a strong desire to walk or pace most of the time.

Distress Related to Restlessness

0 = No distress

1 = Mild

2 = Moderate   _____

3 = Severe

(*continued*)

Table 4 (*continued*)

Barnes Akathisia Scale

GLOBAL CLINICAL ASSESSMENT OF AKATHISIA

0 = Absent. No evidence of awareness of restlessness. Observation of characteristic movements of akathisia in the absence of report of compulsive desire to move the legs should be classified as pseudoakathisia.

1 = Questionable. Nonspecific inner tension and fidgety movements.

2 = Mild Akathisia. Awareness of restlessness in the legs and/or inner restlessness worse when required to stand still. Fidgety movements present but characteristic restless movements of akathisia not necessarily observed. The condition causes little or no distress.

3 = Moderate Akathisia. Awareness of restlessness as described for mild akathisia above, combined with characteristic restless movements such as rocking from foot to foot when standing. The patient finds the condition distressing.

4 = Marked Akathisia. Subjective experience of restlessness includes a compulsion to walk or pace. However, the patient is able to remain seated for short periods of at least 5 minutes. The condition is obviously distressing.

5 = Severe Akathisia. The patient reports a strong compulsion to pace up and down most of the time. Unable to sit or lie down for more than a few minutes. Constant restlessness which is associated with intense distress and insomnia.

____

---

include global assessments of akathisia), unlike the ESRS and the modified Simpson/Angus EPS scale, which were designed to examine extrapyramidal symptoms in general. Advantages of the Barnes scale are that it: (1) is brief and easy to use, (2) separately rates subjective and objective akathisia, (3) gives reliable anchor points for lower levels of objective ratings (i.e., more or less than one-half the time), (4) divides subjective ratings into awareness and distress subsets, (5) uses ratings in naturalistic settings, and (6) assesses global akathisia with defined anchor points.

Clearly, further studies are needed to validate these scales and correlate their results. Only one study to date has compared the ratings between scales. Adler et al.[120] compared changes in subjective and objective akathisia from the 100-mm line corresponding to perceived restlessness and the akathisia item of the modified Simpson/Angus EPS scale, respectively, with ratings from the Barnes akathisia scale after treatment with metoprolol. Pearson correlations were as follows: (1) subjective akathisia: 100-mm line versus Barnes subjective sum (awareness + distress subscales): n = 8, r = 0.68, p≤0.10, and (2) objective akathisia: Simpson/Angus EPS scale versus the Barnes objective akathisia: n = 9, r = 0.77, p≤0.02.

Objective electromechanical measurement of NIA is currently being explored. Lipinski et al. (personal communication) have had some preliminary encouraging results using activity monitors to quantify the restlessness of Alzheimer's disease and of NIA. Adler et al.[120] have used a running shoe with a built-in sensor that measures the number of impacts/unit time in patients with NIA. About one-half the patients from the ICI 118,551 study had decrements in the number of impacts that paralleled decreases in objective (modified Simpson/Angus EPS scale) and subjective (100-mm line) akathisia ratings. Ratings did not correlate well for those patients who did not pace. Therefore, activity monitors would generally be more useful for the general study of akathisia than the running shoe, as the latter will only measure restlessness in those patients who actually pace (and not in those who "leg waggle" or rock from foot to foot).

Types of Akathisia

Acute Akathisia Versus Akathisia Variants

Differentiation of acute akathisia, akathisia variants, and tardive dyskinesia is difficult and is an area where additional studies are needed. Stahl[46] has proposed attempting to understand the relationship of these syndromes by examining the pharmacological responsivity of akathisia variants to a variety of agents. We are currently conducting a study along these lines that compares the effects of serial 1-day treatment epochs of benztropine, propranolol, amantadine, and increased neuroleptic in patients with acute neuroleptic-induced akathisia versus others with akathisia variants and tardive dyskinesia.[121] Premilinary results have shown that improvement in akathisia has led to an amelioration in tardive dyskinetic movements. Similarly, we have found in a study of propranolol treatment of idiopathic Parkinson's disease akathisia[105] that improvements in akathisia correlated with decrements in dyskinetic (presumably dopa-related) movements. This indicates that akathisia may in some way drive dyskinetic movements, when the two co-exist.

Akathisia With and Without Coexistent Parkinsonian EPS

Braude et al.[27] have suggested that there may be two forms of akathisia: (1) one that occurs with parkinsonian EPS and is responsive to anticholinergics and (2) another that occurs without parkinsonian EPS and which is less anticholinergic-responsive. Such a differentiation may allow investigation of subsets of acute akathisia and further insights into the pathophysiology of the syndrome.

Mechanisms of the Therapeutic Effect of β-Blockers in Akathisia

The Role of Membrane Stabilizing Effects

Membrane stabilizing effects (MSE) do not appear to be critical for the therapeutic effect, as d-propranolol (which does have MSE, but is without clinically significant β-blocking effects), was ineffective in treating NIA.[98]

Central Versus Peripheral Sites of Action

Both Lipinski et al.[37] and Ratey et al.[104] found evidence suggesting a subacute onset of action of nadolol in akathisia. Adler et al.[105] verified these observations by finding that the onset of nadolol did not occur until at least 9–11 days of treatment. This longer onset of action than propranolol is most likely secondary to delayed penetration across the blood-brain barrier by this hydrophilic β-blocker. A central site of action is also suggested by the fact that one patient with active CNS syphilis infection had a more rapid response to nadolol.

β_1 *Versus* β_2 *Receptors*

The studies performed to date appear to indicate that blockade of either β_1 or β_2 receptors is sufficient for the therapeutic effect. Both β_1-selective (e.g., low-dose metoprolol[113,114] and betaxolol[116,117]) and β_2-selective agents (ICI 118,551[118]) have been shown to improve akathisia. Blockade of either receptor alone may be sufficient for the therapeutic effect as akathisia ratings in patients treated serially with (1) metoprolol and propranolol[113,114] or (2) ICI 118,551 and propranolol[118] have not shown further improvement with the nonselective agent.

The improvement seen in our two studies with low-dose metoprolol (where β_1 selectivity is maintained) differs from Zubenko et al.'s[111] finding that high doses of metoprolol (where both β_1 and β_2 receptors are blocked) were necessary to achieve any therapeutic effect. Possible explanations for this difference are: (1) most of Zubenko et al.'s patients had affective disorders, while our patients were mainly schizophrenic ; (2) most of Zubenko et al.'s patients were also receiving lithium ; and (3) our patients were treated with higher doses of neuroleptics.

The Role of Serotonin

It has been proposed that serotonin might play a role both in the pathophysiology of NIA and in the mechanism underlying the effects of β-blockers.[68] However, the existing data on the effects of serotonergic agents in NIA are sparse and inconsistent.

Serotonin receptors are subclassified into several subsets (5-HT 1A, 5-HT 1B, 5-HT 1C and 5-HT 2).[122,123] Methysergide, a medication used in the treatment of migraine headaches, antagonizes all of these receptors[123] and has been reported to induce an akathisia-like syndrome in a patient being treated for migraine.[65] We found that methysergide did not change akathisia in two schizophrenics with NIA.[66] Two studies have found that the selective 5-HT 2 antagonist ritanserin can ameliorate akathisia.[71,72] Alternatively, an agent that increases serotonergic function (the re-uptake inhibitor fluoxetine HCl) has been reported to induce akathisia.[68] The 5-HT precursor tryptophan has also been reported to improve akathisia.[67] The anxiolytic buspirone, a more selective 5-HT 1A agonist[122] has been reported to ameliorate NIA in three patients;[69] however, Brody and co-workers found that buspirone induced or worsened akathisia in four of seven neuroleptic-treated schizophrenic patients.[70]

In terms of propranolol, the "l" isomer is a moderate to weak antagonist for the 5-HT 1A receptor, while the "d" isomer is a weaker antagonist at this site. Both isomers are without significant effects at other serotonin receptors.[123] It is possible that such 5-HT 1A antagonistic effects may have contributed to the lack of efficacy we saw for d-propranolol,[97] as d-propranolol has (by in vitro estimates) about a 6.5-fold lower affinity for the 5-HT 1A receptor than the racemate.[123] However, there have been mixed results as to the effects of the 5-HT 1A agonist buspirone.

Thus, the data regarding the role of serotonergic mechanisms in NIA are limited and inconsistent; any conclusions are almost certainly premature.

These recent studies contribute to the initial understanding of the mechanisms of action of β-blockers in NIA. It does appear that β-blockade, rather than membrane stabilization or other nonspecific effects, is crucial for the therapeutic effect and that a central site of action at either β_1 or β_2 receptors is involved. Future directions include: (1) better controlled studies of β-blockers with larger sample sizes, (2) the use of more specific agents when they become available, and (3) attempting to provoke or induce akathisia with β-agonists (particularly if selective, lipophilic agonists become available).

A more fundamental question is why β-blockers improve a syndrome thought to be caused by dopamine receptor blockade. Just as poorly understood is the response reported in patients treated with opioids such as propoxyphene and codeine[124] (a particularly interesting observatin in view of the therapeutic benefit obtained with these drugs in the RLS and the beneficial effects of low-dose propranolol in opiate withdrawal[35]). A more basic understanding of the pathophysiology of akathisia and of the interactions between noradrenergic, dopaminergic, and endogenous opiate systems is needed to answer these questions. This in turn may require the development of valid animal models of akathisia.

References

1. Willis T. The London Practice of Physick, 1st edition, London, Thomas Bassett and William Crooke, 1685, p 404.

2. Beard GM. A Practical Treatise on Nervous Exhaustion, 2nd edition, New York, William Wood, 1880, pp 41–42.
3. Haskovec L. Akathisie. Arch Bohemes Med Clin 1902; 3:193–200.
4. Bing R. Ueber Einige bemerkenswerte Begleiterscheinunger der exrapyram idalen Rigiditat (Akathesie—Mikrographie—Kinesia paradoxica). Schweiz Med Wochenschr 1923; 53:167–171.
5. Sachs O. Awakenings. New York, Vintage Books, 1976, pp 30.
6. Sicard JA. Akathisie and tasikinesie. Presse Med 1923; 31:265–266.
7. Ekbom KA. Asthenia crurum paraesthetica ("irritable legs"). Acta Med Scand 1944; 118:197–209.
8. Ekbom KA. Restless leg syndrome. Neurology 1960; 10:868–873.
9. Akathisia and antipsychotic drugs. Lancet 1986; ii:1131–1132. Editorial.
10. Gibb WR, Lees AJ. The restless leg syndrome. Post Grad Med J 1986; 62:329–333.
11. Sigwald J, Grossiord A, Duriel P, Dumont G. Le traitement de la maladie de Parkinson et des manifestations extrpyramidales par le diethyl aminoethy n-thiodiphenylamine (2987 RP): resultats d'une annee d'application. Rev Neurol (Paris) 1947; 79:683–687.
12. Steck H. Le syndrome extrapyramidal et d'encephalique au cours des traitements au largactil et au serapsil. Ann Medico-Psychol 1954; 112:737–743.
13. Freyhan FA. Psychomotility and parkinsonism in treatment with neuroleptic drugs. Arch Neurol Psychiatry 1957; 78:465–472.
14. Gibb WR, Lees AJ. The clinical phenomenon of akathisia. J Neurol Neurosurg Psychiatry 1986; 49:861–866.
15. Van Putten T. The many faces of akathisia. Compr Psychiatry 1975; 16:43–47.
16. Van Putten T. Why do schizophrenic patients refuse to take their drugs? Arch Gen Psychiatry 1974; 31:67–72.
17. Van Putten T, Mutalipassi LR, Malkin MD. Phenothiazine-induced decompensation. Arch Gen Psychiatry 1974; 30:102–105.
18. Keckich WA. Violence as a manifestation of akathisia. JAMA 1978; 240:2185.
19. Kumar BB. An unusual case of akathisia. Am J Psychiatry 1979; 136:1088.
20. Schulte JR. Homicide and suicide associated with akathisia and haloperidol. Am J Forensic Psychiatry 1985; 6:3–7.
21. Shear K, Frances A, Weiden P. Suicide associated with akathisia and depot fluphenazine treatment. J Clin Psychopharmacol 1983; 3:235–236.
22. Weiden P. Akathisia from prochlorperazine. JAMA 1985; 253:635.
23. Drake RE, Ehrlich J. Suicide attempts associated with akathisia. Am J Psychiatry 1985; 142:499–501.
24. Shaw ED, Mann JJ, Widen P, Sinsheimer LM, Brunn RD. A case of suicidal and homicidal ideation and akathisia in a double-blind neuroleptic crossover study. J Clin Psychopharmacol 1986; 6:196–197.
25. Barnes TRE, Braude WM. Toward a more reliable diagnosis of akathisia (in reply). Arch Gen Psychiatry 1986; 43:1016.

26. Van Putten T, Marder SR. Behavioral toxicity of antipsychotic drugs. J Clin Psychiatry 1987; 48(suppl):13–19.
27. Braude WM, Barnes TRE, Gore SM. Clinical characteristics of akathisia. Br J Psychiatry 1983; 143:134–150.
28. Barnes TRE. A rating scale for drug-induced akathisia. Br J Psychiatry 1989; 154:672–676.
28a. Hermesh H, Munitz H. Unilateral neuroleptic-induced akathisia. Clin Neuropharmacol 1990; 13:253–258.
29. Kendler K. A medical student's experience with akathisia. Am J Psychiatry 1976; 133:454–455.
30. Adler LA, Angrist B, Peselow E, Corwin J, Rotrosen J. Efficacy of propranolol in neuroleptic-induced akathisia. J Clin Psychopharmacol 1985; 5:164–166.
31. Adler LA, Angrist B, Peselow E, Corwin J, Maslansky R, Rotrosen J. A controlled assessment of propranolol in the treatment of neuroleptic-induced akathisia. Br J Psychiatry 1986; 149:42–45.
32. Gold MS, Redmond DE, Kleiber HD. Clonidine blocks the acute opiate withdrawal syndrome. Lancet 1978; ii:403–405.
33. Zubenko GS, Cohen BM, Lipinski JF, Jonas JM. Use of clonidine in the treatment of akathisia. Psychiatry Res 1984; 13:253–259.
34. Adler LA, Angrist B, Peselow E, Reitano J, Rotrosen J. Clonidine in neuroleptic-induced akathisia. Am J Psychiatry 1987; 144:235–236.
35. Roehrich H, Gold MS. Propranolol as adjunct to clonidine in opiate detoxification. Am J Psychiatry 1987; 144:1099–1100.
36. Lipinski JF, Zubenko GS, Barriera P, Cohen BM. Propranolol in the treatment of neuroleptic-induced akathisia. Lancet 1983; ii:685–686.
37. Lipinski JF, Zubenko GS, Cohen BM, Barriera PJ. Propranolol in the treatment of neuroleptic-induced akathisia. Am J Psychiatry 1984; 141:412–415.
38. Adler LA, Angrist B, Reiter S, Rotrosen J. Neuroleptic-induced akathisia: a review. Psychopharmacology 1989; 97:1–11.
39. Kramer SM, Gorkin RA, DiJohnson C, Sheves P. Propranolol in the treatment of neuroleptic-induced akathisia (NIA) in schizophrenics: a double-blind, placebo-controlled study. Biol Psychiatry 1988; 24:823–827.
40. Barnes TRE, Braude WM. Akathisia variants and tardive dyskinesia. Arch Gen Psychiatry 1985; 42:874–878.
41. Simpson GM. Neurotoxicity of major tranquilizers. In: Roizin L, Shiroki H, Grcevic N (eds), Neurotoxicology, New York, Raven Press, 1977, p 3.
42. Jeste DV, Wyatt RJ. Understanding and Treating Tardive Dyskinesia. New York and London, The Guilford Press, 1982, p 64.
43. Braude WM, Barnes TRE. Late onset akathisia: an indicant of covert dyskinesia. Two case reports. Am J Psychiatry 1983; 140:611–612.
44. Chouinard G, Annable L, Ross-Chouinard A, Nestoros JN. Factors related to tardive dyskinesia. Am J Psychiatry 1979; 136:79–83.
45. Munetz MR, Cornes CL. Distinguishing akathisia and tardive dyskinesia: a review of the literature. J Clin Psychopharmacol 1982; 3:343–350.

46. Stahl SM. Akathisia and tardive dyskinesia: changing concepts. Arch Gen Psychiatry 1985; 42:915–917.
47. Munetz MR. Akathisia variants and tardive dyskinesia. Arch Gen Psychiatry 1986; 43:1015.
48. Barnes TRE, Braude WM, Hill DJ. Acute akathisia after oral droperidol and metoclopramide preoperative medication. Lancet 1982; ii:48–49.
49. Ayd FJ. A survey of drug-induced extrapyramidal reactions. JAMA 1961; 175:1054–1060.
50. Kruse W. Persistent muscular restlessness after phenothiazine treatment: report of three cases. Am J Psychiatry 1960; 11:152–153.
51. Weiner WJ, Luby ED. Persistent akathisia following neuroleptic withdrawal. Ann Neurol 1983; 13:466–467.
52. Goldman D. Parkinsonism and related phenomena from administration of drugs: their production and control under clinical conditions and possible relation to therapeutic effect. Rev Can Exp Biol 1961; 20:549–560.
53. National Institute of Mental Health. Psychopharmacology survey center collaborative study group. Phenothiazine treatment in acute schizophrenia. Arch Gen Psychiatry 1964; 10:246–261.
54. Freyhan FA. Extrapyramidal symptoms and other side effects of trifluoperazine: Clinical and pharmacological aspects. Philadelphia, Lea and Febiger, 1958.
55. Van Putten T, May PRA, Marder SR. Akathisia with haloperidol and thiothixene. Arch Gen Psychiatry 1984; 41:1036–1039.
56. Marsden CD, Jenner P. The pathophysiology of extrapyramidal side-effects of neuroleptic drugs. Psycholog Med 1980; 10:55–72.
57. Weiden P, Mann JJ, Haas G, Mattson M, Frances A. Clinical nonrecognition of neuroleptic-induced movement disorders: a cautionary study. Am J Psychiatry 1987; 144:1148–1153.
58. Ayd FJ. Drug-induced extrapyramidal reactions: their clinical manifestations and treatment with akineton. Psychosomatics 1960; 1:143–150.
59. Chouinard G, Ross-Chouinard A, Annable L, Jones BD. Extrapyramidal rating scale. Can J Neurol Sci 1980; 7:233.
60. Fleischhacker EE, Bergmann KJ, Perovich R, Pestreich LK, Borenstein M, Lieberman JA, Kane JM. The Hillside Akathisia Scale: a new rating instrument for neuroleptic-induced akathisia. Psychopharmacol Bull 1989; 25:222–226.
61. Lang AE, Johnson K. Akathisia in idiopathic parkinson's disease. Neurology 1987; 37:477–481.
62. Bartels M, Heide K, Mann K, Schied. Treatment of akathisia with lorazepam: an open trial. Pharmacopsychiatry 1987; 20:51–53.
63. Kutcher SP, Mackenzie S, Galarraga, Szalai J. Clonazepam treatment of adolescents with neuroleptic-induced akathisia. Am J Psychiatry 1987; 144:823–824.
64. Kutcher S, Williamson P, MacKenzie S, Marton P, Ehrlich M. Successful clonazepam treatment of neuroleptic-induced akathisia in older adolescents and young adults: a double-blind study. J Clin Psychopharmacol 1989; 9:403–406.

65. Bernick C. Methysergide-induced akathisia. Clin Neuropharmacol 1988; 11:87–89.
66. Adler LA, Fritz P, Angrist B, Duncan E, Lipinski JF. Psychosis activation without changes in akathisia in two schizophrenic patients treated with methysergide. In preparation.
67. Kramer MS, DiJohnson C, Davis P, Dewey DA, DiGiambattista S. Tryptophan in NIA. Biol Psychiatry 1990; 27:671.
68. Lipinski JF, Mallya G, Zimmerman P, Pope HJ. Fluoxetine-induced akathisia: clinical and theoretical implications. J Clin Psychiatry 1989; 50:339–342.
69. D'Mello DA, McNeil DA, Harris W. Buspirone suppression of neuroleptic-induced akathisia: multiple case reports. J Clin Psychopharmacol 1989; 9:151–152.
70. Brody D, Adler LA, Kim A, Angrist B, Rotrosen J. Effects of buspirone in seven schizophrenic patients. J Clin Psychopharmacol 1990; 10:68–69.
71. Bersani G, Grispini A, Marinia S, Pasini A, Valducci M, Ciani N. Neuroleptic-induced extrapyramidal side effects: clinical perspectives with ritanserin (R55667), a new selective 5-HT2 receptor-blocking agent. Curr Ther Res 1986; 40:492–499.
72. Fleischhacker W, Miller C, Ehrmann H, Kane J. Ritanserin in the treatment of neuroleptic-induced akathisia. Presented at the 28th Annual Meeting of the American College of Neuropsychopharmacology (ACNP), Maui, Hawaii, December 10–15, 1989.
73. Hermesh H, Aizenberg D, Friedberg G, Zemishlani Z, Munitz H. Low dose clomipramine for refractory akathisia. Presented at the Annual Meeting of the American Psychiatric Association, New York, May 15, 1990.
74. Dahlstrom A, Fuxe K. Evidence of the existence of monoamine neurons in the central nervous system. Acta Physiol Scand 1965; 64:37–85.
75. Weisel FA. Effects of high dose propranolol treatment on dopamine and norepinephrine metabolism in regions of rat brain. Neurosci Lett 1976; 2:35–38.
76. Fuxe K, Bolme P, Agnati L and Everitt BJ. The effect of d,l and d-propranolol on central monoamine neurones; 1. Studies on dopamine mechanisms. Neurosci Lett 1976; 3:45–52.
77. Wilbur R, Kulik F, Kulik V. Noradrenergic effects in tardive dyskinesia: akathisia and pseudoparkinsonism via the limbic system and basal ganglia. Prog Neuro-Psychopharmacol Biol Psychiatry 1988; 12:849–864.
78. Sandy K, Fisher H. Serotonin in involuntary movement disorders. Int J Neurosci 1988; 42:185–205.
79. Lipinski JF, Keck PE, McElroy SL. Beta-adrenergic antagonists in psychosis: Is improvement due to treatment of neuroleptic-induced akathisia? J Clin Psychopharmacology 1988; 6:409–416.
80. Zubenko GS, Barreira P, Lipinski JF. Development of tolerance to the therapeutic effect of amantadine on akathisia. J Clin Psychopharmacol 1984; 4:218–219.
81. Kruse W. Treatment of drug-induced extrapyramidal symptoms. Dis Nerv System 1960; 21:79–81.

82. Neu C, DiMascio A, Demirgian E. Antiparkinsonian medication in the treatment of extrapyramidal side-effects: single or multiple doses? Curr Ther Res 1972; 4:246–251.
83. Friis T, Christensen TR, Gerlach J. Sodium valproate and biperiden in neuroleptic-induced akathisia, parkinsonism and hyperkinesia: a double-blind cross-over study with placebo. Acta Psychiatrica Scand 1982; 67:178–187.
84. Merrick EM, Schmitt PP. A controlled study of the clinical effects of amantadine hydrochloride (symmetrel). Curr Ther Res 1973; 15:552–558.
85. DiMascio A, Bernardo DL, Greenblatt D, Marder JE. A controlled trial of amantadine in drug-induced extrapyramidal disorders. Arch Gen Psychiatry 1976; 33:559–602.
86. Stenson RL, Donlon PT, Meyer JE. Comparison of benztropine meslyate and amantadine HCl in neuroleptic-induced extrapyramidal symptoms. Compr Psychiatry 1976; 17:763–768.
87. Donlon P. The therapeutic use of diazepam for akathisia. Psychosomatics 1973; 14:222–225.
88. Gagrat D, Hamilton J, Belmatier R. Intravenous diazepam in the treatment of neuroleptic-induced dystonia or akathisia. Am J Psychiatry 1978; 135:1232–1233.
89. Cruickshank DM. The clinical importance of cardioselectivity and lipophilicity in beta blockers. Am Heart J 1980; 100:160–178.
90. Shanks RG. The properties of beta-adrenoceptor antagonists. Postgrad Med J 1976; 52(Suppl 4):14–20.
91. Frishman WM, Sonnenblick EH. Beta-adrenergic blocking drugs. In: Hurst JW, Logue RB, Rackley CE, Sonnenblick EH, Wallace AG, Wenger NK (eds), The Heart (6th edition), New York, McGraw Hill, 1986, pp 1606–1621.
92. Guidicelli JF, Richer C, Ganansia J, Warrington S, Abriol C, Rulliere R. Betaxolol: beta-adrenoceptor blocking effects and phamacokinetics in man. In: Morselli PL, Kilborn JR, Cavero I, Harrison DC, Langer SZ (eds), Betaxolol and Other Beta-Adrenoceptor Antagonists. New York, Raven Press, 1983, pp 89–99.
93. Shanks RG. Clinical pharmacology of beta-adrenoceptor drugs. In: Morselli PL, Kilborn JR, Cavero I, Harrison DC, Langer SZ (eds), Betaxolol and Other Beta-Adrenoceptor Antagonists, New York, Raven Press, 1983, pp 73–78.
94. Strang RR. The symptom of restless legs. Med J Australia 1967; 24:1211–1213.
95. Kulik AV, Wilbur R. Case report of propranolol (Inderal) pharmacotherapy for neuroleptic-induced akathisia and tremor. Prog Neuro-Psychopharmacol Biol Psychiatry 1983; 7:223–225.
96. Adler LA, Reiter S, Corwin J, Hemdal P, Angrist B, Rotrosen J. Differential effects of benztropine and propranolol in akathisia. Psychopharmacol Bull 1987; 23:519–521.
97. Lipinski JF, Mallya G, Cohen B, Waternaux CW. A double-blind, placebo controlled study of propranolol in neuroleptic-induced akathisia. In preparation.

98. Adler LA, Angrist B, Fritz P, Rotrosen J, Mallya G, Lipinski JF. Lack of efficacy of d-propranolol in neuroleptic-induced akathisia. Neuropsychopharmacology 1991; 4:109–115.

99. Howe R, Shanks RG. Optical isomers of propranolol. Nature 1966; 210:1336–1338.

100. Fitzgerald JD. Perspectives in adrenergic beta-receptor blockade. Clin Pharmacol Ther 1969;10:292–306.

101. Rahn KH. Relationship between adrenergic blocking and antihypertensive effects of beta receptor antagonists. Adv Clin Pharmacol 1976; 11:14–18.

102. Reiter S, Adler L, Erle S, Duncan E. Neuroleptic-induced akathisia treated with pindolol. Am J Psychiatry 1987; 144:383–384.

103. Adler LA, Reiter S, Angrist B, Rotrosen J. Pindolol and propranolol in neuroleptic-induced akathisia. Am J Psychiatry 1987; 144:1241–1242.

104. Ratey JJ, Sorgi P, Polakoff S. Nadolol as a treatment for akathisia. Am J Psychiatry 1985; 142:640–642.

105. Adler LA, Angrist B, Weinreb H, Rotrosen J. Studies on the time course and efficacy of beta-blockers in neuroleptic-induced akathisia and the akathisia of idiopathic parkinson's disease. Psychopharmacol Bull 1991; 27:107–111.

106. Derom E, Elinck W, Buylaert W, Van Der Straeten M. Which beta-blocker for the restless leg? Lancet 1984; i:857.

107. Reiter S, Adler L, Angrist B, Corwin J, Rotrosen J. Atenolol and propranolol in neuroleptic-induced akathisia. J Clin Psychopharmacol 1987; 7:279–280.

108. Patterson JF. Pseudoakathisia associated with atenolol. J Clin Psychopharmacol 1986; 6:390.

109. Silver JM, Yudofsky SC, Kogan M, Katz BI. Elevation of thioridazine plasma levels by propranolol. Am J Psychiatry 1986; 143:1290–1292.

110. Greendyke RM, Kanter DR. Plasma propranolol levels and their effect on thioridazine and haloperidol concentrations. J Clin Psychopharmacol 1987; 7:178–182.

111. Zubenko GS, Lipinski JF, Cohen BM, Barriera PJ. Comparison of metoprolol and propranolol in the treatment of akathisia. Psychiatry Res 1984; 11:143–148.

112. Koch-Weser J. Metoprolol. N Engl J Med 1979; 301:698–703.

113. Kim A, Adler L, Angrist B, Rotrosen J. Efficacy of low-dose metoprolol in neuroleptic-induced akathisia. J Clin Psychopharmacol 1989; 9:294–296.

114. Adler LA, Angrist B, Rotrosen J. Metoprolol versus propranolol. Biol Psychiatry 1990; 27:673–675.

115. Dupuis B, Catteau J, Dumon J-P, Libert C, Petit H. Comparison of propranolol, sotalol, and betaxolol in the treatment of neuroleptic-induced akathisia. Am J Psychiatry 1987; 144:802–805.

116. Barrett AM. Therapeutic applications of beta-adrenoceptor antagonists. In: Morselli PL, Kilborn JR, Cavero I, Harrison DC, Langer SZ (eds), Betaxolol and Other Beta-Adrenoceptor Antagonists, New York, Raven Press, 1983, pp 65–72.

117. Adler LA, Angrist B, Rotrosen J. Efficacy of betaxolol in neuroleptic-induced akathisia. Psychiatry Res 1991; 39:193–198.

118. Adler L, Duncan E, Angrist B, Hemdal P, Rotrosen J, Slotnick V. Effects of a specific beta-2 receptor blocker in neuroleptic-induced akathisia. Psychiatry Res 1989; 27:1–4.
119. Langer SZ. Presynaptic receptors and their role in the regulation of transmitter release. Br J Pharmacol 1977; 60:481–497.
120. Adler L, Duncan E, Kim A, Hemdal P, Rotrosen J, Angrist B. Akathisia: selective beta-blockers and rating instruments. Psychopharmacol Bull 1989; 25(3):451–456.
121. Duncan E, Angrist B, Adler L, Corwin J, Rotrosen J. Pharmacologic challenge in akathisia and akathisia variants. Schizophrenia Bull 1989, 2:242.
122. Peroutka SJ. Serotonin receptors. In: Meltzer HY (ed), Psychopharmacology: The Third Generation of Progress, New York, Raven Press, 1987, pp 303–311.
123. Peroutka SJ. Antimigraine drug interactions with serotonin receptor subtypes in human brain. Ann Neurol 1988; 23:500–504.
124. Walters A, Hening W. Chokroverty S, Fahn S. Opioid responsiveness in patients with neuroleptic-induced akathisia. Mov Disord 1986; 1:119–127.

5

Neuroleptics and Classic Tardive Dyskinesia

Vikram Khot, M.D., Michael F. Egan, M.D.,
Thomas M. Hyde, Ph.D., M.D.,
Richard Jed Wyatt, M.D.

Introduction

The introduction of neuroleptics for the treatment of psychotic disorders was a major landmark in medicine. While the clinical efficacy of these agents was well established within 10 years of their introduction, the emergence of a sometimes persistent involuntary movement disorder (tardive dyskinesia) associated with their long-term use gradually invited more cautious use. In this chapter we will review tardive dyskinesia (TD), including its clinical aspects, epidemiology, pathophysiology, and treatment.

History

Five years after the introduction of chlorpromazine,[1] Schonecker described what were probably the first reported cases of tar-

Lang AE, Weiner WJ (editors): *Drug-Induced Movement Disorders*, Mount Kisco, NY,
© Futura Publishing Co., Inc., 1992.

dive dyskinesia.[2] After 2 to 8 weeks of exposure to chlorpromazine, three elderly women developed lip-smacking dyskinetic movements. For two patients, movements lasted 11 weeks after neuroleptic discontinuation, while the third patient, who remained on the neuroleptic, had movements lasting for at least 3 months. The dyskinesias reported by Schonecker contrasted with the acute transient dyskinesias described earlier.

In 1959 Sigwald and associates[3] used the term "facial-buccolinguo-masticatory dyskinesia" to describe involuntary movements of the tongue, lips, jaw, and facial muscles which followed at least 3 months of phenothiazine treatment. Uhrbrand and Faurbye[4] reported orofacial dyskinesias persisting even after neuroleptics were discontinued. A few years later, Faurbye and his associates introduced the term "tardive dyskinesia."[5]

Tardive dyskinesia was first described in the American literature in 1960.[6] In 1962, Druckman and co-workers[7] reported severe truncal dystonia, today referred to as "tardive dystonia." Several years later, Hunter and associates[8] described dyskinesias in 13 female in-patients with chronic psychiatric illness, all of whom had been treated with phenothiazines. Since some of these patients had coexisting medical and neurological illnesses, they were felt to be particularly at risk for developing dyskinetic movements. The consensus, however, was that since so many patients were treated with neuroleptics, the actual percentage of patients with dyskinesia was very small.

The notion that TD was uncommon persisted until studies in the late 1960s began to reveal relatively high prevalence rates. General acceptance of the association of TD with long-term neuroleptic treatment occurred in the early 1970s. The first therapeutic trials followed shortly thereafter.[9,10] At about the same time, the FDA required package inserts for neuroleptics stating, "Tardive dyskinesia may appear in some patients on long-term treatment or may occur after drug treatment has been discontinued . . . The symptoms are persistent and in some patients appear to be irreversible." In the 1970s, reports of severe, disabling TD[11-13] in adults and TD in children began to appear.[14]

In 1980, the American Psychiatric Association task force report[15] emphasized the importance of using long-term neuroleptics only when there was a clear indication, such as in chronic schizophrenia. The 1980s also witnessed additional studies on treatment.[16]

Even though these studies were methodologically superior to the earlier ones, no effective treatment was reported.

While epidemiologic data point to neuroleptic exposure as being the most significant etiologic factor in the development of TD, a few authors continue to question its importance.[17,18] In a study comparing chronic schizophrenic in-patients treated with neuroleptics with a neuroleptic-naive group, Owens and associates did not find a significant difference between prevalence rates of spontaneous dyskinesia (53.2%) and TD (67%).[17] When the data were re-analyzed adjusting for a difference in the age of the two groups, a slightly higher prevalence in the neuroleptic-treated patients was found. Seventy-nine percent of the treated patients were on neuroleptics at the time of evaluation, which might have masked some cases of TD. Recently,[19] Waddington et al. suggested that abnormal movements in psychotic patients may be a manifestation of subtle brain damage, rather than neuroleptic treatment. In support, they pointed out that dyskinetic movements are seen in patients with classic organic brain syndromes, regardless of exposure to neuroleptics. Furthermore, they noted additional signs of brain disease in patients with TD, such as cognitive impairment, and enlarged ventricles on neuroimaging scans.

Epidemiology

The most compelling evidence supporting the association between neuroleptics and TD has come from epidemiologic studies.[20] These studies have also uncovered risk factors, including age, duration of treatment, and gender. We will review these studies and address important methodological issues.

Prevalence

The first epidemiological studies were cross-sectional, providing point prevalence rates. Later studies were longitudinal and prospective, providing period prevalence rates.[21–23] As the number of studies increased, so did the prevalence rates. In 1965 the prevalence appeared to be about 5%, while studies published between 1976 and 1980 found a prevalence of 25%.[24] Thus the prevalence seemed to increase by approximately 1% a year. The reasons for this increase, while unclear, may be related to longer exposure to neuroleptics, as their benefits became well established.

Estimates of the prevalence of TD have ranged from 0.5 to 57%.[20] Several factors may complicate these estimates and explain the differences between studies. These, among others, include variability of diagnostic criteria and assessment methods, differences in patient age and gender, the possibility of coexisting medical and neurological illnesses, and variability in duration of neuroleptic exposure. An additional complicating factor is that TD is masked by ongoing neuroleptic treatment, which may reduce the number of patients exhibiting TD. Despite these methodological problems, recent reviews have shown consistency in prevalence estimates. Based on minimum methodological criteria, Jeste and Wyatt[24] selectively reviewed 37 studies and, using a weighted mean, found a prevalence of 17.6%. Kane and Smith[25] reviewed 56 studies and found a prevalence of 20%, using unweighted means. More recent estimates (1981–1986) have been higher, with an average prevalence of 30%.[26] Overall, the average prevalence of TD has been estimated as 15–20%.[27–29]

Spontaneous dyskinesia is phenomenologically similar to TD but occurs independently of neuroleptic treatment. To estimate the true prevalence of TD, the frequency of these dyskinesias should be taken into account. The prevalence of spontaneous dyskinesia has been reported to range from 0 to 53%.[28] From a series of 18 studies carried out between 1966 and 1983, Casey and Gerlach[30] calculated the prevalence rate of TD to be 19.8% and spontaneous dyskinesia as 5.9%. The net difference of 13.9% may be a better estimate of the "true" prevalence of TD. Unfortunately, studies comparing neuroleptic-treated and non-neuroleptic-treated cohorts seldom match patients for variables such as diagnosis, age, and gender.

Incidence

While prevalence figures are generally useful in determining the needs for treatment, incidence figures are more useful for understanding etiology. Retrospective studies have limitations. They usually provide point prevalence rates but do not describe the natural history of TD. This drawback has led to the emergence of more informative prospective studies in the 1980s.

The risk for a schizophrenic in-patient developing tardive dyskinesia during 1 year of continuous neuroleptic exposure was estimated by Gardos and Cole to be 4% to 5%.[31] In one of the largest prospective studies,[32–34] Kane and associates reported the cumulative incidence of tardive dyskinesia among individuals exposed to neuroleptics to be 5% after 1 year, 10% after 2 years, 15% after 3 years, and 19% after 4 years. This linear increase in the cumulative incidence of TD over the first 4–5 years does not support the idea of a period of maximal risk, as others have hypothesized. Incidence estimates in other prospective studies have ranged from 3% to 7%,[35,36] with an average of 5%. Studies involving elderly patients on neuroleptics have found incidence rates four times as high as those in young adults.[37] The association between age and TD will be further discussed in the following section.

Risk Factors

In assessing the risk of developing TD, a number of variables related to both the patient and the treatment must be considered.

Patient-Related Variables

Age

The most consistent risk factor associated with TD is age. The older the patient, the greater the patient's risk for developing TD.[37] Smith and Baldessarini[38] also found a direct relationship between age and severity and an inverse correlation between the spontaneous remission rate and age. In a prospective longitudinal study, Saltz, Kane, et al.[39] found that for any given level of exposure to neuroleptics, the incidence of TD was higher among older than younger patients. Additionally, the relationship between age and TD was curvilinear, with a fairly stable risk between 20 and 40 years of age and a dramatic rise after age 40.

Gender

Several studies have shown that the prevalence of TD is higher in women than in men,[24] and particularly higher in older women.[34,40]

Primary Psychiatric Illness

Patients with affective disorders are more susceptible to TD than patients with schizophrenia, given the same degree of exposure to neuroleptics.[37,41] In schizophrenia, earlier studies found a positive correlation between severity of psychotic symptoms and tardive dyskinesia. Subsequent reports, however, have not found this correlation, and instead have tended to find an association with negative symptoms and cognitive impairment. With the exception of affective illness and a subset of schizophrenia (see the section entitled *Incidence*), there does not appear to be a relationship between TD and primary psychiatric illness.

Susceptibility to Parkinsonism (Neuroleptic-Induced)

Crane first suggested that TD was more likely to develop in patients with neuroleptic-induced parkinsonism.[42] While this association was not seen initially,[23,43,44] two recent prospective studies[26,37] have found that patients with neuroleptic-induced parkinsonism have up to a twofold greater risk of developing TD.

Organic Brain Disease

While early studies of chronically hospitalized patients found a clear association between TD and organic brain disease, electroconvulsive therapy (ECT), and lobotomy, more recent studies have not been as certain.[45] Patients with TD may have more negative symptoms, cognitive impairment, neurological soft signs, and ventricular enlargement compared to patients without TD.[66,67] These associations may be more characteristic of older patients while possibly absent in younger ones. These features have been considered to be evidence of brain damage, supporting the hypothesis that a subset of schizophrenics with organic impairment (type II) may be predisposed to develop TD.[67] Alternatively, the processes responsible for the development of TD may contribute to the expression of these associated features.

Other Factors

Since a number of movement disorders, such as Huntington's disease, idiopathic torsion dystonia, and Tourette's syndrome are genetically transmitted, it is possible that there may be a genetic component to TD. However, there is no evidence to support this concept at present.

Treatment-Related Variables

Treatment-related variables such as type of neuroleptic, dose, duration of treatment, and concurrent drug treatment may influence incidence.

Type of Neuroleptic

Early reports suggested that piperazine phenothiazines were more likely to result in TD,[46] but subsequent studies[47,48] did not validate this. Most authors[45,50,51] have not reported a difference between low potency and high potency neuroleptic groups (except Kane and associates).[49] Several retrospective studies[45,50,52] have found that depot fluphenazine increases the prevalence of TD. One prospective study reported that the risk of developing TD on depot fluphenazine was 5% in 1 year and 40% after 11 years.[53] While there may be an increased risk of TD in patients given depot preparations, these studies have not adequately controlled for other risk factors such as neuroleptic blood levels, dose, compliance and severity of psychiatric illness.

Dose of Neuroleptic

A common assumption is that neuroleptic dosage contributes to the risk of developing TD. This view was probably based on early reports[15,21,42] which did find such an association. A number of subsequent studies[40,50,54] mostly in the late 1970s, have not found a correlation between neuroleptic dose and incidence of TD.

Duration of Neuroleptic Exposure

Several studies have found a positive relationship[23,24,55] between the duration of neuroleptic therapy and TD, while others have not.[24,56] The lack of correlation in the negative studies may be secondary to differing rates of development of TD in different subgroups of patients. For example, older patients may develop TD after brief neuroleptic exposure while younger patients may not, even after much longer treatment. Crane and Smeets[57] showed that moderate to severe TD was more common in patients treated for 6 to 8 years than in those who had received either shorter or longer courses of treatment. Chouinard and colleagues[26] found that duration of neuroleptic exposure appeared to be a risk factor, with more than 5 years of exposure being a critical period. In Kane and associates' prospective sample,[34] younger subjects (age<3O) were slightly more likely to develop TD with longer exposure to neuroleptics, while for older subjects, TD prevalence increased sharply with increased exposure. Thus, while length of neuroleptic administration may be a risk factor for the development of TD, the relationship may not be linear.

Drug-Free Periods

There have been suggestions that drug-free periods may predispose patients to TD. However, this is far from clear.[45,54]

Antiparkinsonian Agents

Kiloh and associates[58] and Klawans[59] first suggested that anticholinergic drugs may predispose patients to develop TD. While two studies[60,56] have found a positive correlation between TD and anticholinergics, a third[45] did not. Chouinard and associates[61] found that benztropine, as opposed to procyclidine or ethopropazide, increased the risk of developing TD. Since patients receiving anticholinergic medications usually have drug-induced parkinsonism, either factor could be responsible for this association with TD.

Electroconvulsive Therapy

Early reports noted that in addition to being treated with neuroleptics, patients with TD also had undergone physical treatments such as ECT and leukotomy. The possibility that somatic therapies might predispose to TD by causing brain damage was raised. While one recent study[50] found an association between TD and ECT in chronic psychotic in-patients, most studies have not. There are, however, published reports of improvement in TD after electroconvulsive treatment[45]

Clinical Aspects

Tardive dyskinesia usually begins to appear after several years of treatment with antipsychotic medications, and almost never before 3 months. Neurological causes need to be carefully excluded when the onset is earlier. Symptoms of TD consist primarily of athetotic and choreiform movements, and are sometimes associated with dystonia (see Chapter 6). The lack of pathognomonic signs or symptoms make the diagnosis of TD primarily one of exclusion. TD must be distinguished from other abnormal movements commonly seen in psychiatric populations. A wide number of medical conditions present with choreoathetotic movements and should be excluded before making the diagnosis of TD.

Description of Movements

The facial muscles, particularly the perioral and oral muscles, are most commonly affected in TD. Muscles of the extremities and trunk can also be involved, and may form a separate subsyndrome,[62] although this possibility has not been clearly demonstrated.[63] The movements of TD are generally athetotic (slow writhing) or choreic (rapid, irregular, jerking) or a combination of the two. In mild cases, TD may appear to be an exaggeration of normal movements, such as occasional lip-wetting with the tongue. It may be difficult to determine if such movements are abnormal. An increase in the severity of movements during an activating task, as in the Abnormal Involuntary Movement Scale (AIMS) exam (see below), supports the diagnosis. A brief description of the types of movements seen in different body areas is given in Table 1.

Associated Features

Mild dyskinetic movements may appear transiently and then disappear. It is not clear if they are harbingers of more severe and

Table 1

Abnormal Movements in Tardive Dyskinesia

Area	*Movements*
1. Muscles of Facial Expression	Frowning, or furrowing of forehead, increased blink rate, blepharospasm (spasmodic contraction of the orbicularis oculi). Cheeks retract, puff, suck, grimace; blowing movements.
2. Lips and Perioral Area	Pouting, puckering, lip smacking, sucking.
3. Jaw	Lateral and horizontal movements in a variety of combinations including chewing, clenching, or repeated, irregular opening and closing of mouth.
4. Tongue	Fine vermicular movements, writhing, thrusting irregularly out of mouth ("fly catching") or against the buccal mucosa producing a bulge in the cheek, as if holding a piece of candy (bonbon sign), repeated lip licking. Over time, may see tongue hypertrophy.
5. Upper Extremities	One or more fingers slowly writhe or "dance," or show almost rhythmic movements involving extension and fanning of one or more fingers. May merge into dystonic posture. Irregular, jerky flexion, or more commonly, extension of hand at the wrist and/or elbow. Ballismus.
6. Lower Extremities	Toes may "dance," or show slow irregular extension, flexion, and/or fanning. Foot squirming, inversion and eversion, stamping. Irregular flexion and extension or lateral movements around ankle or knee. Marching in place.
7. Trunk	Includes muscles of the neck, shoulder, diaphragm, and pelvis. Common movements are lateral neck movements merging into a dystonic posture; shoulder shrugging or rotation, pelvic twisting or rotation. Diaphragmatic movements could be involved in whistling, sucking, or irregular breathing.

persistent movements. Schooler and Kane[64] have suggested that the diagnosis of TD be reserved for those cases that exhibit movements rated at least mild in two body areas (see Table 1) or moderate in one area. "Transient" TD persists for less than 3 months. TD that lasts more than 3 months is "persistent." TD may be "masked" by increases in neuroleptics. Conversely, TD-like movements may occur within a few weeks following the decrease or withdrawal of neuroleptics, but disappear within 3 months. This has been defined as "withdrawal" TD,[64] although how these movements are related to persistent TD is unclear. Anxiety or activating tasks such as rapid alternating movements usually worsen symptoms. This feature helps to distinguish TD from somatoform disorders and unusual voluntary movements. Walking is an excellent activating task for bringing out movements in the upper extremities. TD may become worse during the performance of certain neuropsychological tests. Dyskinetic movements usually disappear during sleep, but severe movements can sometimes awaken patients. Patients with schizophrenia are often unaware of their symptoms, whereas patients with affective disorders or dystonias tend to be very aware of and complain about them. Tardive dyskinesia responds to pharmacological manipulations in predictable ways. Increasing neuroleptic doses rapidly suppresses TD, while decreasing doses may worsen movements for weeks. Manneristic movements can also improve with neuroleptics and may be difficult to distinguish from TD. In contrast, parkinsonian symptoms become worse with increasing doses. Anticholinergics do not help and may gradually worsen TD. Because these drug effects are not always seen in acute challenge studies,[65] it is possible that TD is a pharmacologically heterogeneous disorder.

Other features that may be associated with TD in schizophrenic patients, particularly older patients, include cognitive impairment, negative symptoms, prominent ventricular enlargement, and neurological soft signs.[66,67] TD may be accompanied by a supersensitivity psychosis during neuroleptic withdrawal.[68] Both the association of TD with possible "organic features" and the existence of a supersensitivity psychosis have not been found in all studies. TD has also been associated with abnormalities in other biological variables, such as saccadic eye movements,[69] psychophysiological measures,[70] and neurochemical levels.[71] These abnormalities do not yet have implications for clinical practice.

Differential Diagnosis

Neuroleptic-Induced Movement Disorders

TD is most commonly confused with acute extrapyramidal side effects such as parkinsonism or dystonia. Symptoms of the former include tremor, cogwheel rigidity, bradykinesia, and akinesia. Tremors are regular and rhythmic shaking movements occurring 3 to 12 times per second. Some tremors attenuate with movement (rest tremors) while others are only present with sustained posture (postural tremor). TD is irregular, writhing, or jerky. Parkinsonian tremor (usually 4–7 Hz) is most commonly seen in the hands and arms, but can also affect the head, jaw, lips, and tongue. The rabbit syndrome is a regular and rhythmic tremor of the upper lip and perinasal area, suggestive of the rapid facial movement movements a rabbit makes. The lip pursing and other facial movements of TD, on the other hand, are irregular. Akathisia is a subjective feeling of restlessness accompanied by pacing or fidgeting of the feet. Acute dystonias are sustained, forceful muscle contractions of the axial or appendicular musculature and often are painful. These abnormal movements develop shortly after the initiation of neuroleptics or after a significant increase in the dose. They respond to treatment with anticholinergic medications or to lower neuroleptic doses. This medication response is, in a sense, the pharmacological opposite of TD.

About 2% of patients develop dyskinesias shortly after the initiation of neuroleptic therapy. These movements are similar to TD except they start suddenly and remit spontaneously while the patient remains on a constant neuroleptic. Like other acute extrapyramidal symptoms, initial dyskinesias respond to treatment with anticholinergic drugs.

Abnormal Movements in Psychiatric Disorders

Several reports have described TD-like movements in patients with schizophrenia who have never been treated with neuroleptics. These movements are virtually indistinguishable from TD. In clinical practice, dyskinetic movements are classified as TD when they occur after 3 or more months of exposure to neuroleptics, and after organic factors have been excluded. Because of the frequency of spontaneous movement disorders in some groups, however, such a diagnosis may imply we know more about the etiology of their dyskinesias than is justified.

Manneristic and stereotyped movements can be difficult to distinguish from or can be confused with TD. These movements include rubbing, picking, bizarre arm gestures, or grimacing related to psychotic communications. These movements suggest fragments of more organized motor activity, yet are purposeless. Tardive akathisia (Chapter 6) may result in very similar stereotyped movements. Tics tend to be quicker and simpler movements than mannerisms, and include shoulder shrugging, blinking, coughing, or even grunting. Compulsions are more complex behaviors, such as repetitive hand-washing. In unusual cases, abnormal movements may be included as part of a somatoform disorder, such as conversion reactions, factitious disorders, and malingering. While these can look remarkably similar to TD, they do not worsen with activation or neuroleptic withdrawal. Furthermore, they disappear with distracting tasks.

Abnormal Movements in Neurological Disorders

Abnormal movements caused by neurological illnesses may be confused with TD. Tremors may be present in a number of disease states including idiopathic Parkinson's disease, benign familial tremor, cerebellar disease, or lithium therapy. Idiopathic cranial dystonia (Meige's syndrome) is commonly mistaken for "spontaneous orofacial dyskinesia" or TD. Other causes of cranial dystonia result in similar diagnostic confusion. Myoclonus is an isolated, rapid, frequently repetitive, jerking movement of a single muscle or muscle group. Myoclonus may occur normally at the onset of sleep, or pathologically when awake as a manifestation of many possible underlying neurological conditions, including seizure disorders. Other facial movement disorders including hemifacial spasm, facial myokymia, and aberrant regeneration of the facial nerve with synkinetic movements should be ruled out.

Any CNS disorder affecting the basal ganglia can produce dyskinetic movements (see Chapter 1). The common disorders should be excluded before making a diagnosis of TD. A routine evaluation

Table 2

Laboratory Tests Useful in the Differential Diagnosis of TD

Routine	Additional Tests*
Electrolytes	Chest X-ray (e.g., for TB)
CBC with peripheral smear	PPD
Thyroid indices	Drug levels (e.g., Li)
Calcium	Lumbar puncture (infectious causes)
Magnesium	Lyme antibody titer
Liver enzymes	Drug screens
Erythrocyte sedimentation rate	Heavy metal screen (urine or serum)
Antinuclear antibody level	
VDRL	
HIV antibody titer	
Serum ceruloplasmin	
EEG	
CT or MRI of the head	

* Test orders under special circumstances.
CBC = complete blood count; PPD = purified protein derivative; VDRL = Venereal Disease Research Laboratory (syphilis test); Li = lithium.

could include tests listed in Table 2. Additional tests may be warranted in specific cases. These tests are expensive, and a cost/benefit analysis has not shown that they are all necessary. MRI scans in particular are expensive, although it has been suggested that an imaging study is needed.[72] For the time being, a good history and physical exam should guide clinical judgment in deciding on the appropriate use of laboratory tests.

Natural History

Tardive dyskinesia typically begins several years after the initiation of antipsychotic drug treatment. Older patients appear to develop symptoms more quickly than younger patients,[39] perhaps as a result of neurobiological changes associated with aging. TD appears to reach its maximal level of severity rapidly, and then stabilizes.[73]

After a few months of relatively stable movements, significant worsening is unusual. Bergen and colleagues[74] found 45% of patients with TD had relatively persistent symptoms over the course of 5 years, while 24% had a fluctuating course. Only 11% improved, while 7% got worse. Remissions usually appear within 1 to 2 years after discontinuation of medication. Occasionally, spontaneous remissions may not occur until 5 years after discontinuation of medications. Some patients may have a state-dependent course—for example, bipolar patients have been described who had remissions during mania and then became worse during depressions.[75,75a]

Five to 10% of patients on long-term neuroleptics develop symptoms that are severe enough to markedly impair functioning.[76] Schizophrenics with TD may have up to twice the mortality rate of schizophrenics without TD,[77] although it is not clear what role TD plays in this elevated rate. Orofacial dyskinesias can present obstacles to returning to the community or work; they may also produce difficulty in eating, leading to marked weight loss, cachexia, or other medical complications. Pharyngeal involvement, more common in Huntington's disease, sometimes results in aspiration pneumonia, while truncal and extremity involvement can lead to difficulty with ambulation. Significant muscle breakdown can occur with marked elevations in creatine kinase (CK), although we know of no case reports of malignant rhabdomyolysis. Finally, diaphragmatic dyskinesias can compromise respiratory function and speech.[77a]

Pathophysiology

Physiology of the Basal Ganglia

The motor cortex and its projections to the spinal cord are the final mediators of voluntary movement. Lesions of the motor cortex abolish voluntary movement and produce spasticity. The basal ganglia are a group of interrelated subcortical structures that are also involved in the regulation of movement. Disorders of the basal ganglia produce motor abnormalities, characterized by rigidity, tremor, bradykinesia, and dyskinesia. In the past, the basal ganglia were thought to perform primarily motor functions. Information from many cortical areas appeared to funnel through the basal ganglia, being refined and integrated. This highly processed information then passed through the thalamus to the prefrontal cortex.

Recently, our understanding of both structure and function has undergone a profound transformation. The basal ganglia have been shown to comprise a system of five parallel circuits that remain separate from one another in their path to the thalamus and cortex. Even within individual loops, it appears that information is segregated into modules that converge minimally. It may be similar, in this respect, to the modular organization of the cortex.[78] These loops have been described according to functions they subserve and include the motor, oculomotor, limbic, dorsolateral prefrontal and lateral orbitofrontal loops,[79] subserving motor, cognitive, emotional, and oculomotor processing, respectively. The primary circuit of interest for movement disorders is the motor circuit.

Anatomically, the basal ganglia consist of several large subcortical structures (Fig. 1), including the caudate, putamen, and globus pallidus. The caudate and putamen, collectively referred to as the striatum, are developmentally and functionally similar and receive most of the input to the basal ganglia. The globus pallidus (GP) consists of two parts, the externa (GPe) and the interna (GPi), each with different outputs. Two small midbrain structures are included: the substantia nigra (SN) and the subthalamic nucleus. The substantia nigra has two divisions, the pars compacta (SNc), which contains dopaminergic neurons, and the pars reticulata (SNr), which is functionally similar to the GPi.

The primary afferents to the basal ganglia originate in the cortical sensory, motor, and association areas. These project to the striatum, retaining their topographic specificity.[79] Most inputs to the motor circuit come from the primary motor and premotor areas, and to a lesser degree from somatosensory areas. They terminate in the putamen. The striatum projects to the neighboring globus pallidus and to the SNr and SNc, all projections retaining topographic organization. Efferents from the GP flow in two pathways.[80] In the indirect loop, neurons of the GPe project to the subthalamic nucleus, which in turn projects back to the GPi. In the direct loop, striatal information goes directly to the GPi, without processing in the GPe or the subthalamic nucleus. The major basal ganglia efferents originate in the the GPi and the SNr, and project to the ventral anterior and ventral lateral thalamus. These thalamic nuclei, in turn, project back to the prefrontal cortex, completing the loop.[81]

The excitatory cortical projections to the striatum are primarily glutamatergic.[82] The projections synapse on dendritic spines of striatal medium spiny neurons. Spiny neurons comprise 95% of striatal neurons, and probably comprise the primary outflow to the GP and SN. Cortical input to the ends of the dendritic spines appears to be modulated by dopaminergic input to the more medial segments of

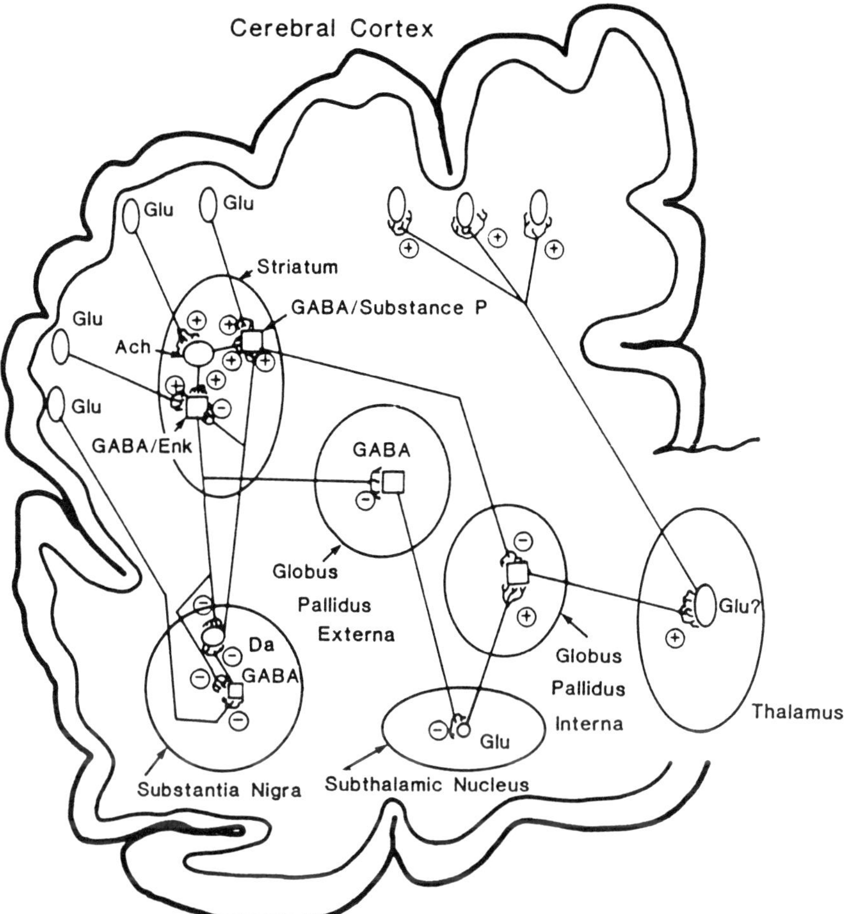

Figure 1: This schematic diagram summarizes basal ganglia circuitry (see references 79, 80, and 83). Excitatory glutamatergic (Glu) projections from the cortex to the striatum synapse on medium spiny GABAergic neurons and ACh interneurons. GABAergic neurons project to a second group of GABAergic neurons in the globus pallidus externa (GP$_e$) or globus pallidus interna (GP$_i$). In the direct pathway (see text), GABAergic GPi neurons inhibit thalamic neurons which project to the cortex. In the indirect pathway, GABAergic GPe neurons inhibit STN glutamatergic neurons which normally excite GPi neurons. The inhibition of STN excitatory input decreases GPi activity, which disinhibits the thalamus. Thus, the two pathways have opposing effects on thalamic output. Striatal GABAergic projections to the GPi may also contain substance P, while projections to the GPe may contain enkephalin. Dopaminergic neurons from the SN project to the striatum. Inhibitory striatonigral GABAergic efferents project back to both SN dopaminergic neurons and GABAergic interneurons. SN = substantia nigra; ACh = acetylcholine.

the same spines.[83] The spiny neurons are GABAergic and also receive input from cholinergic interneurons, and GABAergic inputs from other spiny neurons. The function of the cholinergic interneurons is unclear, but may antagonize the effects of dopamine. This feature is probably responsible for the apparent dopamine-acetylcholine (ACh) balance in striatal-mediated behaviors.

Other structural features of the striatum undoubtedly are related to function, such as its division into an island-like striosomal compartment and a background matrix.[84] The role of many neurotransmitters and modulators, such as norepinephrine, serotonin, neuropeptide Y, somatostatin, and CCK, is unclear. Alterations in any of these could affect function or be involved in the pathophysiology or treatment of TD.

Excitatory cortical input increases striatal GABAergic neuronal firing. This, in turn, inhibits GABAergic neurons of the GPi via the direct loop mentioned above. With a reduction in the activity of GABAergic GPi projection to the thalamus, thalamic neuronal activity is disinhibited, allowing other thalamic inputs to exert excitatory effects.[85] The thalamus, in turn, further stimulates the cortex. A counterbalancing, inhibitory effect on the cortex is produced simultaneously by the indirect loop.[80] Striatal efferents inhibit GPe GABAergic neurons. This reduces the tonic, GABA-mediated inhibition of the GPe on subthalamic neurons, which then increase firing rates. The increased excitatory subthalamic input to the GPi increases GPi GABAergic firing and produces greater inhibition in the thalamus. Thus, cortical stimulation of the striatum activates two opposing circuits that modulate thalamic activity, permitting certain thalamic inputs to stimulate the cortex. Lesions at any point in the circuit can produce abnormal movements. The final common output of the direct and indirect loops is thalamic activity. If this is increased, cortical stimulation is increased and hyperkinetic movements, such as those seen in tardive dyskinesia, may result.

Dopamine appears to serve an important modulatory role in the striatum. Neurophysiological experiments suggest dopamine excites striatal neurons giving rise to the direct pathway, while inhibiting neurons giving rise to the indirect pathway. The overall effect is to reinforce cortically initiated inputs and increase their downstream stimulation of the thalamus.[86] Variability of response is decreased in favor of more stereotyped responses[87] or perhaps dyskinesias.

Striatal dopamine afferents originate in the SNc, which is modulated by a striatonigral feedback pathway. Inhibitory GABAergic striatal efferents synapse onto both dopaminergic neurons and GA-BAergic interneurons. The direct GABA projections inhibit dopamine neurons, while the indirect input to interneurons results in disinhibition. The net control of dopamine firing is determined by the balance between the two inputs.

Dopamine Supersensitivity

The dopamine supersensitivity hypothesis of TD was first proposed in 1970 by Klawans. Based on the similarity between L-dopa-induced dyskinesias and TD, he suggested that chronic neuroleptic treatment produced a supersensitivity of striatal dopamine receptors, similar to denervation-induced supersensitivity seen in peripheral muscles. Supersensitivity has become the predominant theoretical construct guiding TD research and is supported by numerous basic and clinical studies.

Chronic neuroleptic treatment produces an increase in dopamine receptor density in the striatum as well as behavioral supersensitivity to dopamine agonists in both humans and animals. In humans, dopamine agonists such as L-dopa and amphetamine can exacerbate TD.[88] Dopamine antagonists suppress TD, while anticholinergics tend to enhance it.[89] The dyskinesias in other basal ganglia diseases (e.g., Huntington's and Wilson's diseases) are phenomenologically similar to TD. These dyskinesias also improve with neuroleptics, suggesting that dopamine may modulate all dyskinesias. Another version of this hypothesis postulates that TD is caused by a long-term increase in presynaptic dopamine release. Chronic administration of neuroleptics results in increases in dopamine metabolism[90] and release. The degree of dopamine release could be greater in patients with TD. A third version postulates an imbalance between the two major subtypes of dopamine receptors, D_1 and D_2.[91,92] There appears to be an obligatory functional interaction between the two receptors, although this may become uncoupled with the development of supersensitivity. It is possible that restoring the appropriate balance would improve symptoms of TD.

Several observations are difficult to reconcile with the dopamine hypothesis. Dopamine supersensitivity is present in rats within several weeks of neuroleptic treatment,[93,94] whereas TD-like movements take much longer to develop in these animals[95] and patients. When TD finally does develop, only a fraction of animals and patients are affected. Postmortem human studies have shown increased dopamine receptor number in most patients, regardless of the presence of TD.[96] Animals that develop maximal dopamine supersensitivity do not exhibit spontaneous behaviors associated with dopamine excess. Instead, treatment with dopamine agonists is necessary to differentiate between supersensitive and normal rats. This suggests dopamine supersensitivity per se does not have an overt behavioral effect. Rats that develop a TD-like syndrome continue to show signs of the movements long after dopamine supersensitivity has disappeared.[97] Indeed, animal studies demonstrate that dopamine supersensitivity resolves within several weeks, yet TD in animals and man can be persistent. Finally, one would expect that overcoming supersensitive receptors with higher neuroleptic doses would block TD. Clinical reports suggest that in some patients, TD can progress despite long-term treatment with increased doses.

Studies using pharmacological challenges are also not entirely consistent with the dopamine hypothesis. Some but not all patients improve when given dopamine antagonists, while mixed effects are seen with cholinergic agonists and antagonists.[98,99] Furthermore, several studies have found that some dopamine agonists do not exacerbate TD, such as high-dose apomorphine[100] and bromocriptine.[101] Other studies suggest some degree of pharmacological heterogeneity. Some patients seem more susceptible to exacerbation of movements by anticholinergic challenge while others worsen with neuroleptic withdrawal.[102]

It appears that supersensitive dopamine receptors modulate TD to some degree; however, additional factors that are independent of the dopamine receptor are probably involved as well.

GABA Depletion

As a result of deficiencies in the dopamine supersensitivity hypothesis, considerable attention has been focused on the GABA system.[103,104] A number of studies point to decreased GABAergic neuronal activity in one or more areas of the basal ganglia. The strongest evidence comes from animal studies. In rats, long-term treatment with neuroleptics may decrease GABA turnover[105] and increase GABA binding sites[104] in the SN, suggesting a decrease in GABA release or a loss of GABAergic terminals. Neuroleptic treatment also may reduce the activity of glutamic acid decarboxylase (GAD), the rate-limiting enzyme for GABA synthesis, in the SNr, GPi, or subthalamic nucleus,[95,106,107] Furthermore, these reductions are present only in those animals that develop dyskinetic movements.[106] Pharmacological studies also suggest GABA plays a role in modulating dyskinesias. Infusing the GABA antagonist bicuculine into the SN induced acute dyskinesias in rats.[108] The same occurred with isoniazid infusion. In low concentrations, this drug decreases the systhesis of GABA, but at higher levels, it inhibits the enzymatic degradation of GABA. In monkeys, acute treatment with GABA agonists may block neuroleptic-induced dyskinesias, although this evidence is not strong.[109] Not all studies, however, support a role for GABA in TD. Mithani et al.[110] found only a transient decrease in SN GAD after 48 weeks of neuroleptic treatment with no correlation with dyskinetic movements, while Rupniak et al.[111] found no changes at all.

There is evidence that GABAergic activity may be altered in humans with TD. Andersson and colleagues, in a very small postmortem study,[112] found a significant decrease in subthalamic GAD activity in patients with TD compared to patients without TD. A trend towards a decrease was seen in the GPi, while SN GAD activity was normal. This finding requires replication with a larger cohort of patients. Thaker et al.[113] found a decrease in CSF GABA in schizophrenic patients with TD versus schizophrenics without TD, although this was not replicated.[114] Saccadic eye movements are, in part, controlled by GABAergic projections from the SN. Patients with schizophrenia and TD show a twofold greater saccadic distractibility than those without TD. This clinical finding supports the idea that TD is due to a deficiency in GABA in the basal ganglia.[115]

In conclusion, many animal and human studies suggest that TD is related to abnormalities in GABAergic activity in one or more nuclei of the basal ganglia. This is not surprising given the importance of GABA in the neural circuitry of the basal ganglia. In particular, a lesion that decreases GABA-mediated inhibition of the thalamus could produce TD. This effect could originate in either the direct or the indirect GP loop. Although some reports are conflicting, the majority of studies strongly support GABAergic mediation of abnormal movements.

Neurotoxicity

The idea that long-term neuroleptic treatment may have a toxic effect on the brain has led to many studies that look for evidence of neuronal injury. The neurotoxicity hypothesis is particularly engaging given the persistence of TD, in some cases, and the similarity between TD and degenerative diseases of the basal ganglia. Unfortunately, most postmortem studies in animals and man exposed to long-term neuroleptic treatment have been inconsistent or have suffered from methodological problems. Studies on human brains have used very small sample sizes and are poorly controlled (for review see reference 2). Christensen et al.,[116] with the largest published human cohort, found gliosis and degeneration in the substantia nigra in 27 out of 28 cases of TD, with midbrain gliosis in 25 of 28; however, 7 out of 28 normals had similar pathology. Jellinger[117] found striatal neuronal swelling in 5 of 9 patients but only in 1 of 14 controls.

Methodological problems are more easily avoided in animal studies, but the results have also been inconsistent. Two early studies found no evidence of pathology in animals after long-term neuroleptic treatment.[118,119] A more sophisticated quantitative study[120] found a 20% loss of neurons in the basal ganglia with no gliosis in rats treated for 1 year with neuroleptics. This was not seen after 2 months[121] or 6 months.[122] Nielsen and Lyon[123] found a 10% neuronal loss confined to the ventrolateral region of the striatum, concerned with the innervation of the oral musculature.

If neuroleptics do produce pathological changes in the brain, they may be subtle and not evident under light microscopy. Dopamine is known to be a neurotoxin to some cell lines.[124] This may be due to the formation of oxygen-containing free radicals during metabolism.[125] The increase in dopamine turnover produced by neuroleptics could increase the concentration of free radicals, overwhelming the ability of cells to break down these toxic free radicals. This may explain axonal sprouting in the SN induced by treatment with haloperidol.[126] Another line of research has shown that phenothiazines can produce physiochemical changes in rat striatal cell membranes,[127] and cause cell membranes to expand and invaginate.[128] Extremely high concentrations of neuroleptics, as high as 100 to 1000 nM, appear to accumulate in the SN secondary to binding with neuromelanin. These high concentrations may exacerbate the postulated toxic effects. Despite these suggestive studies, more evidence is needed to substantiate the neurotoxicity hypothesis.

Organic Brain Damage

Some researchers have suggested that TD is a symptom of a diffuse organic process.[129] Numerous studies show that schizophrenics with TD have more negative symptoms, poorer premorbid functioning, greater cognitive impairment, more prominent abnormalities on CT or MRI, such as larger ventricles, more prominent eye tracking abnormalities, and more neurological "soft signs." Subtle brain dysfunction could, perhaps, work in conjunction with neuroleptic-induced dopamine supersensitivity to enhance the development of TD. Indeed, animals with prefrontal lesions have a higher incidence of dyskinetic movements after long-term neuroleptic treatment,[130] suggesting that focal organic lesions can contribute to the development of TD. On the other hand, some studies have not found greater evidence of organicity in schizophrenics with TD.[131] Furthermore, it is not clear whether TD is associated with evidence of subtle brain dysfunction in other populations, such as bipolar patients.[132] While subtle brain damage may contribute to or confer additional vulnerability to develop TD, it seems permissive rather than causative.

Norepinephrine

A variety of neurotransmitters other than dopamine and GABA modulate information flow through the basal ganglia, any one of which could play a role in the pathogenesis of TD. One such transmitter is norepinephrine (NE). Central noradrenergic neurons innervate the striatum and appear to influence movement. For example, Hornykiewicz[133] suggested that NE modulates dopamine-induced hyperactivity. The moderate success of some noradrenergic agents in treating TD[16] supports the possibility of NE involvement. Clinical evidence of NE overactivity, however, is inconsistent. Activity of dopamine beta-hydroxylase, the enzyme that converts dopamine to NE, was higher in plasma of schizophrenics with TD compared to those without TD in three studies,[134–136], but not others.[137] Jeste et al.[138] have reported increased CSF NE levels in patients with TD. Kaufmann et al.[136] found a correlation between platelet alpha$_2$ adrenergic receptor binding, CSF levels of NE, and symptom severity in patients with TD. Unfortunately, treatment with an alpha$_2$ antagonist failed to ameliorate TD.[139]

Serotonin

Serotonin is another striatal neurotransmitter that may be involved in regulating abnormal movements, perhaps by modulating dopamine release. Animal studies suggest that serotonergic agents affect abnormal movements, although results have been conflicting. Both agonists and antagonists have been reported to reduce dyskinetic movements in a monkey model of TD.[140] Boosting serotonergic neurotransmission in human patients with tryptophan is usually ineffective, although newer reuptake inhibitors have not yet been studied. Measures of striatal serotonin activity in humans have not yielded consistent findings. Jeste and colleagues[141] found no difference in plasma levels of serotonin between patients with TD and controls. Chase et al.[142] found low CSF levels of 5–hydroxyindoleacetic acid (5HIAA), the major metabolite of serotonin, in patients with TD, while Nagao[144] did not. As with NE, serotonin may play a role in the altered basal ganglia function underlying TD, but this role remains to be elucidated.

Miscellaneous Theories

Acetylcholine (ACh) is important in striatal function, counterbalancing, in some way, the effects of dopamine. Dopamine overactivity could be related to a hypocholinergic state. While basic animal work indicates that cholinergic function returns to normal after prolonged neuroleptic exposure,[143] results from human studies are less clear. It is difficult to assess central ACh activity. While CSF cyclic GMP levels have been used,[144] their validity is unclear. One study using this method found no differences between patients with and without TD. Numerous therapeutic trials have attempted to boost brain ACh activity, but these have generally been unsuccessful.[16]

Virtually any effect of long-term neuroleptic treatment is a potential candidate for mediating their dyskinetogenic properties. One line of research compares antipsychotics that produce TD with one that does not, such as clozapine. Classic neuroleptics such as haloperidol produce an inactivation of nigrostriatal dopamine neurons when given chronically. This has been referred to as "depolarization inactivation" and is mediated by feedback excitation from striatonigral projections. Clozapine does not produce depolarization inactivation, leading to speculation that depolarization inactivation may be involved in the pathogenesis of TD.[145] Clearly, clozapine has unique effects on the nigrostriatal system, and the lack of depolarization inactivation is one aspect of this. Its importance remains to be determined.

A particularly exciting new area of basal ganglia research concerns the function of neuropeptides. A variety of neuropeptides are colocalized in afferent and efferent striatal projections. Cholecystokinin (CCK), for example, is colocalized in nigrostriatal dopaminergic neurons. CCK administration increases D_2 receptor number[146] and stimulates dopamine-mediated striatal neurotransmission.[147] Paradoxically, CCK also has neuroleptic-like activity, as it antagonizes dopamine agonist-induced behaviors.[148] Levels of CCK have not been measured in humans with TD or in animal models. The existence of other neuropeptides, such as substance P in the tachykinin family, dynorphin B of the prodynorphine family, somatostatin, and proenkephalins is expanding our awareness of the complexity of the basal ganglia. These peptides offer new areas to explore in the search for the cause of TD.

Treatment

Currently, the best treatment for many psychiatric disorders is the long-term administration of antipsychotic agents. To forestall the development of TD in patients who require neuroleptics, one should use the minimal dose required for a therapeutic effect. Furthermore, long-term use of these medications is indicated only in patients with a therapeutic response. Some patients can be maintained on other agents that are much less likely to produce TD. These include lithium, anticonvulsants (e.g., carbamazepine, and valproic acid), tricyclics, and benzodiazepines. Prevention is still the treatment of choice for TD.

While there is no generally effective treatment of TD, a number of therapeutic strategies have emerged based on the increasingly sophisticated understanding of the neurobiology of the basal ganglia. Unfortunately, this understanding has far outpaced clinical applications. When approaching a patient with TD, the first issue to address is whether to continue treatment with neuroleptics. While the benefits may be obvious, the risks are also significant. A second issue is whether additional medications are needed to suppress the dyskinesias. If suppressive therapy is needed, a wide choice of mildly to moderately successful suppressive drug therapies is available.

Some evidence indicates that once TD has been present for several months, continued administration of neuroleptics does not worsen movements. However, this evidence is far from conclusive.

Therefore, neuroleptic withdrawal is the usual recommended course of action, and probably the safest and most conservative with respect to TD. In the first several weeks following withdrawal, patients often get worse, but, within 3 months, 36% to 55% of patients will improve;[16] improvement may not occur for up to 5 years afterwards.[149] Jus and colleagues,[150] for example, found improvement in 49 of 62 patients by slowly tapering neuroleptics over 4 years. Significant risks, however, are associated with neuroleptic discontinuation, including increased rates of psychotic decompensation and increased likelihood of injury to self or others. Furthermore, untreated patients with schizophrenia may have a worse long-term prognosis than patients treated with neuroleptics.[151]

There is no simple formula for assessing a patient's ability to tolerate neuroleptic withdrawal. Clearly, a wide variety of other factors need to be considered, such as past history of dangerous behavior, susceptibility to relapse from particular stressors, current living and working environment, and family relationships. There are many patients who, unfortunately, will not be able to tolerate neuroleptic withdrawal. Patients who have had only a marginal response to neuroleptics may be good candidates for withdrawal. TD in patients over 65[38] or with organic brain damage[4] may not improve following neuroleptic withdrawal. Intermittent treatment or use of "drug holidays" probably does not improve[152] or prevent the development of TD.[23] Intermittent drug treatment may even exacerbate TD.[63] It has been suggested that depot neuroleptics may have a higher tendency to cause TD,[153] although this needs additional study.

In our experience, suppressive therapy should be considered if TD poses health risks (e.g., problems with breathing, eating, walking, or sleeping), or is otherwise bothersome, disfiguring, or impairing. Assessment by an occupational therapist can give insight into functional impairment and may suggest strategies to cope with disabilities. Many patients with TD are not aware of their abnormal movements and are not adversely affected by them. Additional treatment in these cases may not be worth the risk and effort.

Several comprehensive reviews[16,63] have surveyed most of the published data on treatment of TD. This discussion will briefly describe the effectiveness, benefits, and risks of the more successful or commonly used agents. There are no clear guidelines to follow when choosing a suppressive agent. In general, therapeutic trials have attempted to manipulate one of the following neurotransmitter systems: dopamine, GABA, acetylcholine, and norepinephrine.

It is helpful to involve both the patient and their family from the outset, if possible, so that informed decisions can be made. Patients educated with printed information sheets appear better informed than those educated verbally.[154] Routine monitoring of TD is essential to quantitatively track the changes and response to medications. The most popular rating procedure is the AIMS examination.[155] Ratings should be performed every 4 to 6 months in patients with TD and perhaps more often if vigorous treatment is being pursued. Moreover, an exam should also be performed at least annually on patients at risk for developing TD.

Dopamine

Suppressive Therapy with Neuroleptics

Neuroleptics suppress TD. This has been found in both short-term and long-term (more than 8 weeks) studies. A review of 50 studies, totaling 501 patients, found that 67% of patients improved with neuroleptics.[156] This included 13 long-term studies where 77% of patients improved; of those, tolerance to the therapeutic effects was reported in only two cases out of 117. A more recent review[16] indicated a lower rate of response. The major concern is the possible exacerbation of the movements with continued exposure to neuroleptics. While the safety of this approach has not been demonstrated, it may be the only effective treatment in severe cases with life-threatening complications. More potent neuroleptics such as haloperidol may be more effective at suppressing movements than low potency or atypical neuroleptics such as molindone.[157] Glazer et al.[157] were able to suppress 66% of patients with withdrawal TD using haloperidol, but only 39% with molindone. If withdrawal dyskinesias are similar pharmacologically to persistent dyskinesias, then they may also be suppressed more effectively by high-potency neuroleptics. In addition, Glazer's report raises the possibility that less potent neuroleptics are less dyskinetogenic. Giving medications in divided doses throughout the day may also be helpful in masking symptoms of TD. In a variation of this suppressive strategy, we have seen improvement in several patients after stopping neuroleptic for several weeks and then restarting at a lower dose. This has not been studied under controlled conditions. The two patients that improved had a marked parkinsonian tremor in addition to TD.

Clozapine

Clozapine is a newly available antipsychotic medication that has only minimally been associated with the development of tardive dyskinesia.[158] This may be related to its unique effects on the nigrostriatal dopaminergic system.[145] Surprisingly, clozapine seems to markedly improve symptoms in up to 44% of patients.[158-160] While further research is needed to verify its effectiveness, clozapine is emerging as an important drug in the treatment of TD. Two drawbacks are its association with agranulocytosis and its expense, due to the required blood monitoring. Clozapine should be considered for any patient who requires chronic antipsychotic medication, particularly those with moderate to severe symptoms. It is also a reasonable alternative for bipolar patients with early or mild signs of TD who cannot be managed off neuroleptics. These patients are often more aware of and disturbed by their movements, and are more compliant with the required weekly blood counts.

Dopamine Depleters

Reserpine (.75 to 3.0 mg/d) and tetrabenazine (up to 200 mg/d; not available in the US) are antipsychotics that work by depleting dopamine from presynaptic vesicles, rather than by blocking D_2 dopamine receptors. Alpha-methyldopa (750 to 1,500 mg/d) also depletes dopamine neurons by competitive inhibition of dopa decarboxylase and the formation of a false neurotransmitter. Dopamine-depleting agents have been reported to alleviate symptoms in up to 50% of patients with TD,[161] although some studies have not found this degree of improvement. Side effects, including hypotension (reserpine, alpha-methyldopa), impotence, and depression, as well as parkinsonism and akathisia, may limit the clinical utility of these agents. Depression may be treated with the addition of antidepressants. Although often used by neurologists to treat tardive dyskinesia, it has been our experience that these agents are not very effective in treating the movement disorder of tardive dyskinesia and are associated with multiple side effects. We do not routinely use dopamine-depleting agents to treat tardive dyskinesia. This discrepancy in usage of dopamine-depleters between neurologists and psychiatrists deserves further study.

Dopamine Agonists

Dopamine agonists, in animal studies, down-regulate dopamine receptors, and therefore could be useful in TD. A major drawback is that they can initially exacerbate both TD and psychotic symptoms. Direct (apomorphine and bromocriptine) and indirect (amantadine and levodopa) agonists have been studied.[162] Some positive case reports have been published, but most double-blind studies show little improvement.[16] One exception is a recent report of 35 in-patients with severe orofacial TD who showed marked improvement on L-dopa after 2 months. Symptoms returned when L-dopa was discontinued, and again responded when treatment was restarted.[163] This finding needs to be replicated in a double-blind crossover study, but is encouraging nonetheless.

Dopamine autoreceptor agonists (e.g., 3-PPP) decrease the release of dopamine and present another possible mechanism to treat TD. 3-PPP has been shown in monkeys to improve TD,[164] but it has not been tried in humans. In low doses, apomorphine is an autoreceptor agonist, while in high doses it is a postsynaptic receptor agonist. Theoretically, low doses should decrease dopamine release and improve symptoms of TD, while high doses should do the opposite. Paradoxically, one study showed that high doses, up to 6.0 mg, reduced TD movements.[165] The usefulness of apomorphine may be limited by side effects such as nausea and vomiting at therapeutic doses; however, these can be managed quite effectively by the peripheral dopamine receptor blocker, domperidone.

Noradrenergic Antagonists

Noradrenergic innervation of the striatum offers another site for therapeutic intervention. Beta-adrenergic antagonist propranolol may partially suppress TD in up to 73% of patients,[63,166] although depression can be a side effect, and some of this suppressing effect may simply be due to the ability of propranolol to increase neuroleptic blood levels. Clonidine, an alpha$_2$ agonist, decreases release of norepinephrine by autoreceptor stimulation, and has been reported to have antidyskinetic properties in a majority of patients.[167–169] Clonidine may also have antipsychotic properties and has relatively few side effects (hypotension, sedation). Other norepinephrine antagonists with some clinical benefit include disulfiram[170] and fusaric acid, both of which are dopamine beta hydroxylase inhibitors. Oxypertine depletes NE and may also improve dyskinesias.[171] The success of these agents needs to be demonstrated with larger controlled studies. At the present time, NE antagonists, particularly clonidine and propranolol, appear to be among the safest and most effective treatments and are reasonable choices for a first-line agent.

Anticholinergics

Dopamine and acetylcholine appear to have opposite effects on striatal-mediated behaviors. One would predict that anticholinergics in the presence of dopamine supersensitivity should make TD worse. While this has been found in some reports,[172] surprisingly, the opposite has also been found. In an acute challenge study using intravenous administration, benztropine (Cogentin) tended to improve movements while physostigmine made them worse.[65] This suggests that dopamine and ACh are not simply functional antagonists in the basal ganglia. In general, however, long-term treatment with anticholinergics either do not help or may actually worsen TD.[173,174] Withdrawal is sometimes helpful, perhaps in 60% of patients.[16] Anticholinergics may predispose patients to develop TD,[175] although this is not clear.[176] While much is still unknown about the effects of anticholinergics, the available data suggest that patients with TD should not receive them if possible.

Cholinergics

Just as anticholinergics theoretically should worsen TD, cholinergic agonists should improve it. Several ACh precursors, which increase synthesis of ACh, have been tried with generally disappointing results. These agents include deanol, choline, and lecithin (a naturally occurring precursor of choline). Physostigmine, a centrally acting cholinesterase inhibitor, has been used to investigate the pharmacology of TD, with mixed results.[65,177] An encouraging preliminary study using ACh releasing agent meclofenoxate found improvement in 5 out of 11 patients.[178] Cholinergic agents do not currently play a significant role in the treatment of TD, but future studies with agents such as meclofenoxate may change this.

GABA Agonists

A variety of experimental and commercially available GABA agonists have been used with limited success. Jeste and Wyatt's 1982 review[174] describes 19 studies totaling 204 patients, with 54% having greater than 50% improvement, the most effective non-neuroleptic class of drugs they reviewed. In their 1988 review of nine additional studies,[16] the efficacy of GABA agonists fell to about 30%. On the other hand, in a selective review of the effects of benzodiazepines, Thaker and colleagues[179] found that, in 15 reports involving a total of 158 patients, 83% of patients improved to some degree. There are significant problems with side effects for many of these agents, including sedation, ataxia, and addiction. They are probably best used as second-line agents for the suppression of TD.

The most-studied commercially available GABA agonists include valproate, diazepam, clonazepam, and baclofen. Sodium valproate has produced mixed results, with improvement in 3 of 6 patients in one study,[180] but 0 of 10 in a second.[181] Diazepam, in a single-blind study, was helpful in 11 of 20 patients[182] and in 26 of 29 in four studies prior to 1979,[56] but can cause sedation, addiction, and perhaps impulsiveness and belligerence.[182] Clonazepam, which may have antipsychotic effects, helped 26.5% of patients with choreoathetosis and 41.5% of patients with dystonia in a double-blind, controlled study of TD.[179] In two open studies, 2 out of 18 reported benefit in one,[184] while all 42 patients benefited in the other.[185] Tolerance can develop to the therapeutic effects, but this may be overcome.[179] In eight studies with baclofen, only two showed significant results.[186] In one of these, 3 out of 13 improved,[186] while in the second, 9 of 13 improved.[187] Efficacy may decrease with long-term use, and side effects, including sedation, nausea, vomiting, and ataxia, can also limit use. Abrupt discontinuation can produce psychosis and seizures. Baclofen may act primarily on $GABA_B$ receptors,[188] which may not be as important to TD. To summarize, select patients may benefit from clonazepam or diazepam, while valproate and baclofen may be less effective.

Experimental agents have produced mixed results. THIP, a $GABA_A$ agonist,[189] and gamma-vinyl-GABA (GVG), a GABA-transaminase inhibitor,[190] improve TD but to a minor degree. Muscimol, another $GABA_A$ agonist, produced a 45% reduction in seven patients.[177] Several reports suggest that progabide, a mixed $GABA_A$ and $GABA_B$ agonist, may have significant therapeutic effects, but more studies are needed. While the efficacy of these agents supports a role for GABA in the pathophysiology of TD, they are not currently useful in clinical management.

Antioxidants

One of the more promising new agents to treat TD is vitamin E, an antioxidant and free radical scavenger. This compound was originally used to test the hypothesis that neuroleptics produce toxic free radicals which cause neuronal dysfunction or cell death. Two published reports have shown beneficial effects in patients with TD.[191,192] These two studies used 1200 IU per day, in divided doses. Its prophylactic use could theoretically prevent the development of TD. Generally, vitamin E is safe, producing few side effects. Rarely, patients report abdominal pain, headaches, muscle cramps, nausea, or fatigue. Vitamin E may elevate triglycerides and cholesterol, and decrease thyroid indices, although it has not been reported to cause hypothyroidism. These abnormalities and symptoms all disappear after discontinuation of the drug. Vitamin E may interact with coumadin to prolong bleeding time. Additional research is needed to establish its therapeutic effects and to clarify its use in prevention.

Miscellaneous Therapeutic Agents

A number of other medications have been reported to attenuate symptoms of TD. Calcium channel blockers have been successful in a few cases. Verapamil in doses up to 80 mg q.i.d. produced mild improvement,[193] while diltiazem produced minimal improvement.[194] Lithium, which reportedly prevents dopamine supersensitivity when used with neuroleptics,[195] has not been effective in treating TD in clinical trials. Cerulitide, a CCK antagonist, has been beneficial in one study.[196] A very low dose (5 mg/d) of prednisolone surprisingly produced a complete remission after 2 days in two patients with severe TD.[197] Again, more research is needed to clarify the effectiveness of these agents.

Serotonin modulates striatal dopamine release and may thereby influence dyskinetic movements. A recent case report describes high doses (40–60 mg/t.i.d.) of buspirone (Buspar), a serotonin 1A agonist, markedly improving TD. Buspirone has also been reported to cause akathisia and a persistent oral dyskinesia in one case,[119] although the latter has been questioned due to the prior use of neuroleptics. Buspirone is weakly antidopaminergic, which could account for its therapeutic effect on TD. Fluoxetine, a serotonin reuptake inhibitor, has been reported to reduce dopamine synthesis in a variety of brain areas, including the striatum,[200] and to exacerbate parkinsonian symptoms.[201] Theoretically, it might improve symptoms of TD. Studies with other serotonergic agents are underway and will help to illuminate this issue.

Nondrug treatments may be beneficial under certain circumstances. The use of dentures and correction of other dental problems can markedly reduce oral TD. Canes, braces, or biofeedback may offer some limited benefit in severe cases. ECT has had a variable therapeutic effect in TD (see Chapter 8). Finally, neurosurgical intervention, while theoretically possible, has not been tried to our knowledge.

Summary of Treatment Recommendations

Prevention of TD is still the best therapeutic intervention. This may be achieved by restricting the use of long-term antipsychotics to appropriate patients and by using the lowest dose possible. In the future, clinicians may be able to use safe clozapine-like agents that do not produce TD. At present, clinicians should consider alternative treatments, such as lithium, carbamazepine, or valproic acid before planning a course of long-term neuroleptic treatment. Once TD is present, the diagnosis should be confirmed with repeated examinations and with the exclusion of organic causes. The patient and/or family should be consulted about continued neuroleptic exposure and presented with treatment alternatives. Movements should be monitored periodically and functional impairment assessed when needed. Neuroleptic dose should be lowered if possible. In some cases, switching to a lower potency, atypical neuroleptic such as loxapine, molindone, or mesoridazine may be of benefit. These atypical agents may be less dyskinetogenic. Clozapine is a unique agent that can sometimes suppress TD without leading to exacerbation. In the future, it may become the drug of choice for psychotic patients with marked TD. Anticholinergics often can be discontinued.

If marked impairment, disfigurement, or discomfort exists, one should consider suppressive therapy. Apart from dopamine antagonists, the greatest success has been found with noradrenergic antagonists (propranolol, clonidine) and GABA agonists (clonazepam, diazepam, valproate, or baclofen). One's choice should be based on the profile of side effects that are most easily tolerated by the patient. For example a patient with hypertension might do well on clonidine. Other medications should be considered as second-line agents. These include vitamin E, buspirone, and calcium channel blockers. For more severe or treatment-resistant cases, purely experimental agents such as prednisolone, cerulitide, or fluoxetine might be tried. The role of dopamine agonists is also unclear, although in our experience, they have not been particularly helpful. Neuroleptics will usually give quick relief and may be needed, but one must bear in mind the potential for long-term exacerbation. In disabling, persistent TD, dopamine depletors such as reserpine or tetrabenzine may be effective in controlling the abnormal movements. However, drug-induced parkinsonism and akathisia may be dose-limiting and a patient with a history of depression with suicide attempts should probably limit the use of these drugs.

Future Trends in Research

As our understanding of the structure and function of the basal ganglia grow, so too will our understanding of the pathophysiology of movement disorders and TD. Advances are coming in a number of areas, such as in our understanding of the organization of the striatum, the physiology of individual circuits, and the role of neuropeptides and modulators. One important area of basic research involves the exploration of the long-term effects of antipsychotic drugs, including possible toxic actions and structural changes, and their effects on neurotransmitters and neuropeptides. Combining behavioral studies with postmortem neurochemical and neuropathological studies will clarify associations between movement disorders and specific changes in the brain. Pharmacological studies in animals with movement disorders using more specific ligands for a variety of receptors may suggest new therapeutic agents for human use.

The most important clinical advances are likely to come as new antipsychotics, such as clozapine, become available. Understanding the differences between these new medications and traditional neuroleptics will lead to additional agents. A number of medications with promising effects in pilot studies need additional testing, such as NE antagonists, GABA agonists, vitamin E, calcium channel blockers, and serotonergic agents. New drugs selectively targeting specific receptors, such as the D_1 receptor, subpopulations of serotonin receptors, or peptide receptors may also prove beneficial. Finally, as the techniques of molecular biology are brought to bear on neuropsychiatric disorders, understanding which genes regulate neuronal firing rates, receptor number, and overall activity of the neural circuits involved may lead to an ability to make more fundamental alterations in abnormal information processing.

References

1. Delay J, Deniker P. Trente-huit cas de psychoses traites par la cure prolongee et continue de 4568 R. Ann Med Psychol 1952; 110:364.
2. Schonecker M. Ein eigentumliches syndrom im oralen bereich bei megaphen applikation. Nervenartz 1957; 28:35.
3. Sigwald J, Bouttier D, Raymondeaud Cl. Quatre cas de dyskinesie facio-bucco-lingui-masticatrice a evolution prolongee secondaire a un traitment par les neuroleptiques. Rev Neurol 1959; 100:751–755.
4. Uhrbrand L, Faurbye A. Reversible and irreversible dyskinesia after treatment with perphenazine, chlorpromazine, reserpine, and electroconvulsive therapy. Psychopharmacologia 1960; 1:408–418.
5. Faurbye A, Rasch PJ, Petersen PB, Brandborg G, Pakkenberg H. Neurological symptoms in pharmacotherapy of psychoses. Acta Psychiatr Scand 1964; 40:10–27.
6. Kruse W. Persistent muscular restlessness after phenothiazine treatment: report of 3 cases. Am J Psychiatry 1960; 117:152–153.
7. Druckman R, Seelinger D, Thulin B. Chronic involuntary movements induced by phenothiazines. J Nervous Mental Dis 1962; 135:69–76.
8. Hunter R, Earl JC, Thornicroff S. An apparently irreversible syndrome of abnormal movements following phenothiazine medication. Proc R Soc Med 1964; 57:758–762.
9. Jeste DV, Wyatt RJ. Understanding and Treating Tardive Dyskinesia, New York, Guilford Press, 1982, p 8.
10. Kazamatsuri H, Chien C, Cole JO. Treatment of tardive dyskinesia: I and II. Arch Gen Psychiatry 1972; 27:95–103.
11. Keegan DL, Rajput AH. Drug-induced dystonia tarda: treatment with L-dopa. Dis Nerv Syst 1973; 38:167–169.
12. Tarsy D, Granacher R, Bralower M. Tardive dyskinesia in young adults. Am J Psychiatry 1977; 134:1032–1034.
13. Casey DE, Rabins P. Tardive dyskinesia as a life-threatening illness. Am J Psychiatry 1978; 135:486–488.
14. Tarsy D. History and definition of tardive dyskinesia. Clin Neuropharmacol 1983; 6:91–99.
15. American Psychiatric Association Task Force on Late Neurological

Effects of Antipsychotic Drugs. Tardive dyskinesia. Am J Psychiatry 1980; 137:1163–1172.

16. Jeste DV, Lohr JB, Clark K, Wyatt RJ. Pharmacological treatments of tardive dyskinesia in the 1980s. J Clin Psychopharmacol 1988; 8(suppl):38–48.

17. Owens DG, Johnstone EC, Frith CD. Spontaneous involuntary disorders of movement. Arch Gen Psychiatry 1982; 39:452–461.

18. Waddington JL. Abnormal involuntary movements and psychosis in the preneuroleptic era and in unmedicated patients: implications for the concept of tardive dyskinesia. In: The Neurobiology of Dopamine Systems. Manchester, England, Manchester University Press, 1986, pp 51–66.

19. Waddington JL, Youssef HA, O'Boyle KM, et al: A reappraisal of abnormal, involuntary movements ("tardive dyskinesia") in schizophrenia and other disorders. In: Winlow W, Markstein R (eds), The Neurobiology of Dopamine Systems, Manchester, England, Manchester University Press, 1986, pp 266–286.

20. Kane JM. Tardive dyskinesia. In: Jeste DV, Wyatt RJ (eds), Neuropsychiatric Movement Disorders, Washington, DC, American Psychiatric Press, 1984, pp 68–95.

21. Crane GE. Tardive dyskinesia in patients treated with major neuroleptics: a review of the literature. Am J Psychiatry 1968; 124 (suppl):40–48.

22. Crane GE. High doses of trifluoperazine and tardive dyskinesia. Arch Neurol 1970; 22:176–180.

23. Jeste DV, Potkin SG, Sinha S, et al. Tardive dyskinesia: Reversible and persistent. Arch Gen Psychiatry 1979; 36:585–590.

24. Jeste DV, Wyatt RJ. Understanding and Treating Tardive Dyskinesia, New York, Guilford Press, 1982.

25. Kane JM, Smith JM. Tardive dyskinesia. Arch Gen Psychiatry 982; 39:473–481.

26. Chouinard G, Annable L, Ross-Chouinard A, Mercier P. A 5-year prospective longitudinal study of tardive dyskinesia: factors predicting appearance of new cases. J Clin Psychopharmacol 1988; 8(suppl)21–26.

27. Baldessarini RJ, Cole JO, Davis JM, et al. Tardive dyskinesia: a task force report. Washington, DC, American Psychiatric Association, 1980.

28. Casey DE, Hansen TE. Spontaneous dyskinesia. In: Jeste DV, Wyatt RJ (eds), Neuropsychiatric Movement Disorders, Washington, DC, American Psychiatric Press, 1984, pp 68–95.

29. Kane JM, Woerner M, Lieberman J. Tardive dyskinesia: Prevalence, incidence, and risk factors. In: Casey DE, Chase T, Christensen AV, Gerlach J (eds), Dyskinesia Research and Treatment (Psychopharmacology suppl 2), Berlin, Springer, 1985, pp 72–78.

30. Casey DE, Gerlach J. Tardive dyskinesia. Acta Psychiatr Scand 1988; 77:369–378.

31. Gardos G, Cole JO. Overview: public health issues in tardive dyskinesia. Am J Psychiatry 1980; 137:776–781.

32. Kane JM, Woerner M, Weinhold P. A prospective study of tardive dyskinesia development: preliminary results. J Clin Psychopharmacol 1982; 2:345–349.
33. Kane JM, Woerner M, Weinhold P. Incidence of tardive dyskinesia: five-year data from a prospective study. Psychopharmacol Bull 1984; 20:387–389.
34. Kane JM, Woerner M, Borenstein M, Wegner J, Lieberman J. Integrating incidence and prevalence jof tardive dyskinesia. Psychopharmacol Bull 1986; 22:254–258.
35. Barron ET, McCreadie RG. One year follow-up of tardive dyskinesia. Br J Psychiatry 1983; 143:423–424.
36. Yassa R, Nair V, Schwartz G. Tardive dyskinesia: a two-year follow-up study. Psychosomatics 1984; 25:852–855.
37. Kane JM, Woerner M, Lieberman J. Tardive dyskinesia: prevalence, incidence, and risk factors. J Clin Psychopharmacol 1988; 8(suppl)52–56.
38. Smith JM, Baldessarini RJ. Changes in prevalence, severity and recovery in tardive dyskinesia with age. Arch Gen Psychiatry 1982; 37:1368–1373.
39. Saltz BL, Kane JM, Woerner MG, Lieberman JA, Alvir JJ, Kahaner K, et al. Prospective study of tardive dyskinesia in the elderly. Psychopharmacol Bull 1989; 25:52–56.
40. Smith JM, Oswald WT, Kucharski LT, Waterman LJ. Tardive dyskinesia: age and sex differences in hospitalized schizophrenics. Psychopharmacology 1978; 58:207–211.
41. Gardos G, Casey D (eds). Tardive Dyskinesia and Affective Disorders, Washington, DC, American Psychiatric Press, 1983.
42. Crane GE. Persistent dyskinesia. Br J Psychiatry 1973; 122:395–405.
43. Degwitz R, Wenzel W. Persistent extrpyramidal side effects after long-term application of neurolpetics. In: Brill H (ed), Neuropsychopharmacology, Amsterdam, Excerpta Medica, 1967, pp 608–615.
44. Pandurangi AK, Ananth J, Channabasavanna SM. Dyskinesia in an Indian mental hospital. Indian J Psychiatry 1978; 20:339–342.
45. Klawans HL, Tanner CM, Goetz CG. Epidemiology and pathophysiology of tardive dyskinesias. In: Jankovic J, Tolosa E (eds), Advances in Neurology, Vol. 49: Facial Dyskinesias, New York, Raven Press, 1988, pp 185–197.
46. Marsden CD, Tarsy D, Baldessarini RJ. Spontaneous and drug-induced movement disorders in psychotic patients. In: Benson DF, Blumer D (eds), Psychiatric Aspects of Neurologic Disease, New York, Grune & Stratton, 1975, pp 219–265.
47. Klawans HL, Goetz CG, Perlik S. Tardive dyskinesia: review and update. Am J Psychiatry 1980; 137:900–908.
48. Tarsy D, Baldessarini RJ. The tardive dyskinesia syndrome. In: Klawans HL (ed), Clinical Neuropharmacology, Vol 1, New York, Raven Press, 1976, pp 29–61.
49. Kane JM, Wenger J, Stenzler S, Ramsey P. The prevalence of presumed tardive dyskinesia in psychiatric inpatients and outpatients. Psychopharmacology 1980; 69:247–251.

50. Gardos G, Cole JO, LaBrie RA. Drug variables in the etiology of tardive dyskinesia: application of discriminant function analysis. In: Fann WE, Smith RC, Davis JM, Domino EF (eds), Tardive Dyskinesia: Research and Treatment, New York, SP Medical and Scientific Books, 1980, pp 291–296.
51. Perris C, Dimitrijevic P, Jacobsson L, Paulson P, Rapp W, Froberg H. Tardive dyskinesia in psychiatric patients treated with neuroleptics. Br J Psychiatry 1979; 135:509–514.
52. Smith RC, Strizich M, Klass D. Drug history and tardive dyskinesia. Am J Psychiatry 1978; 135:1402–1403.
53. Gibson AC. Depot fluphenazine and tardive dyskinesia in an outpatient population. In: Fann WE, Smith RC, Davis JM, Domino EF (eds), Tardive Dyskinesia: Research and Treatment, New York, SP Medical and Scientific Books, 1980, pp 315–324.
54. Jus A, Pineau R, Lachance R, et al. Epidemiology of tardive dyskinesia. Dis Nerv Sys 1976; 37:210–213, 257–261.
55. Gardos G, Cole JO, LaBrie RA. Drug variables in the etiology of tardive dyskinesia: application of discriminant function analysis. Progr Neuropsychopharmacol 1977; 1:147–154.
56. Mallya A, Jose C, Baig M. Antiparkinsonics, neuroleptics and tardive dyskinesia. Biol Psychiatry 1979; 14:645–649.
57. Crane GE, Smeets RA. Tardive dyskinesia and drug therapy in geriatric patients. Arch Gen Psychiatry 1974; 30:341–343.
58. Kiloh LG, Smith JS, Williams SE. Antiparkinsonian drugs as causal agents in tardive dyskinesia. Med J Australia 1973; 2:591–593.
59. Klawans HL. The pharmacology of tardive dyskinesia. Am J Psychiatry 1973; 130:82–86.
60. Csernansky JG, Grabowski K, Cervantes J, Kaplan J, Yesavage JA. Fluphenazine decanoate and tardive dyskinesia: a possible association. Am J Psychiatry 1981; 138(10):1362–1365.
61. Chouinard G, Annable L, Ross-Chouinard A. Ethopropazine benztropine in neuroleptic-induced parkinsonism. J Clin Psychol 1979; 40:147.
62. Karson CN, Jeste DV, LeWitt PA, Wyatt RJ. A comparison of two iatrogenic dyskinesias. Am J Psychiatry 1983; 140:1504–1506.
63. Jeste DV, Wyatt, RJ. Understanding and Treating Tardive Dyskinesia, New York, Guilford Press, 1982, pp 72–170.
64. Schooler NR, Kane, JM. Research Diagnosis for tardive dyskinesia (letter). Arch Gen Psychiatry 1982; 39:486–487.
65. Lieberman JH, Pollack S, Lesser MS, Kane JM. Pharmacological characterization of tardive dyskinesias. J Clin Psychopharmacol 1988; 8:254–260.
66. Waddington JL. Tardive dyskinesia in schizophrenia and other disorders: association with aging, cognitive dysfunction, and structural brain pathology in relation to neuroleptic exposure. Hum Psychopharmacol 1987; 2:11–22.
67. Waddington JL, Youssef HA, Dolphin C, Kinsella A. Cognitive dysfunction, negative symptoms, and tardive dyskinesia in schizophrenia. Arch Gen Psychiatry 1987; 44:907–912.
68. Chouinard G, Jones BD. Neuroleptic-induced supersensitivity psy-

chosis: clinical and pharmacological characteristics. Am J Psychiatry 1980; 137:16–20.

69. Thaker GK, Nguyen JA, Tamminga CA. Increased saccadic distractability in tardive dyskinesia: functional evidence for subcortical GABA dysfunction. Biol Psychiatry 1988; 1:49–59.

70. Adler LE, Pecevich M, Nagamoto H. Bereitshaftspotential in tardive dyskinesia. Mov Disord 1989; 9:105–112.

71. Glazer WM, Boers MB, Charney DS, Henninger GR. The effect of neuroleptic discontinuation on psychopathology, involuntary movements and biochemical measures in patients with persistent tardive dyskinesia. Biol Psychiatry 1989; 26:224–233.

72. Weinberger DR. Brain disease and psychiatric illness: when should a psychiatrist order a CAT scan. Am J Psychiatry 1984; 141:1521–1527.

73. Tarsy D, Baldessarini RJ. Tardive dyskinesia. Annu Rev Med 1984; 605–623.

74. Bergen JA, Eyland EA, Campbell JA, Jenkings P, Kellehear J, Richards A, Beumont PJ. The course of tardive dyskinesia in patients on long-term neuroleptics. Br J Psychiatry 1989; 154:523–528.

75. Cutter NR, Post RM, Rey RC, et al. Depression-dependent dyskinesias in two cases of manic-depressive illness. N Engl J Med 1981; 304:1088–1089.

75a. Weiner WJ, Werner TR. Mania-induced remission of tardive dyskinesia in manic-depressive illness. Ann Neurol 1982; 12:229–230.

76. Yassa R. Functional impairment in tardive dyskinesia: medical and psychosocial dimensions. Acta Psychiat Scand 1989; 80:108–109.

77. Yagi G, Takamuja M, Kauba S, Kanijima K. Mortality rates of schizophrenic patients with tardive dyskinesia during 10 years: a controlled study. Keio J Med 1989; 38:70–72.

77a. Weiner WJ, Goetz CG, Nausieda PA, Klawans HL. Respiratory dyskinesias: extrapyramidal dysfunction and dyspnea. Ann Intern Med 1978; 88:327–333.

78. Graybiel AM. Neurotransmitters and neuromodulators in the basal ganglia. Trends Neurosci 1990; 13:244–254.

79. Alexander GE, DeLong MR, Strick PL. Parallel organization of functionally segregated circuits linking basal ganglia and cortex. Annu Rev Neurosci 1986; 9:357–381.

80. DeLong MR. Primate models of movement disorders of basal ganglia origin. Trends Neurosci 1990; 13:281–289.

81. Schell GR, Strick PL. The origin of thalamic inputs to the arcuate premotor and supplementary motor areas. J Neurosci 1984; 4:539–560.

82. Divac I, Fonnum F, Storm-Mathisen J. High affinity uptake of glutamate in terminals of corticostriatal axons. Nature 1977; 266:377–378.

83. Smith AD, Bolam JP. The neural network of the basal ganglia as revealed by the study of synaptic connections of identified neurons. Trends Neurosci 1990; 13:259–265.

84. Graybiel AM. Dopamine-containing innervation of the striatum: subsystems and striatal correspondents. In: Fahn S, et al. (ed), Recent Developments in Parkinson's Disease, New York, Raven Press, 1986.

85. Chevalier D, Denian JM. Disinhibition as a basic process in the expression of striatal functions. Trends Neurosci 1990; 13:277–280.

86. Alexander GE, Crutcher MD. Functional Architecture of basal ganglia circuits: neuralsubstrates of parallel processing. Trends Neurosci 1990; 13:266–271.
87. Servan-Schreiber D, Printz H, Cohen JD. A network model of catecholamine effects: gain, signal to noise ratio, and behavior. Science 1990; 249:892–895.
88. Smith RC, Tamminga CA Harasgti J, Pandey G, Davis J. Effects of dopamine agonists in tardive dyskinesia. Am J Psychiatry 1977; 134:763–768.
89. Gerlach J, Reisby N, Randrup A. Dopaminergic hypersensitivity and cholinergic hypofunction in the pathophysiology of TD. Psychopharmacologia 1974; 34:21.
90. Scatton B. Differential regional development of tolerance to increase in dopamine turnover upon repeated neuroleptic administration. Eur J Parmacol 1977; 46(4):363–369.
91. Gerbach J. Tardive dyskinesia; pathophysiologic mechanisms and clinical trials. Encephale 1988; 14:227–232.
92. Rosengarten H, Schweitzer JW, Friedhoff AJ. Selective dopamine D_2 receptor reduction enhances a D_1 mediated oral dyskinesia in rats. Life Sci 1986; 39:29–35.
93. Jenner P, Marsden CD. Adaptive changes in brain dopamine function as a result of neuroleptic treamtent. Adv Neurol 1988; 49:417–431.
94. Burt DR, Creese I, Snyder SH. Antischizophrenic drugs: chronic treatment elevates dopamine receptor binding in brain. Science 1977; 196:326–328.
95. Gunne LM, Haggstrom JE. Reduction of nigral glutamic acid decarboxylase in rats with neuroleptic-induced oral dyskinesia. Psychopharmacology 1983; 81:191–194.
96. Cross AJ, Crow TJ, Ferrier IN, et al. Dopamine receptor changes in schizophrenia in relation to the disease process and movement disorder. J Neurol Transm 1983; 18(suppl):265–272.
97. Waddington JL, Cross AJ, Gamble SJ, Bourne RL. Spontaneous orofacial dyskinesia and dopaminergic function in rats after 6 months of neuroleptic treatment. Science 1983; 220:530–532.
98. Casey DE, Denney D. Pharmacologic characterization of tardive dyskinesia. Psychopharmacology 1977; 54:1–8.
99. Lieberman JA, Pollack S, Lesser MS, Kane JM. Pharmacologic characterization of tardive dyskinesia. J Clin Psychopharmacol 1988; 8:254–260.
100. Carroll BJ, Curtis GC, Kokeman E. Paradoxical response to dopamine agonists in tardive dyskinesia. Am J Psychiatry 1977; 134:285–289.
101. Poldinger W. Therapy of extra-pyramidal side effects, with particular reference to persistent dyskinesia and lithium tremor. Int Pharmacopsychiatry 1978; 13:230–233.
102. Gardos G, Cole JV, Rapkin RM, LaBrie RA, et al. Anticholinergic challenge and neuroleptic withdrawal. Arch Gen Psychiatry 1984; 41:1030–1035.
103. Gale K. Chronic blockade of dopamine receptors by antischizophrenic drugs enhances GABA binding in substantia nigra. Nature 1980; 283:569–570.

104. Fibiger HC, Lloyd KG. Neurobiological substrates of tardive dyskinesia: the GABA hypothesis. Trends Neurosci 1989; 12:462–464.
105. Mao CC, Cheney DC, Marco E, Revuelta A, Costa E. Turnover times of gamma aminobutyric acid and acetylcholine in nucleus caudatus, nucleus accumbens, globus pallidus, and substantia nigra: effects of repeated administration of haloperidol. Brain Res 1977; 132:375–399.
106. Gunne LM, Haggstrom JE, Sjokvist B. Association with persistent neuroleptic-induced dyskinesia of regional changes in the brain GABA synthesis. Nature 1984; 309:347–349.
107. Itoh M. Effect of haloperidol on glutamate decarboxylase activity in discrete brain areas of the rat. Psychopharmacology 1983; 79:169–172.
108. Gunne LM, Bachus SE, Gale K. Oral movements induced by interference with nigral GABA neurotransmission: relationship to tardive dyskinesia. Exp Neurol 1988; 100:459–469.
109. Andersson U, Haggstrom JE. GABA agonists in cebus monkeys with neuroleptic-induced persistent dyskinesias. Psychopharmacology 1988; 94:298–301.
110. Mithani S, Atymadja A, Bainbridge KG, Fibiger HC. Neuroleptic-induced oral dyskinesias: effects of progabide and lack of correlation with regional changes in glutamic acid decarboxylase and choline acetyltransferase activities. Psychopharmacology 1987; 93:94–100.
111. Rupnick NMJ, Prestwick SA, Horton RW, Jenner P, Marsden CD. Alterations in cerebral glutamic acid decarboxylase and [^{3}H]-flunitrazepam binding during continuous treatment of rats for one year with haloperidol, sulpiride, or clozapine. J Neurol Transm 1987; 68:113–125.
112. Andersson U, Haggstrom JE, Levi ED, Bondessan U, Valverius M, Gunne LM. Reduced glutamate decarboxylase activity in the subthalamic nucleus in patients with tardive dyskinesia.   Mov Disord 1989; 4:37–46.
113. Thaker GK, Tamminga CA, Alphs LA, Lafferman J, Ferraro TN, Hare TA. Brain gamma-aminobutyric acid abnormality in tardive dyskinesia. Arch Gen Psychiatry 1987; 44:522–529.
114. Perry TL, Hansen SC, Jones K. Schizophrenia, tardive dyskinesia, and brain GABA. Biol Psychiatry 1987; 25:200–206.
115. Thaker GK, Nguyen JA, Tamminga CA. Increased saccadic distractability in tardive dyskinesia: functional evidence for subcortical GABA dysfunction. Biol Psychiatry 1988; 1:49–59.
116. Christensen E, Moller JE, Faurbye A. Neuropathological investigation of 28 brains from patients with dyskinesias. Acta Psychiatry Scand 1970; 46:14–23.
117. Jellinger K. Neuropathological findings after neuroleptic long-term therapy. In: Roizin L, Shnaki H, Grcevic N (eds), Neurotoxicology, New York, Raven Press, 1977, pp 25–42.
118. Colon RJ. Long-lasting changes in cerebral neurons induced by drugs. Biol Psychiatry 1975; 10:227.
119. Gerlach J. Long-term effects of perphenazine on the substantia nigra in rats. Psychopharmacologia 1975; 45:51.
120. Pakkenberg H, Fog R, Nikkantan B. The long-term effect of perphena-

zine enanthate on the rat brain: some metabolic and anatomic observations. Psychopharmacologia 1973; 29:329–336.

121. Pakkenberg H, Fog R. Short-term effect of perphenazine evantoate on the rat brain. Psychopharmacologia 1974; 40:165–169.

122. Fog R, Pakkenberg H, Jaul P, Bock E, Jorgensen O, Anderssen J. High-dose treatment of rats with perphenazine enanthate. Psychopharmacology 1976; 50:305–307.

123. Nielsen EB, Lyon M. Evidence for cell loss in corpus striatum after long-term treatment with a neuroleptic drug (fluphenthixol) in rats. Psychopharmacology 1978; 59:85–89.

124. Parsons PG. Modification of dopa toxicity in human tumor cells. Biochem Pharmacol 1985; 34:1801–1807.

125. Cadet, JL, Lohr JB. Free radicals and the developmental pathobiology of schizophrenic burnout. Integr Psychiatry 1987; 5:40–48.

126. Benes FM, Pakevich PA, Domesick VB. Haloperidol-induced plasticity of axon terminals in rat substantia nigra. Science 1983; 221:969–971.

127. Cohen BM, Zubenko CS. In-vivo effects of psychotropic agents on the physiochemical properties of cell membranes in the rat brain. Psychopharmacology 1985; 86:365–368.

128. Seeman P. Tardive dyskinesia, dopamine receptors, and neuroleptic damage to cell membranes. J Clin Psychopharmacol 1988; 4:35–85.

129. Waddington JL. Tardive dyskinesia in schizophrenia and other disorders: association with aging, cognitive dysfunction and structural brain pathology in relation to neuroleptic exposure. Hum Psychopharmacol 1987; 2:11–22.

130. Gunne LM, Growden J, Glaeser B. Oral dyskinesia in rats following brain lesions and neuroleptic drug administration. Psychopharmacology 1982; 77:134–139.

131. Bartzokis G, Hill MA, Altshuler L, Cummings JL, Wirshing W, May PR. Tardive dyskinesia in schizophrenic patients: correlates with negative symptoms. Psychiatry Res 1989; 28:145–151.

132. Waddington JL, Brown K, O'Neill J, McKean P, Kinsella A. Cognitive impairments, clinical course, and treatment history in out-patients with bipolar affective disorder. Psychol Med 1989; 9:897–902.

133. Hornykiewicz O. Neurohumoral interactions in the basal ganglia function and dysfunction. In: Yahr MD (ed), The Basal Ganglia, New York, Raven Press, 1976.

134. Jeste DV, Phelps B, Wagner RL, Wise CO, Wyatt RJ. Platelet monoamine oxidase and plasma dopamine beta hydroxylase in tardive dyskinesia. Lancet 1979; 2:850–851.

135. Arato M, Perenyi A, Fekete M, et al. Neuroendocrine investigations in tardive dyskinesia. Neuroendocrin Lett 1980; 6:315–320.

136. Kaufmann CA, Jeste DV, Shelton RC, Linnoila M, Kofka MS, Wyatt RJ. Noradrenergic and neuroradiological abnormalities in tardive dyskinesia. Biol Psychiatry 1986; 21:799–812.

137. Markianos M, Tripodianokis J, Garelis E. Neurochemical studies of tardive dyskinesia. II. Urinary methoxyhydroxyphenylglycol and plasma dopamine beta hydroxylase. Biol Psychiatry 1983; 18:347–354.

138. Jeste DV, Doonagi DR, Linnoila M. Elevated cerebrospinal fluid noradrenaline in tardive dyskinesia. Br J Psychiatry 1984; 144:172–180.

139. Glazer WM, Charney DS, Heninger GR. Noradrenergic function in schizophrenia. Arch Gen Psychiatry 1987; 44:898–904.
140. Gunne LM, Baranyi S. A primate model for tardive dyskinesia. In: Fann WE, Smith RC, Davis JM, Damino EF (eds), Tardive Dyskinesia: Research and Treatment, New York, S.P. Medical and Scientific Books. 1980, p 1.
141. Jeste DV, DeLisi LE, Zakman S, Wise CD, Phelps BH, Rosenblatt JE, Potkin SG, Bridge HS, Wyatt RJ. A biochemical study of tardive dyskinesia in young male patients. Psychiatry Res 1981; 4:327–331.
142. Chase TN, Schur JA, Gordon EK. Cerebrospinal fluid monoamine catabolites in drug-induced extrapyramidal disorders. Neuropharmacology 1970; 9:265–268.
143. Ladinsky H, Consolo S, Saminin R, Algeri S, Ponzio F. Long-term effects of haloperidol, clozapine, and methadone on rat striatal cholinergic and dopaminergic dynamics. In: Cattabeni F, Racagni G, Spano PF, Costa E (eds), Long-term Effects of Neuroleptics, New York, Raven Press, 1980, p 259.
144. Nagao T, Ohshimo T, Mitsunobu K, et al. Cerebrospinal fluid monoamine metabolites and cyclic nucleotides in chronic schizophrenic patients with tardive dyskinesia or drug-induced tremor. Biol Psychiatry 1979; 14:509–523.
145. Chiodo LA, Bunney BS. Typical and atypical neuroleptics: differential effects of chronic administration on the activity of A-9 and A-10 midbrain dopaminergic neurons. J Neurosci 1983; 3:1607–1619.
146. Dumbrille-Ross A, Seeman P. Dopamine receptor elevation by cholecystokinin. Peptides 1984; 5:1207–1212.
147. Worms P, Martinez J, Buet C, Castro B, Bigiere K. Evidence for dopamimetic effect of intrastriatally injected cholecystokinin octapeptide in mice. Eur J Pharmacol 1986; 121:395–401.
148. Zetter G. Antistereotypic effects of cholecystokinin octapeptide (CCK-8), ceruletide, and related peptides on apomorphine-induced gnawing in sensitized mice. Neuropharmacology 1985; 24:251–259.
149. Klawans HL, Tanner CM, Barr A. The reversibility of "permanent" tardive dyskinesia. Clin Neuropsychopharmacol 1984; 7:153–159.
150. Jus A, Jus K, Fontaine P. Long-term treatment of tardive dyskinesia. J Clin Psychiatry 1979; 40:72–77.
151. Wyatt RJ, Alexander RC, Egan ME, Kirsch DJ. Schizophrenia: just the facts. What do we know and how well do we know it. Schizo Res 1988; 1:3–18.
152. Newton JEO, Cannon DJ, Couch L, Fody EP, McMillan DE, Metzer MS, Paige SR, Reid GM, Summers BN. Effects of repeated drug holidays on serum haloperidol concentration, psychiatric symptoms, and movement disorders in schizophrenic patients. J Clin Psychiatry 1989; 50:132–135.
153. Gibson A. Depot injections and tardive dyskinesia. Br J Psychiatry 1978; 132:361–365.
154. Kleinman I, Schacter D, Kouter E. Informed consent and tardive dyskinesia. Am J Psychiatry 1989; 28:117–118.
155. Guy W (ed). ECDEU Assessment Manual for Psychopharmacology:

Publication ADM 76–358. Washington, DC, US Dept. of Health, Education, and Welfare, 1976, pp 534–537.

156. Jeste DV, Wyatt RJ. In search of treatment for tardive dyskinesia: review of the literature. Schizo Bull 1979; 5:253–293.

157. Glazer WM, Hafez HM, Benarroche LL. Molindone and haloperidol in tardive dyskinesia. J Clin Psychiatry 1985; 46:4–7.

158. Lieberman JA. Neuroleptic-induced movement disorders and experience with clozpine in tardive dyskinesia. J Clin Psychiatry 1990; 8:3–8.

159. Small JG, Milstein V, Marhenke JD, Hall DD, Kellams JJ. Treatment outcome with clozapine in tardive dyskinesia, neuroleptic sensitivity, and treatment resistant psychosis. J Clin Psychiatry 1987; 48:263–267.

160. Naber D, Leppig M, Grohmann R, Hippius H. Efficacy and adverse effects of clozapine in the treatment of schizophrenia and tardive dyskinesia. Psychopharmacologia 1989; 99:573–576.

161. Huang CC, Wang RH, Hasegawa A, Alverno L. Reserpine and alpha methyl dopa in the treatment of tardive dyskinesia. Psychopharmacology 1981; 73:359–362.

162. Lieberman JA, Alvin J, Mukherjee S, Kane JM. Treatment of tardive dyskinesia with bromocriptine. A test of the receptor modification strategy. Arch Gen Psychiatry 1989; 46:908–913.

163. Ludatscher JI. Stable remission of tardive dyskinesia by L-dopa. J Clin Psychopharmacol 1989; 9:39–41.

164. Kovacic B, LeWitt P, Clark D. Suppression of neuroleptic-induced persistent abnormal movements in *Cebus apella* monkeys by enantiomers of 3-PPP. J Neurol Transm 1988; 74:97–107.

165. Smith RC, Tamminga CA, Harasgti J, Pandy G, Davis J. Effects of dopamine agonists in tardive dyskinesia. Am J Psychiatry 1977; 134:763–768.

166. Schrodt GR, Wright JH, Simpson R, et al. Treatment of tardive dyskinesia with propranolol. J Clin Psychiatry 1982; 43:328–331.

167. Freedman R, Kirch D, Bell J, et al. Clonidine treatment of schizophrenia. Double-blind comparison to placebo and neuroleptic drugs. Acta Psychiatry Scand 1982; 65:35–45.

168. Nishikawa T, Tanaka M, Tsuda A, Koga I, Uchida Y. Clonidine therapy for tardive dyskinesia and related syndromes. Clin Neuropharmacol 1984; 7(3):239–245.

169. Browne J, Silver H, Martin R, Hart R, Mergener M, Williams P. The use of clonidine in the treatment of neuroleptic-induced tardive dyskinesia. J Clin Psychopharmacol 1986; 6:88–92.

170. Jeste DV, Lohr JB, Kaufman CA, Wyatt RJ. Pathophysiology of tardive dyskinesia: evaluation of supersensitivity theory and alternative hypotheses. In: Casey D, Gardos G (eds), Tardive Dyskinesia: From Dogma to Reason, Washington, DC, Am Psychiatric Press, 1986, pp 15–32.

171. Soni SD, Freeman HL, Hussein EM. Oxypertine in tardive dyskinesia: an 8-week controlled study. Br J Psychiatry 1984; 144:48–52.

172. Klawans HL. The pharmacology of tardive dyskinesia. Am J Psychiatry 1973; 130:82–86.

173. Friis T, Christensen TR, Gerlach J. Sodium valproate and biperiden in neuroleptic-induced akathesia, parkinsonism, and hyperkinesia. Acta Psychiatry Scand 1983; 67:178–187.
174. Jeste DV, Wyatt RJ. Therapeutic strategies against tardive dyskinesia. Arch Gen Psychiatry 1982; 39:803–816.
175. Klawans HL. Therapeutic approaches to neuroleptic-induced tardive dyskinesia. In: Yahr MD (ed), The Basal Ganglia, New York, Raven Press, 1976, pp 447–457.
176. Yassa R. Tardive dyskinesia and anticholinergic drugs: a critical review of the literature. Encephale 1988; 14:233–239.
177. Tamminga CA, Crayton J, Chase T. Improvement in tardive dyskinesia after muscimol therapy. Arch Gen Psychiatry 1979; 36:595–598.
178. Izumi K, Tamminaga H, Koja T, Nomoto M, Shimizu T, Sonoda H, Imamura K, et al. Meclofenoxate therapy in tardive dyskinesia. Biol Psychiatry 1986; 21:151–160.
179. Thaker GK, Nguyen JA, Strauss ME, Jacobson R, Kaup BA, Tamminga CA. Clonazepam treatment of tardive dyskinesia: a practical GABA-mimetic strategy. Am J Psychiatry 1990; 147:445–451.
180. Friis T, Christensen TR, Gerlach J. Sodium valproate in neuroleptic-induced akathisia, parkinsonsism, and hyperkinesia. Acta Psychiatry Scand 1983; 67:178–187.
181. Nasrallah HA, Smith RE, Bunner FJ, McKalley-Whittier M. Pharmacologic probes of neurotransmitter systems in tardive dyskinesia: implications for clinical management. J Clin Psychiatry 1986; 47:56–59.
182. Singh MM, Becker RE, Pitman RK, Nasrallah HA, Kal H. Sustained improvement in tardive dyskinesia with diazepam: indirect evidence for corticolimbic involvement. Brain Res Bull 1983; 11:179–185.
183. Klawans HL, Weiner WJ, Nausieda PA. The effects of lithium on an animal model of tardive dyskinesia. Prog Neuropsychopharmacol 1977; 1:53–60.
184. Sedman G. Clonazepam in the treatment of tardive oral dyskinesia. Br Med J 1976; 2:583.
185. O'Flannagan PM. Clonazepam in the treatment of drug-induced dyskinesia. Br Med J 1975; 1:269–270.
186. Glazer WM, Moore DC, Bowers MB, Bunney BS, Roffman M. The treatment of tardive dyskinesia with baclofen. Psychopharmacology 1985; 87:480–483.
187. Stewart RM, Robbin J, Beckham B. Baclofen in tardive dyskinesia patients maintained on neuroleptics. Clin Neuropharmacol 1982; 5:365–373.
188. Bowery NG, Hill DR, Hudson AL, et al. (-)Baclofen decreases transmitter release in the mammalian CNS by an action at a novel GABA receptor. Nature 1983; 283:92–94.
189. Thaker GK, Tamminga CA, Alphs LD, Lafferrman J, Ferraro TN, Hare TA. Brain gamma-aminobutyric acid abnormality in tardive dyskinesia. Arch Gen Psychiatry 1987; 44:522–529.
190. Stahl SW, Thornton JE, Simpson ML, Berger PA, Napolielle MS. Gamma-vinyl-GABA treatment of tardive dyskinesia and other movement disorders. Biol Psychiatry 1985; 20:888–893.

191. Lohr JB, Cadet JL, Lohr MA, Jeste DV, Wyatt RJ. Alpha-tocopherol in tardive dyskinesia. Lancet 1987; 1:913–914.
192. Elkashef AM, Ruskin PE, Bacher N, Barrett D. Vitamin E in the treatment of tardive dyskinesia. Am J Psychiatry 1990; 147:505–506.
193. Reiter S, Adler L, Angrist B, Perelow E, Rotrosen J. Effects of verapamil on tardive dyskinesia and psychosis in schizophrenic patients. J Clin Psychiatry 1989; 50:26–27.
194. Adler L, Duncan E, Reiter S, Angrist B, Perelow E, Rotrosen J. Effects of calcium-channel antagonists on tardive dyskinesia and psychosis. Psychopharmacol Bull 1988; 24:421–425.
195. Klawans HL, Weiner WJ, Nausieda PA. The effects of lithium on an animal model of tardive dyskinesia. Prog Neuropsychopharmacol 1977; 1:53–60.
196. Nishikawa T, Tanaka M, Tsuda A, Koga I, Uchida Y. Treatment of tardive dyskinesia with ceruletide. Prog Neuropsychopharmacol Biol Psychiatry 1988; 12(5):803–812.
197. Benecke R, Conrad B, Klingehhofer J. Successful treatment of tardive and spontaneous dyskinesias with corticosteroids. Eur Neurol 1988; 28:146–149.
198. Neppe VM. High dose buspirone in case of tardive dyskinesia (letter). Lancet 1989; 2:1458.
199. Strauss A. Oral dyskinesia associated with buspirone use in an elderly woman. J Clin Psychiatry 1988; 49:322–323.
200. Baldessarini RJ, Marsh E. Fluoxetine and side effects (letter). Am J Psychiatry 1990; 147:191–192.
201. Bouchard RH, Pourcher E, Vincent P. Fluoxetine and extrapyramidal side effects (letter). Am J Psychiatry 1989; 146:1352–1353.
202. Gosek E, Weller RA. Improvement of tardive dyskinesia associated with electroconvulsive therapy. J Nerv Ment Dis 1988; 176:120–122.

6

Neuroleptic-Induced Tardive Dyskinesia Variants

Robert E. Burke, M.D.

Introduction

Since the earliest reports of tardive dyskinesia (TD), a variety of involuntary movements, in addition to the now well-known oral-buccal-lingual masticatory movements, have been described, including dystonia, akathisia, and myoclonus. However, it is only within the past 10 years or so that there has been widespread recognition that these variant forms of tardive dyskinesia exist. It is difficult to know why historically these forms have taken longer to gain wide recognition. One probable reason is that while definitive prevalence studies have yet to be done, it appears that these forms are less common than oral-buccal-lingual dyskinesia. In addition, some of the clinical features of two major variant forms, tardive dystonia and tardive akathisia, are quite variable, sometimes subtle, and not widely known among neurologists and psychiatrists. In spite of the delayed recognition of these variants, there now seems to be a consensus that they do exist as distinct forms of tardive dyskinesia. Although they may coexist with oral dyskinesia, they also occur in isolation. In addition, although they have a clinical pharmacology

Lang AE, Weiner WJ (editors): *Drug-Induced Movement Disorders,* Mount Kisco, NY, © Futura Publishing Co., Inc., 1992.

167

similar to that of oral dyskinesia, in that they are suppressed by antidopaminergic drugs, there is some evidence that they have their own unique pharmacology as well. With further study, they may prove to have their own unique pathophysiology. Most importantly, these variants deserve distinct recognition by the practicing neurologist or psychiatrist because, unlike oral dyskinesia, they are usually quite disabling, particularly tardive dystonia and akathisia. Therefore, the main emphasis here will be on the clinical recognition, differential diagnosis, and treatment of these disorders.

The term *tardive dyskinesia* is used differently by different authors. In this chapter, the term is used to encompass all forms of persistent dyskinesia due to neuroleptics, and it therefore includes not only classic oral dyskinesia, but also the variant forms described here. The reader should be aware that often in the literature, especially earlier literature, the term is used to refer strictly to the oral-lingual form of dyskinesia. Although the term *tardive* was originally intended to emphasize the late appearance of these disorders during neuroleptic treatment, it has become clear with more recent analysis that these disorders may appear early in the course of therapy, and there is no fundamental distinction between cases appearing early and those appearing late. The current definition emphasizes what is a more important characteristic shared by these disorders, their *persistence*. It is this characteristic that distinguishes these tardive dyskinesias from the other neuroleptic-induced movement disorders, including acute dystonia, acute akathisia, and parkinsonism, which typically remit following cessation of neuroleptics.

Tardive Dystonia

The Nature of Dystonic Movements

Dystonic movements are strikingly different from the classically described oral-lingual masticatory movements of oral tardive dyskinesia, and it is this clear distinction in clinical phenomenology which led investigators at Columbia, and our colleagues in London (Drs. Marsden and Lang) and Houston (Dr. Jankovic), to identify persistent dystonia as a subtype of tardive dyskinesia,[1] although many earlier reports had noted this occurrence.[2-12] Formally defined, dystonia is "a syndrome of sustained muscle contractions, frequently causing twisting and repetitive movements, or abnormal postures."[13] Dystonic movements take on a variable appearance according to the body region involved. For example, dystonia affecting the muscles about the eyes (blepharospasm) appears as frequent blinking in mild form, and sustained spasms of eye closure in more severe form. Dystonia of lower facial muscles appears as facial grimacing, sustained jaw closure, or jaw opening. Sustained, forceful protrusion of tongue may also occur. Neck involvement may appear as twisting about the long axis of neck (torticollis), backward pulling (retrocollis), or forward pulling (anterocollis). Further examples of dystonic movements affecting other body regions in tardive dystonia will be discussed below in relation to its specific clinical features.

Two general features of dystonic movements deserve mention. First, many dystonic movements are action-specific, meaning that they occur with some actions but not with others. For example, some individuals with dystonia affecting the hand will develop their involuntary movements only during the act of writing ("writer's cramp"). We have observed an individual who had pronounced tardive dystonia of the arms and trunk with walking, but who showed minimal dystonia during dancing. Second, many patients with dystonia note that their movements can be partially controlled by small tactile maneuvers, such as touching the chin to control torticollis, or the brow to control blepharospasm. These "sensory tricks" are quite characteristic. Both the action-specific nature and partial control by sensory tricks often mislead neurologists and psychiatrists to an erroneous diagnosis of hysteria or malingering in patients with true dystonia.

The Evidence that Chronic Dystonia is Associated with Neuroleptic Drug Use

For the oral-buccal-lingual form of tardive dyskinesia, a number of retrospective epidemiologic studies have convincingly demonstrated an association between the use of neuroleptics and the involuntary movements.[14] These data are important to establish a causal relationship between drug use and the oral movements, because oral, masticatory movements apparently can occur in elderly patients spontaneously. Dystonic movements may also occur spontaneously, and therefore it is important to consider the evidence to support an association between neuroleptic drug use and persistent dystonia.

Unfortunately, formal epidemiologic studies have not been done. In their stead, there is a widespread impression among neurologists who treat patients with movement disorders that there is a frequent history of ongoing neuroleptic use among patients who present with dystonic movements in the absence of any other identifiable cause. Little is known of the epidemiology of the dystonias themselves, but these are not common disorders, and the frequent association between them and neuroleptic use is suggestive. Table 1 lists a number of reports of dystonia occurring during neuroleptic drug use. There have been 218 patients described among 41 reports. This list is undoubtedly not complete, because some authors do not use the term *dystonia* to characterize the involuntary movements; for example, the term *Pisa syndrome* appears to refer to a truncal dystonia that causes leaning. Furthermore, movement disorder neurologists now consider the association between neuroleptic use and persistent dystonia to be so commonplace that these cases are no longer reported, unless there is some aspect of interest.

In addition to the frequently reported association between neuroleptic use and dystonia, a number of other observations suggest a causal relationship. First, there are close temporal relationships between the use of neuroleptics and the occurrence of dystonia in a given individual. We have reported a 12% remission rate of dystonia following withdrawal of neuroleptics.[24] The majority of these individuals had nonfocal dystonias. It is distinctly unusual for idiopathic, nonfocal dystonias to spontaneously remit. Furthermore, in a few individuals who have undergone remission following withdrawal of neuroleptics, they have then again developed persistent dystonia when re-exposed to the drugs. Second, when dystonia occurs during treatment with neuroleptics, it occurs with oral-lingual dyskinesia in 55% cases or with tardive akathisia in 31% of cases. Strong evidence indicates that both oral-lingual dyskinesia and tardive akathisia (as discussed below) are due to neuroleptic drugs, and their co-occurrence with dystonia strongly suggests that it is also due to the drugs. Idiopathic dystonia and dystonia due to other identifiable causes do not cause the simultaneous occurrence of oral dyskinesias or akathisia. Third, it is clear that neuroleptics cause acute dystonia, and in a few instances, these occurrences have continued as a persistent dystonia.[1] Fourth, the clinical pharmacology of persistent dystonia which develops during neuroleptic drug treatment is distinctive; it fairly consistently can be suppressed by dopamine receptor-blocking drugs.[24] In this respect, it is like other forms of tardive dyskine-

Table 1

Reported Cases of Persistent Dystonia Associated with Dopamine Antagonist Treatment

Authors (Ref.)	Year	Patients (No.)	Age of Onset
Druckman et al.[2]	1962	1	46
Chateau et al.[3]	1966	1	27
Dabbous & Bergman[4]	1966	1	5
Harenko[5]	1967	6	74–89
Angle & McIntire[6]	1968	1	10
Crane[7]	1973	1	34
Keegan & Rajput[8]	1973	1	40
Shields & Bray[9]	1976	1	5
Tarsy et al.[10]	1977	2	25, 25
McLean & Casey[11]	1978	1	12
Weiner et al.[12]	1981	2	17, 59
Burke et al.[1]	1982	42	13–60
Bartels et al.[15]	1982	1	36
Weiner & Werner[16]	1982	1	38
Glazer et al.[17]	1983	1	37
Kwentus et al.[18]	1984	1	52
Nishikawa et al.[19]	1984	3	?
Gimenez-Roldan et al.[20]	1985	9	17–61
Lazarus & Toglia[21]	1985	1	45
Luchins & Goldman[22]	1985	1	26
Wolf & Koller[23]	1985	3	?
Kang et al.[24]	1986	51*	13–72
Saxena[25]	1986	1	37
Yassa et al.[26]	1986	7	21–76
Rosse et al.[27]	1986	1	70
Gardos et al.[28]	1987	2	24, 32
Samie et al.[29]	1987	1	66
Corbin et al.[30]	1987	1	21
Friedman et al.[31]	1987	5	?
Girion[32]	1987	1	30
Lal et al.[33]	1988	1	42
Falk et al.[34]	1988	1	?
Anath et al.[35]	1988	2	39, 29
Chin et al.[36]	1989	3	23–24
Cooper et al.[37]	1989	1	25
Gureje[38]	1989	2	26, 32
Miller & Jankovic[39]	1990	1	37
Lang[40]	1990	20	22–50
Adityanjee et al.[41]	1990	1	37
Miller & Jankovic[42]	1990	30	13–89
Yadalan et al.[43]	1990	5	x27, M x34, F

* In the series of 67 patients, 16 had been reported earlier.

sia (both oral-lingual dyskinesia and tardive akathisia) and is unlike other forms of dystonia.[44] These considerations have led many movement disorder neurologists to conclude that neuroleptics are capable of causing persistent dystonia.

Diagnostic Criteria

Our current criteria for a diagnosis of tardive dystonia include the following: (1) The patient must have dystonia, as defined above. (2) The dystonia must develop either during or within 3 months of a course of neuroleptic treatment. We chose this 3-month cutoff somewhat arbitrarily, in recognition of the fact that neuroleptics themselves may suppress tardive dyskinesia and often movements do not become apparent until some time after drugs have been stopped. On the other hand, in the absence of direct evidence, it seems difficult to claim that a movement disorder due to neuroleptics could first appear more than 3 months after their use. (3) Wilson's disease must be excluded by a serum ceruloplasmin level and a slit-lamp examination for Kayser-Fleischer rings. In addition, there must be no other neurological signs to suggest one of the many known causes of secondary dystonia.[45] (4) There must be a negative family history for dystonia. In the presence of a positive family history, it would not be possible to know whether the affected individual had neuroleptic-induced dystonia or had simply expressed an inherited form coincident with neuroleptic use.

In the diagnosis of tardive dystonia by the above criteria, the presence of dystonia is sufficient. We do not require that dystonia be the dominant movement disorder. We do not force a single unitary diagnosis on a patient; thus, a given patient may have not only tardive dystonia, but also classic oral-lingual dyskinesia or tardive akathisia. If all are present, all are diagnosed; we do not apply a single diagnosis depending on which is predominant. Among patients with tardive movement disorders, there frequently is a mixture of abnormal movements, and to attempt to choose one as "predominant" is subjective and arbitrary.

Epidemiology

There are few rigorous epidemiologic data available about tardive dystonia; it has not been the subject of prospective or case-controlled studies. It is undoubtedly less common than oral-buccal-lingual tardive dyskinesia. In a survey of 555 psychiatric in- and out-patients, Yassa and colleagues found a prevalence of 34% for oral tardive dyskinesia, and only 1.4% for tardive dystonia.[46] Similarly, Friedman and co-workers found a prevalence of only 1.5% among 352 psychiatric inpatients.[31] Estimates of the prevalence of oral dyskinesia among psychiatric patients have varied, but often are about 20%.[14]

One recent study indicated a prevalence of 21% for tardive dystonia among chronically institutionalized veterans.[47] However, the majority of these cases were mildly affected; only 20% were symptomatic. Nevertheless, this study indicates that the prevalence of tardive dystonia depends on the diagnostic criteria used, and more data are needed.

Although patient characteristics for oral dyskinesia and tardive dystonia have rarely been compared within the same patient population, it appears that tardive dystonia usually has an earlier mean age of onset. In Yassa's study,[46] 11 patients with severe oral dyskinesia had a mean age of onset of 64 years whereas 8 patients with tardive dystonia had a mean age of onset of 40.5 years. Other investigators have likewise noted an early mean age of onset, ranging from 34 to 39 years.[1,20,24] In a single patient population referred for neurological evaluation, Miller and Jankovic reported a mean onset of 45 years among 30 tardive dystonics, and 59 years among 79 patients with predominantly oral dyskinesia.[42] In that series, the majority of patients with oral dyskinesia had onset in the sixth to eighth decades, whereas patients with tardive dystonia had a uniform distribution of age of onset. Similarly, Kang et al.[24] found in a series of neurological referrals that age of onset of tardive dystonia was uniformly distributed across a range spanning from 13 to 72 years.

Data on the male:female ratio of tardive dystonia are conflicting. In our original report, we noted a slight male preponderance at 1.6:1.[1] Subsequently, however, three retrospective reviews of neurological referrals failed to note a significant male predominance.[20,24,42] However, neurological referrals are a select group and may not be representative. In the only studies of unselected, psychiatric populations, a male predominance was found: 4:1 in Friedman's study[31] and 3:1 in Yassa's.[46] The numbers of patients in these studies were small. This issue needs more study in large, unselected populations exposed to neuroleptics.

Virtually all of the dopamine (DA) receptor antagonists that have been reported to cause oral tardive dyskinesia have also been reported to cause tardive dystonia. These include the aliphatic, piperazine, and piperidine classes of phenothiazines; butyrophenones (e.g., haloperidol); thioxanthenes (chlorprothixene, thiothixene); dibenzazepines (loxapine); diphenylbutylpiperidines (pimozide); and an indolone (molindone).[1,24,42] Amoxapine, an antidepressant with DA receptor-blocking properties, has been implicated in cases of tardive dystonia. Several antiemetics with DA receptor-blocking properties have also been associated with tardive dystonia, including prochlorperazine,[24] promethazine,[1] and metoclopramide.[42] There have been no studies to indicate that any particular class of antipsychotics is more (or less) likely to induce tardive dystonia. However, to the author's knowledge, there have been no reports to date of tardive dystonia in association with the atypical antipsychotic clozapine.

As there have been no prospective studies, there has been no careful assessment of any possible relationship between duration or dose of antipsychotics and the likelihood of occurrence of tardive dystonia. Retrospective studies have shown, however, that although tardive dystonia usually occurs, on the average, following years of neuroleptic exposure, it can occur within a few days or weeks.[1,24] In fact, in our most recent series, 20% of patients developed dystonia within the first year of exposure (Fig. 1).[24] The same was true of 43 patients reported in the literature at that time (Fig. 1). Thus, there does not appear to be a minimum "safe" period of exposure to neuroleptics during which time tardive dystonia will not occur.

The occurrence of acute dystonia does not appear to be a significant risk factor for the occurrence of tardive dystonia. In our most recent series of 67 patients, only four (6%) had a history of an acute dystonic reaction, which is not much different from the incidence in the general population exposed to neuroleptics.

In our original description of 42 cases of tardive dystonia, we noted that 7 of 18 patients with onset prior to 30 years had a history of an abnormal birth or development.[1] Subsequently, in a retrospective analysis of neurological referrals, Gimenez-Roldan and co-workers noted mental retardation in 3 of 9 tardive dystonia patients.[20] However, it is difficult to know the significance of these observations made in selected patient groups, referred for neurological evaluation, and in the absence of controls. In the absence of prospective or case-controlled observations, it is uncertain whether pre-existing brain damage constitutes a risk factor for tardive dystonia.

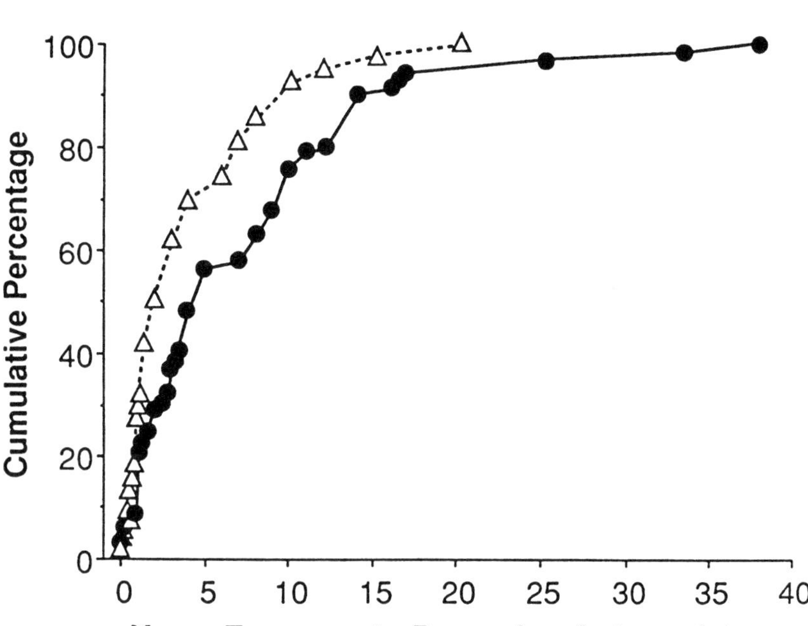

Figure 1: Duration of exposure to dopamine antagonists among patients with tardive dystonia (from reference 24). The cumulative percentage of patients with tardive dystonia is shown in relation to years of exposure to dopamine antagonists, for both the 67 patients in reference 24 (black circles) and 43 patients in the literature as of 1986 (open triangles) (see reference 24 for citations). Instances of tardive dystonia occurred soon after exposure, seen as a rapidly rising cumulative percentage curve arising from the origin. Thus, there was no "safe" minimum exposure less than which this condition was unlikely to occur. (Reproduced with permission.[24])

It is also unknown in the absence of adequate epidemiologic data whether any particular psychiatric diagnosis constitutes a risk factor for the development of tardive dystonia. It is clear from retrospective analysis, however, that the full range of psychiatric, and many nonpsychiatric, diagnoses are represented among these patients. In our series of 67 patients, 12 (18%) had been treated with neuroleptics for questionable, or at best secondary, indications as outlined by the American Psychiatric Association:[14] eight for nervousness or anxiety, three for aggressive behavior, and one for multiple somatic complaints.[24] Three additional patients developed tardive dystonia following treatment with antiemetics.

Clinical Features

Onset

Tardive dystonia uniformly affects various age groups. We reported ages of onset ranging from 13 to 72 years, with a mean of 39 years.[24] Although it is unclear whether males are more likely to develop tardive dystonia, they do appear to develop it at an earlier age. In our series, men had an average age of onset of 34 years; women had an average onset of 44 years—a significant difference. Whether this difference represents a difference in susceptibility to tardive dystonia or a difference in prescription patterns of neuroleptics for men and women is unclear.

In most patients, tardive dystonia begins in the face or neck. In our series, 67% of patients did so. Less commonly, the dystonia may begin in one of the arms (11% in our series). In the author's experience, tardive dystonia never begins as a focal foot dystonia. In this respect, it differs from the primary torsion dystonias which commonly, in children, begin in a foot.

Clinical Course

Since tardive dystonia has never been the subject of a prospective analysis, it is difficult to describe how it typically evolves, either in patients maintained on neuroleptics or in those taken off them. We do know, based on retrospective analysis, that it usually begins in one location and then spreads to other body regions. It is also our impression that following an initial period of progression, tardive dystonia stabilizes whether or not the patient is maintained on neuroleptics, and neither spreads further nor worsens in severity.

Among our 67 patients, only 15% remained focal. Most (72%) developed dystonia in multiple regions; an additional 13% developed generalized dystonia. All of those with strictly focal dystonia had involvement of the cranial musculature, either the neck, upper face (blepharospasm), or lower face. There was a tendency for patients with generalized dystonia to be younger (mean age 31 years at onset) than those with focal dystonia (mean age of 44 years). Interestingly, a similar observation has been made for the primary dystonias. A longer duration of exposure to neuroleptics did not correlate with more severe dystonia. On the contrary, patients who developed generalized dystonia had been treated for shorter periods by the time of dystonia onset (4.9 years) than patients with focal dystonia (13.6 years).

At the time of maximum severity of their illness, 83% of our patients had involvement of cranial regions. The neck was involved in 80% of cases. Retrocollis was characteristic, occurring in 50% of those with neck involvement. The trunk was affected in 35% of patients. Most of them had back-arching movements. The arms were affected in 42% of patients, often in the form of sustained extension at the elbow, especially when walking. The legs were affected in a minority.

In keeping with the infrequent involvement of the legs, and the rare occurrence of generalized dystonia, tardive dystonia rarely leads to a bedridden state. In our original series of 42 patients, only one was bedridden.[1] Among reports in the literature, only a few patients are described[20,43] with this severe degree of disability. In spite of the rarity of this degree of disability, it does occur, and in some instances can become life-threatening. Lazarus and Toglia described a young woman with tardive dystonia who, 3 months after withdrawal of neuroleptics, developed severe dystonic movements that resulted in elevation of serum muscle enzymes, myoglobinuria, renal failure, and death.[21] We have also observed patients with long-standing tardive dystonia who suddenly develop a severe dystonic state with elevation of serum muscle enzymes, either following abrupt neuroleptic withdrawal or in the setting of systemic infection. It can be difficult to differentiate such severe exacerbations of tardive dystonia from neuroleptic malignant syndrome (NMS). A key point of distinction is that a tardive dystonia patient will have a history of chronic dystonic movements, whereas a patient with NMS will develop severe dystonia (and/or rigidity) acutely.

In general, the dystonic movements observed in tardive dystonia are identical to those seen in primary torsion dystonia. Like the primary dystonias, tardive dystonias can sometimes be relieved briefly by "sensory tricks," such as a touch to the chin to relieve torticollis, a touch above the brow to relieve blepharospasm, or a hand lightly resting on the hip to straighten severe axial torsion. In addition, the tardive dystonias, like the primary dystonias, can be remarkably action-specific. For example, a patient with truncal dystonia may have difficulty walking and yet be able to run or dance reasonably well. These aspects of dystonia frequently lead to a misdiagnosis of hysteria, especially in a population of patients with a prior psychiatric diagnosis.

The clinical diagnosis of tardive dystonia is often aided by the co-existence of other tardive involuntary movements. Classic oral-buccal-lingual tardive dyskinesia occurred sometime during the course of 55% of our patients with tardive dystonia. Tardive akathisia, characterized by subjective and motor restlessness, was present in 31% of patients.[24] The presence of these additional involuntary movements would exclude primary dystonia as the sole diagnosis.

On rare occasions, tardive dystonia may cause "oculogyric crisis," a deviation of the eyes, usually upward.[48] These ocular deviations are more commonly observed in acute dystonic reactions. They never occur in the primary dystonias.

We have analyzed the clinical course of patients with tardive dystonia following discontinuation of neuroleptics. In our 67 patients, neuroleptics were discontinued in 42. Among these patients, five (12%) underwent remission, defined as prolonged cessation of dystonic movements in the absence of ongoing therapy. The cohort of 42 patients was followed for a mean of 2.8 years (and up to 6.7 years) following neuroleptic withdrawal. In comparing the few who underwent remission to the majority who did not, the former had an earlier age of onset (mean of 28 versus 39 years), a shorter total duration of exposure to neuroleptics (3.1 versus 7.7 years), and earlier withdrawal of neuroleptics after dystonia onset. However, in view of the small number of patients who achieved remission, these differences can only be considered tentative, pending further study. Among these patients, remission occurred 1 to 5 years after neuroleptic withdrawal.

Differential Diagnosis and Diagnostic Evaluation

In movement disorders, diagnosis is performed in two steps: first the type of involuntary movement is identified; then, for that particular type of movement, various possible etiologies are considered. In the diagnosis of tardive dystonia, it is usually possible to readily distinguish the sustained, twisting movements of dystonia from other dyskinesias. Choreic movements are quick, brief, and random in their timing and location. Myoclonic movements are brief and shock-like. Tremors are regular, oscillatory movements. Some motor tics can resemble dystonic movements, being sustained or twisting.

Tics can usually be identified on the basis of their timing. They occur intermittently, sometimes in flurries. Tics are characteristically preceded by a subjective urge to perform the movement and are followed by a sense of relief. Tics can often be entirely suppressed by the patient for prolonged periods, whereas dystonia usually cannot. Finally, patients with tics often have variety of them, and it is frequently possible to identify a sustained tic (also called a "dystonic tic") by the company it keeps.

One difficulty that many neurologists have in diagnosing dystonia is that they think of it as consisting *exclusively* of slow, sustained movements. While dystonia is always sustained, there can be superimposed rapid, jerking, or even oscillatory movements. These rapid movements are especially likely to be seen when the patient attempts to move against the direction of the sustained, dystonic pull; for example, when some patients attempt to turn their head away from the direction of their torticollis, they develop a rapid, oscillatory movement resembling a tremor. Such rapid movements affecting lower facial muscles can lead to difficulty in distinguishing dystonic facial involvement from the repetitive, chewing movements of oral tardive dyskinesia. Usually dystonia can be identified as a sustained contraction in association with the rapid movements; there may be sustained facial grimacing or sustained jaw closure. The distinction between tardive dystonia and oral-buccal lingual TD affecting the face is of more than academic interest; identification of the type of movement has implications for therapy.

Once a diagnosis of dystonia is made, consideration must be given to the possible causes. In a patient on neuroleptics, an acute dystonic reaction must be considered. Acute dystonia almost always occurs within the first 5 days of beginning neuroleptics; the only exception is if a substantial increase in dose is made during the course of therapy. Acute dystonia is much more likely to be accompanied by oculogyric crisis. Finally, acute dystonia universally responds to administration of diphenhydramine or benztropine (Cogentin). As mentioned earlier, NMS may present with prominent dystonia. Generally, the associated alteration in mental status, fever, and serum biochemical evidence of muscle injury make that diagnosis clear. Only rarely in our experience does tardive dystonia become so severe as to cause fever and muscle injury, and in these instances it is typically preceded by a history of chronic dystonia, unlike NMS, which is acute and fulminant in its onset.

After acute causes of dystonia are excluded, we always proceed next to evaluate for Wilson's disease by obtaining a serum ceruloplasmin and a slit-lamp examination by an ophthalmologist. Wilson's disease can present with dystonia (or other movement abnormalities) and any of a number of psychiatric disorders that may encourage the initial inappropriate use of neuroleptic drugs. As it is

Table 2

Some Causes of Dystonia*

I. The Primary Dystonias
  A. Familial
    1. Non-Jewish (autosomal dominant)
    2. Jewish (Ashkenazic) (autosomal dominant)
    3. L-dopa responsive (may also be sporadic)
    4. X-linked recessive
  B. Sporadic
II. The Secondary Dystonias
  A. Causes of acquired dystonia
    1. Perinatal injury (asphyxia or kernicterus): early onset or delayed onset
    2. Encephalitis
    3. Head injury (concussive or nonconcussive): early or delayed onset
    4. Stroke
    5. Tumor
    6. Drugs
  B. Metabolic or inherited causes
    1. Huntington's disease
    2. Wilson's disease
    3. Hallervorden-Spatz syndrome
    4. Freidreich's ataxia
    5. Olivopontocerebellar atrophy
    6. Ceroid lipofuscinosis
    7. Juvenile dystonic lipidosis
    8. GM_1 and GM_2 gangliosidoses
    9. Ataxia telangiectasia
    10. Lesch-Nyhan syndrome
    11. Leigh's syndrome
    12. Metachromatic leukodystrophy
    13. Glutaric acidemia
  C. Degenerative disease
    1. Parkinson's disease
    2. Progressive supranuclear palsy

* This is a partial list. See Calne and Lang[45] and Table 7, Chapter 1, in this volume for more complete lists.

treatable, it must always be carefully sought. Beyond this evaluation for Wilson's disease, further evaluation depends on the presence or absence of other neurological signs besides dystonia. If there are no other signs and no evidence for Wilson's disease, we do no further studies and make a diagnosis of tardive dystonia. If there are other neurological signs, the differential diagnosis is lengthy (see Table 2). Diagnostic studies to differentiate among these numerous causes may need to be extensive and will not be detailed here. If there are other neurological signs besides dystonia that are *progressive*, then tardive dystonia cannot be the sole diagnosis, as neuroleptics do not induce progressive changes in intellect, sensory function, pyramidal motor systems, cerebellar function, and so on. If, however, there are other neurological signs that are entirely static (e.g., mental retardation) then once appropriate studies have been performed to rule out metabolic and degenerative conditions listed in Table 2, it is possible to diagnose tardive dystonia associated with a static encephalopathy. In any patient, a diagnosis of tardive dystonia is supported by the presence of other tardive movements such as oral-buccal-lingual tardive dyskinesia, or tardive akathisia.

Treatment

When a diagnosis of any form of tardive dyskinesia is made, the first therapeutic step should be to taper and discontinue the causative drugs if possible. Many times, severe psychiatric illness will make it impossible to do so. Nevertheless, it is imperative to carefully reconsider the indications for DA antagonists in a given patient and to consider alternate therapy. Many patients are given these drugs chronically for inappropriate indications. Discontinuation of these drugs is an important first therapeutic step because the ideal therapeutic outcome is to have a complete remission of involuntary movements without need for continued drug treatment. To our knowledge, this ideal therapeutic response requires discontinuation of the offending drugs; we are not aware of tardive dyskinesia remitting during DA antagonist treatment and *remaining in remission after discontinuation of these drugs*. There is evidence for tardive dyskinesia of the classic oral choreic type that less DA antagonist exposure after the onset of movements is associated with an enhanced likelihood of complete remission. It is difficult to obtain this type of evidence retrospectively, because often patients are not aware when the condition began and it is difficult to quantitate drug exposure. Data of this type are not available for tardive dystonia. We have observed patients who had complete remissions of their dystonia after discontinuation of DA antagonists who after subsequent re-exposure developed persistent dystonia that did not remit after again stopping drugs. This observation supports the need to minimize drug exposure after the first appearance of tardive dystonia.

After a decision has been made to continue or discontinue DA antagonists, the degree of disability caused by the involuntary movements must be considered. If DA antagonists cannot be discontinued for psychiatric reasons and they sufficiently suppress the involuntary movements such that they are not disabling, then we do not treat with additional drugs. If the patient is disabled by the involuntary movements, we then recommend drug treatment. The treatment depends on the type of dyskinesia.

We initially treat patients with tardive dystonia with either DA-depleting drugs (either reserpine or tetrabenazine [TBZ]) or anticholinergics (either trihexyphenidyl or ethopropazine). In the United States, TBZ is available as an investigational drug only. Tardive dystonia resembles classic oral tardive dyskinesia in its response to DA-depleting drugs but differs in its response to anticholinergics. Classic oral tardive dyskinesia is said to be exacerbated by anticholinergics. Tardive dystonia patients vary in their response to DA depletors and anticholinergics, and unfortunately we have no way of predicting who will respond to which class of drug. We recently compared patients who responded to anticholinergics to those who responded to DA depletors. We found no difference between these patient groups in age at onset of dystonia, sex, distribution of dystonia at onset or at maximum severity, duration of exposure to DA antagonists before dystonia, or presence of classic oral dyskinesia.[24] Without a means of predicting which drug a patient will respond to, our choice is often guided by anticipated side effects. Older patients are more likely to suffer confusion or memory loss from anticholinergics so we will often opt for DA depletors. Patients with a history of depression, however, are at risk for recurrence due to DA depletors, so we choose anticholinergics.

Our general approach to the use of these drugs is similar for each of them. We start with a low dose and gradually increase until either adequate benefit is obtained, or intolerable side effects intervene, or a judicious maximum is reached. We start reserpine at a dose of 0.25 mg per day and gradually increase. If symptomatic hypotension occurs, we decrease the dose as needed and consider using mineralocorticoids. We have used up to 9.0 mg per day, although our average dose is 5.0 mg per day. We use trihexyphenidyl and ethopropazine as described for the treatment of dystonia, starting with 5.0 mg per day of the former or 50.0 mg per day of the latter and gradually increase the dose.[49] In treating dystonia, we have used up to 120 mg per day of trihexyphenidyl but our average dose in treating tardive dystonia has been 20 mg per day.

If a tardive dystonia patient does not respond to either DA depletors or anticholinergics, other drugs can be tried, but it is difficult to make a specific recommendation as no other drug has emerged as a next-best therapy. We have found benzodiazepines, including diazepam, clonazepam, and lorazepam to be occasionally helpful. Baclofen is also occasionally helpful.

For patients with focal cranial dystonias, botulinum toxin injections into affected muscles are a valuable alternative. Blepharospasm responds well, as does torticollis.[85]

Although we believe it is therapeutically ideal to discontinue DA antagonists in patients with tardive dystonia, there are two situations in which we use them therapeutically for their ability to suppress the dystonic movements. We use them when a patient has severe, generalized tardive dystonia that is either painful or causes muscle damage (evidenced by an elevated serum CPK). In the latter circumstance, tardive dystonia is potentially life-threatening. In this setting, we will suppress the dystonic movements with a parentally administered DA antagonist. The second situation in which we will use DA antagonists to suppress the movements is when DA depletors, anticholinergics, and other drugs have failed, and the patient has either been successfully maintained off DA antagonists for 4 to 5 years without remission or has not tolerated withdrawal. The possibility of a remission would at this point seem remote, and with the failure to find other drugs to alleviate the movements, we turn to DA antagonists to suppress them.

Tardive Akathisia

The Nature of Akathisia

Many of the early reports of classic oral-buccal-lingual tardive dyskinesia contain very clear descriptions of motor restlessness associated with the oral movements,[50-53] and yet persistent akathisia, as a subtype of tardive dyskinesia, has received only recent recognition.[54] A possible reason for this delayed recognition is that a consensus on the definition of akathisia does not emerge from the literature. Many authorities have considered the term *akathisia* to refer strictly to an abnormal subjective state, characterized by restlessness.[55] Others, however, consider the motor phenomena of akathisia to be characteristic and important for diagnosis.[54,56] Some even consider the characteristic movements as sufficient for a diagnosis of akathisia[57] or at least "pseudoakathisia."[58] It has been our opinion that the most satisfactory "gold standard" definition of akathisia for the present must rest on both the subjective and objective features.[59] The degree to which more partial manifestations of the condition may be sufficient to define it remains to be determined by more complete study of its spectrum. The subjective state of akathisia is reported as an aversion to being still. The patient may or may not use the term "restless." They may instead refer to "nervousness," or "jitteriness," and so on, but they must report discomfort related to being still, which can be relieved by movement. The objective motor signs of akathisia consist of an increased, abnormal frequency of movements. The movements are often complex and stereotyped, i.e., repeated in the same pattern over and over. Examples include repetitive crossing/uncrossing or rapidly abducting/adducting the legs while sitting, or marching in place while standing. The combination of these subjective and motor features defines akathisia.

Evidence that Chronic Akathisia is Due to Neuroleptic Drug Use

Like tardive dystonia, tardive akathisia has not been the subject of case-controlled studies to investigate its relationship to neuroleptic drug use. Unlike dystonia, however, akathisia rarely, if ever, occurs on an idiopathic basis. Today, other than parkinsonism, there are few other causes of akathisia besides treatment with neuroleptic drugs. Thus, there is a broad consensus that persistent akathisia is a complication of treatment with these agents.

The association between neuroleptic drugs and akathisia is further strengthened by a number of observations. As for tardive dystonia, there are close temporal relationships between the use of these drugs and the occurrence of akathisia. In a number of patients, discontinuation of the drugs has led to remission.[59] In addition, we are aware of an instance in which a patient who had gone into remission developed persistent akathisia a second time, during re-exposure to a neuroleptic. Tardive akathisia is even more frequently associated with oral-buccal-lingual tardive dyskinesia (90% of our cases[59]) than tardive dystonia. Tardive akathisia not infrequently appears to evolve from acute akathisia, which is clearly a complication of neuroleptics. These occurrences have been called "acute persistent" akathisia.[54] Finally, the clinical pharmacology of tardive akathisia, as will be discussed, is like that of oral-lingual tardive dyskinesia, further indicating a close relationship between these disorders.

Diagnostic Criteria

To diagnose tardive akathisia, we use the following criteria: (1) akathisia, defined as above on the basis of both the subjective and motor features of restlessness, must be present; (2) the akathisia must not have preceded, and must develop during (or within 3 months of cessation of) neuroleptic treatment; (3) the akathisia must be *persistent,* i.e., present for at least 1 month's duration. We do not include any stipulation about the duration of neuroleptic treatment prior to onset in making this diagnosis. Although tardive akathisia usually develops late in the course of therapy, it can, like tardive dystonia and oral-lingual dyskinesia, develop early. The more critical feature is its persistence. We do not distinguish between "acute persistent" and late onset (or "tardive" akathisia) as did Barnes and Braude, because we find that individual patients often have difficulty pinpointing when their akathisia began in relation to therapy. In addition, since there is a smooth continuum for onset in relation to duration of therapy, it seems arbitrary to try to divide between early-onset and late-onset persistent neuroleptic-induced akathisias. We also do not use treatment response to DA antagonists as a necessary diagnostic criterion. It is, however, helpful to attempt to discontinue DA antagonists and observe the response in one situation, where a patient develops akathisia early in the course of DA antagonist therapy, and has persistent akathisia (>1 month) while on a constant dose. The patient may have acute akathisia that is persistent due to ongoing therapy, or may have a chronic akathisia, i.e., tardive akathisia. The only way to determine which type of akathisia the patient has is to attempt to stop the drugs. If the akathisia promptly abates on drug withdrawal, then the patient had acute akathisia. If, however, the akathisia persists (or worsens) for more than a month following drug withdrawal, then the patient has tardive akathisia. If the patient cannot be taken off neuroleptic drugs, then it is not possible to know for certain which form of akathisia the patient has.

Epidemiology

In his classic monograph, Ayd found acute akathisia to have a prevalence of 21%, making it the most common drug-induced movement disorder.[60] There have been few studies, but tardive akathisia may also be common. Braude and Barnes examined 82 schizophrenic outpatients to determine the presence of restless movements.[54] They found that 39 patients (48%) had such movements. Of these 39 patients, 6 (7% of the total) apparently had acute akathisia. An additional 10 (12%) had "pseudoakathisia," i.e., restless movements in the absence of subjective complaints. The remaining 23 (28%) had chronic akathisia (i.e., what we have defined as tardive akathisia); 12 of these patients (15% of the total group) had acute persistent akathisia and 11 patients (13% of the total) had late-onset, chronic akathisia. Thus, chronic akathisia was quite common. A prevalence of 28% is close to an observed prevalence of 20% of late-onset akathisia among 65 schizophrenic out-patients reported by Schilkrut and colleagues.[61] These estimates are similar in magnitude to typical estimates of the prevalence of oral dyskinesia, and they require confirmation in larger patient groups.

Among our 52 patients with tardive akathisia, the mean age of onset was 58.4 years, ranging from 21 to 82 years. Women outnumbered men by almost 2 to 1. Men tended to have an earlier age of onset (54.1 years) than women (60.9 years).

Like tardive dystonia and oral tardive dyskinesia, tardive akathisia has been reported following treatment with a wide variety of classes of DA receptor-blocking drugs: all three classes of phenothiazines, butyrophenones, dibenzoxazepines, and metoclopramide.[62]

There have been no prospective studies of the onset of tardive akathisia in relation to the duration or dose of neuroleptic therapy. In our retrospective review, the average duration of therapy prior to onset was 4.5 years. However, like tardive dystonia, tardive akathi-

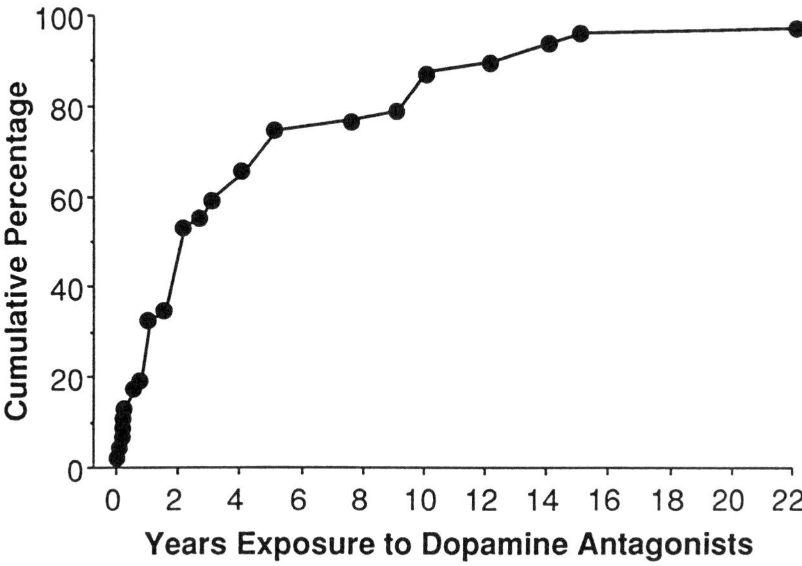

Figure 2: This figure demonstrates the relationship between years of treatment with dopamine antagonists and the cumulative onset of tardive akathisia in our group of patients (N = 45; reference 59). It can be seen that cases begin to occur within the first year of exposure; there is no period of minimum safe exposure to DA antagonists free of risk from inducing tardive akathisia. The first point on the curve is a patient who developed persistent akathisia following 2 weeks of neuroleptic therapy. (Reproduced with permission.[59])

sia can occur early in the course of therapy. Figure 2 shows the time of onset in relation to duration of neuroleptic treatment; it can be seen that many cases develop within the first year of treatment. Some of our cases in this group would include instances of what Barnes and Braude term "acute persistent" akathisia. As mentioned earlier, we include such cases under the diagnosis of tardive akathisia because they are persistent. It can be seen in Figure 2 that onset in relation to duration of therapy is a smooth and continuous function; there is no clear separation between early-onset and late-onset persistent cases. The average age of onset (60.4 years) among our early-onset (≤1 year of neuroleptic exposure) patients was no different than the others.

Like the other tardive syndromes, tardive akathisia occurs among patients with a variety of psychiatric and nonpsychiatric diagnoses. In fact, 36% of our patients had been treated with neuroleptics for secondary or even questionable indications: anxiety, nausea, gastrointestinal distress, pain. A notable proportion of our patients, 46%, had been treated for an affective disorder. However, ours was a neurological referral population, and referral patterns may influence these data.

Clinical Features

The Subjective State of Akathisia

Patients suffering from akathisia frequently complain of an unbearable inner torment and beg repeatedly for relief. There is evidence that akathisia may be associated with suicide.[63] Many patients do not know how to describe what they feel, and they may use a variety of terms other than "restless"; they may complain of "jitteriness," "a tortured sort of feeling," "fidgety," "nervous," "about to jump out of my skin," "all revved up," and so on. Patients who are floridly psychotic or impaired intellectually will be especially unlikely to clearly express their subjective condition. Akathisia may therefore be confused with a variety of psychiatric states that lead to agitation, such as mania, agitated depression, or severe anxiety.[64,65] In addition, the emotions associated with akathisia, including fright or anger, can be associated with a spectrum of abnormal behaviors and "acting out."[66,67] Patients with mild akathisia complain of impatience, irritability, or inability to concentrate.

It has been suggested that patients with acute akathisia suffer more severe subjective distress and that the subjective component becomes less severe in the chronic setting. Braude and Barnes have suggested that in the chronic setting, akathisia may evolve to a state of "pseudoakathisia" in which there are motor features of restlessness but no subjective restlessness.[54] Whether this is true, and how often it occurs, will require prospective analysis. In our retrospective survey, there certainly did exist patients who had severe subjective distress that continued for years without abatement.

Among our patients, the position most frequently identified as the most uncomfortable was sitting. The most preferred position was lying down. Thus, patients would often complain that they could no longer sit through a meal, or sit for TV or the movies. Inability to stand in one place for a prolonged period also interfered with activities of daily living; many of these patients could not stand in line for shopping or banking.

Motor Features

In general, patients with akathisia show an increased frequency of movement, and they make movements that are complex and stereotyped, i.e., repeated in the same pattern over and over. Patients can often suppress the movements, if asked to do so, for at least brief periods of time. During the time they suppress the movements, they build a greater inner sense of restlessness or "tension," which is then relieved by performing the movements. The type of movements the patient makes depends on their position; for example, when sitting, they may cross and uncross the legs, whereas on standing, they will march in place.

In our analysis of movements in 52 patients with tardive akathisia, we found that the legs are the most frequently affected. Marching in place while standing and crossing/uncrossing the legs while sitting occurred in 58% and 48%, respectively, of our patients. Other common leg movements included pumping the leg up and down or rapidly adducting/abducting it while sitting.

Truncal movements were also common and included rocking back and forth and frequent shifts of position while sitting. Somewhat less common, but more distinctive, were complex arm and hand movements, including face rubbing, hair rubbing, head or face scratching, folding/unfolding the arms, and picking at clothes.

Many of these patients also complain of respiratory irregularities such as panting or grunting. In addition, some of our most severely affected patients would moan or even shout.

Movements of the facial region were less common, in our experience, but they may occur. We have observed repetitive, lateral tongue movements and repetitive head nodding.[68]

In our series of 52 patients, tardive akathisia was associated with either oral-buccal-lingual dyskinesia or tardive dystonia in all but one patient. Sixty-three percent had oral dyskinesia, 8% had tardive dystonia and 27% had both. The few patients with tardive akathisia and tardive dystonia had an earlier age of onset (39 years) than those with akathisia and oral dyskinesia (62.2 years).

Clinical Course

Among our patients, 67% had persistent akathisia at last follow-up for a mean duration of 4.2 years. Most of these patients had discontinued neuroleptics several years earlier. Among the 33% of our patients who did not have akathisia at last follow-up, 6% were in true remission; that is, they had been weaned from therapy without recurrence of akathisia. The other patients who did not have akathisia at follow-up were receiving ongoing therapy that suppressed it. The patients who did not have akathisia at follow-up had an earlier age of onset. Thus, younger patients appear to have a more reversible or treatable condition.

Differential Diagnosis

Akathisia can be difficult to differentiate from psychiatric conditions that cause agitation. It is helpful to recall that the subjective distress of akathisia is an aversion to remaining still and is at least partially relieved by movement. Subjective distress due to psychiatric disease does not necessarily show this relationship to movement. In the case of agitation due to psychiatric illness, other aspects of the patient interview will generally reveal other features consistent with exacerbation of the psychiatric condition, such as hallucinations or delusions. An additional differentiating point is that the movements we have described tend to be characteristic of akathisia.

Neuroleptic-induced akathisia must be distinguished from Ekbom's restless legs syndrome. The latter consists of uncomfortable dysesthesias in the legs that occur nocturnally as the patient lies down to go to sleep. The dysesthesias are relieved by pacing about. The sensory complaints, the nocturnal occurrence, the predominant leg involvement, and the worsening rather than improvement in the supine position all help to distinguish restless legs syndrome from akathisia.

One of the few other causes of akathisia today, besides neuroleptic drug treatment, is Parkinson's disease (PD).[69] In Lang and Johnson's series, 26% of Parkinson patients had true akathisia. In some, it was an early symptom of PD, but in most it developed later, when the diagnosis of parkinsonism was apparent.

Treatment

The general approach to the treatment of tardive akathisia is like that for tardive dystonia and oral dyskinesia. If neuroleptics can be stopped, they should be. A certain percentage of patients (8% in our series) will undergo spontaneous remission. Whether or not neuroleptics are stopped, the next step is to assess the degree of disability. If there is only mild akathisia, then the patient can simply be followed. If, however, there is significant disability, then we treat the akathisia (whether or not the patient has been taken off neuroleptics). In our experience, DA-depleting drugs are the most frequently beneficial. Among 30 patients treated at Columbia, 15 were managed with reserpine; of these, 13 (87%) showed improvement. In 11 of these patients, reserpine gave complete control (N = 3) or marked improvement (N = 8). Tetrabenazine was effective in 7 of 12 (58%) treated patients. Of patients treated with these drugs, about 50% remained on them at follow-up. The approach to using these drugs is similar. One begins with a small dose (0.25 mg/day for reserpine) and very gradually titrates upward. Our mean reserpine dose was 5.0 mg/day.

Opiates have been reported to be effective in the management of acute akathisia.[70] However, we found them rarely to be effective for tardive akathisia. Walters and co-workers have recently reported a similar experience.[71]

While a number of investigators have reported that the β-blocker propranolol is effective for the management of acute akathisia,[72] we have not had much success in the few tardive akathisia patients we have treated. Thus, tardive akathisia differs from acute akathisia in its clinical pharmacology. It has an opposite response to DA depletion (or antagonism); it does not respond to the opiates or β-blockers.

Tardive Myoclonus and Tardive Tics

Myoclonus refers to sudden, brief shock-like jerks. Like dystonia and akathisia, myoclonus was described in early reports of tardive dyskinesia.[73] Several of the patients we described with tardive dystonia also had myoclonus.[1] More recently, pure myoclonus has been reported as a complication of neuroleptic treatment.[74,75] Jankovic's patient demonstrated myoclonic movements of the neck and lower face after discontinuation of neuroleptics; ultimately, they were suppressed by thiothixene. Only one such patient had been observed in a series of 158 patients referred for neurological evaluation of neuroleptic-induced movement disorders.

Tominaga et al. described myoclonic jerks in the arms and shoulders of patients, elicited by holding the hands up and forward.[74] These jerks were observed in 24% of 133 patients. From this brief report, it was not clear that the authors were describing a persistent motor disturbance, particularly whether it persisted following discontinuation of neuroleptics. Thus, it is not clear that they were describing a true tardive disorder. Furthermore, the clinical significance of their observation is unclear, given that the movements were observed in only a single posture and that the authors do not state that the movements were symptomatic. The authors state that the movements were suppressed by clonazepam. We have also observed among tardive dystonia patients with significant myoclonus that clonazepam may be effective.

For a number of reasons, it is difficult to ascribe tics to neuroleptic drug treatment with certainty. Transient tics occur quite commonly among children in the general population. Furthermore, spontaneously occurring Tourette's syndrome is a common neurological disease of childhood. Tics, unlike oral-buccal-lingual dyskinesia, dystonia, akathisia, and myoclonus, quite characteristically occur and remit spontaneously. Thus, it is more difficult to make meaningful temporal connections between the use of neuroleptics and the occurrence of the tics. Finally, a number of reports of "Tourettes" associated with neuroleptic treatment may actually have been cases of tardive akathisia, with repeated complex stereotyped movements and grunting or moaning that resembled motor and vocal tics.

These caveats notwithstanding, there have been a number of reports of tic disorders occurring in patients during or soon following neuroleptic therapy, which, considered together, seem suggestive that in rare instances neuroleptics may induce tics[76–84] (Table 3). Most of these patients developed their tics in adulthood, long after spontaneously occurring Tourette's syndrome would ordinarily occur. In most of them, the described vocal utterances seem to have been more complex or formed than typically occurs in akathisia; there were barks, clicks, coprolalia, and so on. In Table 3, those patients with only nonspecific vocalizations, such as grunting or howling, which may also be observed in tardive akathisia, are noted

Table 3

Reported Cases of Tourette's Syndrome Associated with Dopamine Antagonist Treatment

Authors (Ref.)	Year	Patient (No.)	Age of Onset	Signs	During or After DA Antagonists	Other Tardive Disorder	Comments
Klawans et al.[76]	1978	1	28	Face, arm tics Barking	1 month after	dystonia	
DeVaugh-Geiss[77]	1980	1	65	Facial tics Barking	2 months after	OBLD	
Stahl[78]	1980	1	28	Facial tics Barking Coprolalia	1 month after	none	
Fog & Pakenberg[79]	1980	1	20	"tics of head & body," grunting	after	NS	? Tardive akathisia
		2	54	"Arm movements" Shouting	NS	NS	? Tardive akathisia
		3	50	No tics Howling	NS	OBLD	? Tardive akathisia
Seeman et al.[80]	1981	1	25	"Blepharo-spasm" "Facial grimacing" Grunting	during	NS	? Tardive dystonia & akathisia
Mueller & Aminoff[81]	1982	1	27	Head turning Gutteral noises Barking	3 weeks after	OBLD	
Klawans et al.[82]	1982	1	(Reported in Ref. 76)				
		2	71	Facial tics	after	OBLD	
		3	32	Facial tics Grunting Coprolalia	during	None	
Munetz et al.[83]	1985	1	60	Head and neck tics Coprolalia	after	OBLD	
Karagianis & Nagpurkar[84]	1990	1	10	Shoulder and face tics Coprolalia	during	OBLD	

NS = not specified; OBLD = oral-buccal-lingual dyskinesia; DA = dopamine.

in the final column to have a possible diagnosis of tardive akathisia, in my assessment.

The average age of onset among the 12 reported cases was 39 ± 5 (SEM) years, ranging from 10 to 71. In the majority of these patients (7 of 10 with available information), the tics began after discontinuation of neuroleptics. As in spontaneously occurring Tourette's syndrome, most of the motor tics occurred in the cranial regions (face, head, neck). As in Tourette's syndrome, there was a wide range of vocal utterances: barks, clicks, sniffs, coprolalia, and echolalia. For the nine patients with sufficient information, seven had associated tardive movements, either oral-buccal-lingual dyskinesia or tardive dystonia. These associated movements strengthen the association between the occurrence of the tics and exposure to neuroleptics. Among these 12 patients, adequate information about the clinical course is provided in 10; eight had their tics suppressed by a DA antagonist; two went into spontaneous remission.

Thus, these occasional reports suggest a relationship between neuroleptic treatment and the occurrence of tics, but the strength of this relationship requires further documentation, particularly by videotape analysis.

Acknowledgments: The author is supported by NINDS R29 NS 26836, the Parkinson's Disease Foundation, and The Dystonia Medical Research Foundation.

References

1. Burke RE, Fahn S, Jankovic J, Marsden CD, Lang AE, Gollomp S, et al. Tardive dystonia: late onset and persistent dystonia caused by antipsychotic drugs. Neurology (NY) 1982; 32:1335–1346.
2. Druckman R, Seelinger D, Thulin B. Chronic involuntary movements induced by phenothiazines. J Nerv Ment Dis 1962; 135:69–76.
3. Chateau R, Fau R, Groslambert R, Perret J. A propos d'un cas de torticollis spasmodique irreversible survenu au cours d'un traitement par neuroleptiques. Ann Med Psychol (Paris) 1966; 122:110–111.
4. Dabbous IA, Bergman AB. Neurologic damage associated with phenothiazine. Am J Dis Child 1966; 111:291–296.
5. Harenko A. Retrocollis as an irreversible late complication of neuroleptic medication. Acta Neurol Scand 1967; 43:(Suppl):145–146.
6. Angle CR, McIntire MS. Persistent dystonia in a brain-damaged child after ingestion of phenothiazine. J Pediatr 1968; 73:124–126.
7. Crane GE. Persistent dyskinesia. Br J Psychiatry 1973; 122:395–405.

8. Keegan DL, Rajput AH. Drug-induced dystonia tarda: treatment with L-Dopa. Dis Nerv Syst 1973; 38:167–169.
9. Shields WB, Bray PF. A danger of haloperidol therapy in children. J Pediatr 1976; 88:301–303.
10. Tarsy D, Grancher R, Bralower M. Tardive dyskinesia in young adults. Am J Psychiatry 1977; 134:1032–1034.
11. McLean P, Casey DE. Tardive dyskinesia in an adolescent. Am Psychiatry 1978; 135:969–971.
12. Weiner WJ, Nausieda P, Glantz RH. Meige syndrome (blepharospasm-oromandibular dystonia) after long-term neuroleptic therapy. Neurology 1981; 31:1555–1556.
13. Fahn S. Concept and classification of dystonia. In: Fahn S, Marsden CD, Calne DB (eds), Dystonia 2, Advances in Neurology, 1988, 50:2–8.
14. Tardive dyskinesia: Report of the American Psychiatric Association Task Force on Late Neurological Effects of Antipsychotic Drugs. Washington, D.C., American Psychiatric Association, 1980.
15. Bartels M, Riffel B, Stohr. Neuroleptic-induced dystonia tarda: An uncommon side effect. Nervenarzt 1982; 53:674–676.
16. Weiner WJ, Werner TR. Mania-induced remission of tardive dyskinesia in manic-depressive illness. Ann Neurol 1982; 12:229.
17. Glazer WM, Moore DC, Hansen TC, Brenner LM. Meige syndrome and tardive dyskinesia. Am J Psychiatry 1983; 140:798–799.
18. Kwentus JA, Schulz SC, Hart RP. Tardive dystonia, catatonia, electroconvulsive therapy. J Nerv Ment Dis 1984; 172:171–173.
19. Nishinawa T, Tanaka M, Tsuda A, et al. Clonidine therapy for tardive dyskinesia and related syndromes. Clin Neuropharmacol 1984; 7:239–245.
20. Gimenez-Roldan S, Mateo D, Bartolome P. Tardive dystonia and severe tardive dyskinesia. Acta Psychiatr Scand 1985; 71:488–494.
21. Lazarus AL, Toglia JU. Fatal myoglobinuric renal failure in a patient with tardive dyskinesia. Neurology 1985; 35:1055–1057.
22. Luchins DJ, Goldman M. High-dose bromocriptine in a case of tardive dystonia. Biol Psychiatry 1985; 20:179–181.
23. Wolf ME, Koller WC. Tardive dystonia: treatment with trihexyphenidyl. J. Clin Psychopharmacol 1985; 5:247–248.
24. Kang UJ, Burke RE, Fahn S. Natural history and treatment of tardive dystonia. Mov Disord 1986; 1:193–208.
25. Saxena S. Tardive dystonia and pisa syndrome. Br J Psychiatry 1986; 149:524.
26. Yassa R, Nair V, Dimitry R. Prevalence of tardive dystonia. Acta Psychiatr Scand 1986; 73:629–633.
27. Rosse RB, Allen A, Lux WE. Baclofen treatment in a patient with tardive dystonia. J Clin Psychiatry 1986; 47:474–475.
28. Gardos G, Cole JO, Salomon M, Schniebolk S. Clinical forms of severe tardive dyskinesia. Am J Psychiatry 1987; 144:895–902.
29. Samie MR, Dannenhoffer MA, Rozek S. Life-threatening tardive dyskinesia caused by metoclopramide. Mov Disord 1987; 2:125–130.
30. Corbin DO, Williams AC, White AC. Tardive dystonia: which way do schizophrenics twist? Lancet 1987; 1:268–269.

31. Friedman JH, Kucharski LT, Wagner RL. Tardive dystonia in a psychiatric hospital. J Neurol Neurosurg Psychiatry 1987; 50:801–803.
32. Girion LT. Tardive dystonia after a short course of thioridazine. J Fam Pract 1987; 24:405–406.
33. Lal KP, Saxena S, Mohan D. Tardive dystonia alternating with mania. Biol Psychiatry 1988; 23:312–316.
34. Falk WE, Wojick JD, Glenberg AJ. Diltiazem for tardive dyskinesia and tardive dystonia. Lancet 1988; 1:824–825.
35. Anath J, Edelmuth E, Dargan B. Meige's syndrome associated with neuroleptic treatment. Am J Psychiatry 1988; 145:513–515.
36. Chin HFK, Leung JYW, Lee S. Tardive dystonia in Chinese. Sing Med J 1989; 30:441–443.
37. Cooper SJ, Doherty MM, King DJ. Tardive dystonia: The benefits of time. Br J Psychiatry 1989; 155:113–115.
38. Gureje O. The significance of subtyping tardive dyskinesia: a study of prevalence and associated factors. Psychol Med 1989; 19:121–128.
39. Miller LG, Jankovic J. Sulpiride-induced tardive dyskinesia. Mov Disord 1990; 5:83–84.
40. Lang AE. Clinical differences between metoclopramide- and antipsychotic-induced tardive dyskinesias. Can J Neurol Sci 1990; 17:137–139.
41. Adityanjee, Jayaswal SK, Chan TM, Subramaniam M. Temporary remission of tardive dystonia following electroconvulsive therapy. Br J Psychiatry 1990; 156:433–435.
42. Miller LG, Jankovic J. Neurologic approach to drug-induced movement disorders: A study of 125 patients Southern Med J 1990; 83:525–532.
43. Yadalam KG, Korn ML, Simpson GM. Tardive dystonia: four case histories. J Clin Psychiatry 1990; 51:17–20.
44. Greene P, Shale H, Fahn S. Experience with high dosages of anticholinergic and other drugs in treatment of torsion dystonia. In: Fahn S, Marsden CD, Calne DB (eds), Dystonia 2, Advances in Neurology 1988; 50:547–556.
45. Calne D, Lang AE. Secondary dystonia. In: Fahn S, Marsden CD, Calne DB (eds), Dystonia 2, Advances in Neurology, 1988; 50:9–34.
46. Yassa R, Nair V, Iskandar H. A comparison of severe tardive dystonia and severe tardive akathisia. Acta Psychiatr Scand 1989; 80:155–159.
47. Sethi KD, Hess DC, Harp RJ. Prevalence of dystonia in veterans on chronic antipsychotic therapy. Movement Disorders 1990; 5:319–321.
48. Fitzgerald PM, Jankovic J. Tardive oculogyric crises. Neurology 1989; 39:1434–1437.
49. Fahn S. High dosage anticholinergic therapy in dystonia. Neurology (Cleveland) 1983; 33:1255–1261.
50. Uhrbrand L, Faurybe A. Reversible and irreversible dyskinesia after treatment with perphenazine, chlorpromazine, reserpine and electroconvulsive therapy. Psychopharmacologia 1960; 1:408–418.
51. Druckman R, Seelinger D, Thulin B. Chronic involuntary movements induced by phenothiazines. J Nerv Ment Dis 1962; 135:69–76.
52. Hunter R, Earl CJ, Thornicroft S. An apparently irreversible syndrome of abnormal movements following phenothiazine medication. Proc R Soc Med 1964; 57:758–762.

53. Kruse W. Persistent muscular restlessness after phenothiazine treatment: report of three cases. Am J Psychiatry 1960; 117:152–153.

54. Braude WM, Barnes TRE. Late-onset akathisia—an indicant of covert dyskinesia: two case reports. Am J Psychiatry 1983; 140:611–612.

55. Duvoisin R. Neurological reactions to psychotropic drugs. In: Efron DH (ed), Psychopharmacology: A Review of Progress 1957–1967, US Government Printing Office, 1968, pp 561–573.

56. Gibb WRG, Lees AJ. The clinical phenomenon of akathisia. J Neurol Neurosurg Psychiatry 1986; 49:861–866.

57. Simpson GM. Neurotoxicology of Major tranquilizers. In: Roizin L, Shiraki H, Grcevic N (eds), Neurotoxicology, New York, Raven Press, 1977, pp 1–7.

58. Munetz MR, Cornes CL. Akathisia, pseudoakathisia and tardive dyskinesia: clinical examples. Compr Psychiatry 1982; 23:345–352.

59. Burke RE, Kang UK, Jankovic J, Miller LG, Fahn S. Tardive akathisia: an analysis of clinical features and response to open therapeutic trials. Mov Disord 1989; 4:157–175.

60. Ayd F. A survey of drug-induced extrapyramidal reactions. JAMA 1961; 175:1054–1060.

61. Schilkrut VR, Duran E, Haverbeck C, Katz I, Vidal P. Verlauf von psychopathologischen und extrapyramidalmotorischen symptomen unter einer Langzeit-Neuroleptika behandlung schizophrener Patienten. Drug Res 1978; 28:1494–1495.

62. Shearer RM, Bownes IT, Curran P. Tardive akathisia and agitated depression during metoclopramide therapy. Acta Psychiatr Scand 1984; 70:428–431.

63. Drake RE, Ehrlich J. Suicide attempts associated with akathisia. Am J Psychiatry 1985; 142:499–501.

64. Kumar B. An unusual case of akathisia. Am J Psychol 1979; 136:8.

65. Raskin DE. Akathisia: A side effect to be remembered. Am J Psychiatry 1972; 129:345–347.

66. Van Putten T. The many faces of akathisia. Compr Psychiatry 1975; 16:43–47.

67. Siris S. Three cases of akathisia and "acting out." Clin Psychiatry 1985; 46:395–397.

68. Burke RE, Kang UJ, Fahn S, Jankovic J, Miller LG. Tardive akathisia (letter). Mov Disord 1990; 5:181–182.

69. Lang AE, Johnson K. Akathisia in idiopathic Parkinson's disease. Neurology 1987; 37:477–480.

70. Walters A, Hening W, Chokroverty S, Fahn S. Opioid responsiveness in patients with neuroleptic-induced akathisia. Mov Disord 1986; 1:119–128.

71. Walters S, Hening W, Chokroverty S. Tardive akathisia (letter). Mov Disord 1990; 5:89–90.

72. Adler LA, Angrist B, Peselow E, et al. Noradrenergic mechanisms in akathisia: treatment with propranolol and clonidine. Psychopharmacol Bull 1987; 23:21–25.

73. Degwitz R. Extrapyramidal motor disorders following long-term treatment with neuroleptic drugs. In: Crane GE, Gardner R (eds), Psycho-

tropic Drugs and Dysfunctions of the Basal Ganglia, Public Health Service Publication No. 1938, 1969, pp 22–33.
74. Tominaga H, Fukuzako H, Izumi K, et al. Tardive myoclonus (letter). Lancet 1987; 1:322.
75. Little JT, Jankovic J. Tardive myoclonus. Mov Disord 1987; 2: 307–312.
76. Klawans HL, Falk DK, Nausieda PA, Weiner WJ. Gilles de la Tourette's syndrome after long-term chlorpromazine therapy. Neurology 1978; 28:1064–1068.
77. DeVaugh-Geiss J. Tardive Tourette's syndrome. Neurology 1980; 30: 562–563.
78. Stahl S. Tardive Tourette's syndrome in an autistic patient after long-term neuroleptic administration. Am J Psychiatry 1980; 137:1267–1269.
79. Fog R, Pakenberg H. Theoretical and clinical aspects of the Tourette syndrome (chronic multiple tic). J Neural Trans 1980; (Suppl) 16:211–215.
80. Seeman MV, Patel J, Pyke J. Tardive dyskinesia with Tourette-like syndrome. J Clin Psychiatry 1981; 42:357–358.
81. Mueller J, Aminoff MJ. Tourette-like syndrome after long-term neuroleptic drug treatment. Br J Psychiatry 1982; 141:191–193.
82. Klawans HL, Nausieda PA, Goetz CC, et al. Tourette-like symptoms following chronic neuroleptic therapy. In: Friedhoff AJ, Chase TN (eds), Gilles de la Tourette Syndrome, New York, Raven Press, 1982, pp 415–418.
83. Munetz MR, Slawsky RC, Neil JF. Tardive Tourette's syndrome treated with clonidine and mesoridazine. Psychosomatics 1985; 26:254–257.
84. Karagianis JL, Nagpurkar R. A case of Tourette syndrome developing during haloperidol treatment. Can J Psychiatry 1990; 35:228–232.

7

Neuroleptic Malignant Syndrome

Stewart A. Factor, D.O., Carlos Singer, M.D.

History

Neuroleptic malignant syndrome (NMS) is a potentially fatal drug-induced disorder associated with various movement disorders. It was first described by Delay and associates[1] during the proceedings of the Societé Medico-Psychologique.[1] This presentation was a communication on the efficacy and safety of haloperidol. Initially referred to as the "syndrome malin," in their 1968 chapter in the *Handbook of Clinical Neurology,*[2] the term neuroleptic "malignant" syndrome was introduced. This was the first English report on the subject. They described it as the "most serious but also the rarest and least known of complications of neuroleptic chemotherapy." Three main groups of signs were discussed. Changes in the "general condition" included hyperthermia and pallor. Psychomotor signs included "akinesis with a greater or lesser degree of stupor, or hypertonicity and varying dyskinesias." It was suggested that these signs were seen exclusively in "brain-damaged" individuals. Finally, "signs in the lungs" included congestion and infarction with resultant dyspnea and asphyxia. The poor prognosis was clear . . . "death

Lang AE, Weiner WJ (editors): *Drug-Induced Movement Disorders,* Mount Kisco, NY, © Futura Publishing Co., Inc., 1992.

in hyperthermia supervenes unless appropriate measures are instituted in time." These measures included discontinuation of antipsychotic medications, rehydration, and correction of electrolyte abnormalities. They suggested antipyrexic medication, including chlorpromazine (a drug now known to cause NMS) and antiparkinsonian medications in the later stages, if necessary.

Through 1980, the syndrome was underdiagnosed and rarely reported. Approximately 60 cases were published before 1980 and Caroff[3] reviewed them. Most were from the French literature, and few were from the United States. In addition, NMS received little or no attention in psychiatric and psychopharmacological text books. At this time, NMS was thought to be related to treatment only with high-potency neuroleptics. Caroff's landmark paper stimulated increased interest and recognition and has been followed by numerous reports, studies, and reviews. Approximately 20 neuroleptics have now been shown to cause the disorder. In addition, it is now clear that NMS also occurs in situations where neuroleptics are not utilized. In 1981, Burke and associates[4] reported NMS in a patient with Huntington's disease treated with dopamine-depleting agents, and in the same year NMS was reported in patients with Parkinson's disease after sudden withdrawal of dopaminergic medications.[5] These situations strongly suggest that NMS is related to an alteration in dopaminergic transmission in the CNS.[6] The recent interest in NMS has led to a better understanding of the clinical features and pathophysiology, which has resulted in a rational treatment regimen.

Clinical Aspects

Signs and Symptoms (Table 1)

The principal features of NMS are hyperthermia, muscle rigidity, autonomic dysfunction, and mental status changes. Hyperthermia is present in nearly all cases of NMS.[7-9] Rare afebrile patients have been reported.[9a] Patients may have a low-grade temperature or one as high as 42.2°C.[10] Addonizio et al.[11] reported temperatures above 38°C (100.4°F) in 92% of patients, temperatures equal to or higher than 40°C (104°F) in 40% of patients, and temperatures equal to or higher than 41°C (105.8°F) in 13%. The elevation in temperature usually occurs either at the same time or after the onset of motor signs.[11a] It usually reaches a peak within 48 hours.[8]

Table 1
Clinical Signs of Neuroleptic Malignant Syndrome

Hyperthermia

Muscle rigidity:
  lead pipe, plastic, cogwheel

Autonomic dysfunction:
  Respiratory—tachypnea, dyspnea
  Cardiovascular—arrhythmia, tachycardia, lability of blood pressure, hypotension, hypertension
  Other—diaphoresis, pallor, flushing of the skin, urinary incontinence, dysuria

Mental status change:
  agitation, lethargy, muteness, confusion, delirium, stupor, coma

Movement disorders:
  akinesia, bradykinesia, tremor, dystonia, chorea, myoclonus

Other neurological signs:
  seizures, ataxia, nystagmus, gaze paresis, ocular fluttering, reflex changes, Babinski signs

Muscle rigidity is typically described as being "lead-pipe" or "plastic" in nature.[3,7,10,12] Cogwheel rigidity, as seen in parkinsonism, has also been described.[13] Rigidity is reported in over 90% of patients.[7–9,11,14] It may be severe enough to result in a decrease in chest wall compliance resulting in tachypneic hypoventilation requiring respiratory support.[12,15] The presence of rigidity has led some investigators to conclude that NMS is a severe form of drug-induced parkinsonism.[16] However, the differences between these two drug-induced disorders (including treatment modalities) are significant enough to make this unlikely.[17] Other complications of muscle rigidity include muscle loss with secondary avulsions and orthopedic deformities of the hands and feet if the disorder is prolonged.[18] Rigidity of the muscles of the pharynx and esophagus may also result in dysphagia, dysarthria, and sialorrhea.[9,10,18] Other parkinsonian features that accompany rigidity are often seen. Akinesia (the loss of voluntary movements) and/or bradykinesia (slowness of movement) have frequently been described as features of NMS[3,7,10,12,15] occurring in nearly 40% in one study.[7] Tremor has also been well described with NMS.[8–10,12,19–21] Resting tremor, similar to that seen in Parkinson's disease[9] and, in addition, a coarse tremulousness of the trunk and extremities have been reported.[8] It occurs in approximately half of the patients with this syndrome.[7,9,11] In addition, parkinsonian gait disorder has also been rarely described.[9]

Varying dyskinesias have been reported in early papers on NMS.[1–3] Dystonia is probably the most frequent, occurring in approximately one-third of patients.[7,9,11,20,22] Blepharospasm,[9] opisthotonos,[9,15,23] oculogyric crises,[9,12,15,23] and trismus[9,15,23] may all represent manifestations of this movement disorder. Chorea, including oral-buccal-lingual dyskinesia, has also been well described[9,10,15,23] and is probably less frequent than dystonia.[9] Myoclonus has also been reported.[19] Other less common neurological features include seizures, Babinski signs, reflex changes, ataxia, nystagmus, gaze paresis, and ocular fluttering.[9,9a,11a,15,23–26]

Autonomic abnormalities other than hyperthermia are also frequently present. Cardiovascular autonomic changes include tachycardia, cardiac arrhythmias, and instability of blood pressure. Hypertension, hypotension, and lability of blood pressure have been described.[3,8–12,15,18,23,27] Diastolic hypertension has been found to be common and perhaps a specific early feature of NMS.[11,18] This may allow early detection when monitoring patients at risk. Autonomic changes affecting the respiratory system result in tachypnea and dyspnea.[3,8,9,12,23] Other dysautonomic features include diaphoresis, pallor, flushing of the skin, urinary incontinence, and dysuria.[3,8–12,15,18,23,27]

Alterations in mental status are a hallmark of NMS. In the early stages, there may be various degrees of fluctuating alertness. Patients may go from being alert, responsive, and perhaps even agitated to being more lethargic and mute. During this period, emotional distress, confusion, and delirium may predominate.[8,18] Some suggest that the variations in behavior associated with muteness, immobility, and lack of response may be the result of catatonic behavior.[27] Although mutism is a common manifestation of catatonia, it is not specific. Various combinations of the "classic" features should be present if a diagnosis of catatonia is to be considered. These features include catalepsy, waxy flexibility, automatic obedience, stereotypic mannerisms, and echophenomenon often associated with extremes of hyper- and hypoactivity.[28] At least three of these features should be present. These symptoms are not typically exhibited in NMS.[28] In general, catatonics frequently become withdrawn and lack any desire to cooperate or communicate. However, patients have been described as attempting to communicate but being unable to because of their muteness. In such cases, they are not actually withdrawn.[29] In addition, patients have been described as having "a striking, frightened facial expression." These patients apparently have an inability to speak because of an impending sense of doom and a high level of anxiety.[8] These findings would suggest that true catatonia does not occur in NMS. In the later stages, the fluctuating mental status may lead to depressed consciousness, stupor, and coma.[3,10,12,15,27] Some variation in consciousness occurs in 75% of patients.[9]

Laboratory Features (Table 2)

Laboratory findings in NMS are nonspecific but supportive of the diagnosis. There are two abnormalities, in particular, that are consistently found. The first is an elevation of creatine kinase (CK).[3,8–10,14,15,23,27] In reviews of previously reported cases, elevated CK was found in 44%,[9] 71%[14] 92%,[7] and 97%.[11] In a prospective evaluation of 24 consecutive patients with NMS, CK was elevated in all cases in which it was measured.[8] Elevations vary widely from >200 to hundred thousands. In one study,[8] 86% had elevations above 1,000 IU/L and 33% had elevations higher than 10,000 IU/L. The highest reported level was over 300,000.[7,19] The mechanism of CK elevation probably involves myonecrosis developing during the intense sustained muscle rigidity. Polymorphonuclear leukocytosis is the other consistently reported abnormality.[3,7–11,14,15,23] The elevation can be anywhere from 10,000 to 30,000 cells per mm^3.[15] It occurs

---

Table 2
Laboratory Features of Neuroleptic Malignant Syndrome

Elevated creatine kinase

Polymorphonuclear leukocytosis

Elevated aldolase, alkaline phosphatase, LDH, SGOT, SGPT

Hypocalcemia

Hypomagnesemia

Hypoferremia

Proteinuria

Myoglobinuria

in half to three-quarters of patients with NMS.[8,9,14] It may or may not be associated with a left shift. Other enzyme abnormalities include elevated aldolase,[23] alkaline phosphatase, lactate dehydrogenase, SGOT, and SGPT.[8,9,15,23] Although many of these enzyme abnormalities were thought to be hepatic in origin, in reviews of case reports, Rosebush et al.[8] have discussed the more likely possibility that these changes originate from muscle. All enzymes are elevated to a much lesser extent than CK. Only 14% of cases had an elevation in LDH above 1,000 IU/L. SGOT, which is elevated in about 80% of patients, rarely goes above 700 IU/L, and SGPT, elevated in 64%, is rarely greater than 500 IU/L. Alkaline phosphatase has been elevated in a small number of patients and bilirubin is always normal.[8] Other features include hypocalcemia, which may be due to rhabdomyolysis. This was found to be present in about half of those with NMS and in all patients with CK elevated above 10,000. Hypomagnesemia was also observed in over 60% of patients.[8] Serum iron levels were found to be diminished in 95% of patients within a week. The etiology of this hypoferremia is thought to be related to muscle injury and may turn out to be an important marker for this illness.[8] Urinary changes include proteinuria and myoglobinuria.[8,15]

Neurological studies including CT scan, radionuclide brain scan, and cerebrospinal fluid evaluation are typically normal.[7–9, 11,15,23,27,29] Electroencephalogram may be normal or shows signs of diffuse slowing without focal changes. These findings are usually suggestive of a metabolic encephalopathy.[3,7–11,14,15,23,25,27,29]

Course and Complications (Table 3)

Once NMS develops, it usually progresses at a rapid rate. The syndrome typically reaches peak intensity within 72 hours.[2,3,9–12,15,27] This may vary, however, from 45 minutes to as long as 65 days.[7,11,19] Features of NMS may vary in severity and combination. Some of the less severe forms may represent aborted episodes due to rapid diagnosis and intervention. However, NMS may take on a mild self-limited course that clears quickly with little or no intervention and causes very little in the way of complications or sequelae.[30] Such cases are sometimes associated with or preceded by a mild viral illness. On the other hand, a very malignant course may occur that ultimately will result in death despite rigorous treatment. The overall duration of illness has varied from 8 hours to as

Table 3
Complications of Neuroleptic Malignant Syndrome

Respiratory:
  Tachypneic hypoventilation from decreased chest wall compliance
  Aspiration pneumonia
  Pulmonary embolism
  Pulmonary edema

Cardiovascular:
  Arrhythmia
  Myocardial infarction
  Cardiovascular collapse
  Cardiac Arrest

Renal:
  Prerenal azotemia
  Renal failure secondary to rhabdomyolysis

Neurological (long-term sequelae):
  Parkinsonism
  Tardive dyskinesia
  Dystonia
  Cerebellar degeneration (secondary to hyperpyrexia)
  Peripheral neuropathy
  Dementia progression
  Anoxic complications

long as 40 days.[9–11,15,18] This varies depending on whether oral or depot neuroleptics are the causative agents. With oral medications, NMS typically lasts about 13 days; however, depot drugs increase the duration 2 to 3 times.[10–12,15]

Approximately 40% of patients with NMS suffer from medical complications, many of which are life-threatening. The presence and severity of these complications depends primarily on the severity and duration of NMS. Respiratory complications most commonly result in death of the patients.[10,27] These include tachypneic hypoventilation from decreased chest wall compliance, aspiration pneumonia probably resulting from dysphagia, pulmonary embolism secondary to phlebitis and immobility, and pulmonary edema.[9,9a,10,12,14,15,27] Approximately 20% of patients require endotracheal intubation and respiratory support.[8,9a] Cardiovascular complications include arrhythmia, myocardial infarction, cardiac arrest, cardiovascular collapse, and phlebitis.[3,9,9a,10,14,15] Renal complications include prerenal azotemia and renal failure.[3,8–10,14,15] Renal failure is generally the result of myoglobinuria from rhabdomyolysis and hemodynamic factors.[7,9a] If death occurs, it usually does so within 30 days.[3,15,19] Early reviews reported a mortality rate between 11% and 30% in NMS.[3,7,9,9a,11,19] This seems to be changing as the result of increased recognition of the syndrome and early, aggressive treatment.

Long-term sequelae have rarely been reported in patients recovering from NMS. Levenson[31] reported four patients followed 2 to 11 years and found no cognitive or neurological sequelae and no chronic changes in serum CK or white blood cell measures. Of those abnormalities described, parkinsonism is the most frequent. It was observed in three patients followed for 5 months[8] and in four others after 10 months.[32] Permanent dystonia has also been described.[7] Tardive dyskinesia (oral-buccal-lingual dyskinesia) was observed in three patients after 3, 5, and 6 months.[32,33] Peripheral neuropathy[34] and cerebellar degeneration, perhaps from hyperpyrexia,[35] have also been reported. In two patients, anomia lasted several weeks but eventually cleared.[8] One patient had a worsening of dementia that lasted 3 months before the patient returned to baseline.[8] In two others, the worsened dementia was still present after 10 months.[32] Should anoxia occur during an episode, complications such as memory deficits and alterations in level of consciousness may be observed.[7]

Situations Resulting in NMS (Table 4)

NMS was originally described in psychiatric patients treated with neuroleptics[1-3] It is now clear that NMS is not confined to psychiatric patients only.[6] All groups of neuroleptics have been associated with NMS, including phenothiazines, butyrophenones, and thioxanthenes. The drugs most commonly associated with this disorder are haloperidol and fluphenazine alone or in combination with other neuroleptics.[3,8-10,12,14,15,27] Levenson[9a] has suggested that the high association with haloperidol may be related to its frequent use. This needs further evaluation. In addition, clozapine, a new antipsychotic drug that causes few extrapyramidal side effects, has been implicated in a case of NMS.[36] In most cases, serum levels are therapeutic and not toxic, suggesting that this is not an overdose phenomenon.[10,29,37] Despite these findings, other studies have indicated that it still may be a dose-related phenomenon.[8] Allan and White[21] revealed a clear relationship between drug concentrations and NMS.

Table 4

Situations Resulting in Neuroleptic Malignant Syndrome

Psychiatric patients (any diagnosis):
    Treated with neuroleptic for the first time
    Treated with neuroleptic after a drug-free period
    Increase in neuroleptic dose or potency
    Dehydrated, metabolic disturbance, stable doses of neuroleptics
    Sudden withdrawal of amantadine

Nonpsychiatric, non-neurological patients:
    Treated with neuroleptics for sedation
    Treated with metoclopramide
    Cocaine abuse

Neurological patients:
    AIDS dementia treated with neuroleptics
    Huntington's disease treated with dopamine depletors
    Parkinson's disease:
        Sudden withdrawal of dopaminergic medications
        Treatment with neuroleptics
        "Off" periods
        "On-Off" treated with lithium

In their case, signs improved as concentrations of urinary fluphenazine metabolites decreased. Neuroleptic potency may also play an important role given the more frequent occurrence of NMS with more potent agents.

Many patients (60%) have a history of earlier uncomplicated neuroleptic exposure before the onset of NMS.[8] The disorder usually occurs when patients are treated for the first time, when neuroleptics are reintroduced after a drug-free interval, or if the dose is increased within a short period of time.[3,7,8,11] In a small number of cases, NMS may develop while the patient receives a stable dose of neuroleptic.[38] In these patients, it is possible that other risk factors such as agitation and dehydration may play an important role in the onset of the syndrome.[8] Psychiatric patients are frequently given amantadine to treat or prevent extrapyramidal side effects. In two reports, NMS occurred with cessation of this drug.[39,40] An unusual picture is the apparent occurrence of NMS in psychiatric patients who experience the sudden reduction or cessation of neuroleptics.[41,42] In these patients, the syndrome probably began before the drug doses were diminished and continued to progress to a clearly recognizable stage after the drugs were stopped.[41]

Any patient on neuroleptics is at risk for NMS. Evaluation of psychiatric diagnoses preceding the onset of NMS indicates that approximately 50% of patients have a diagnosis of schizophrenia.[7,9,9a,11] Affective disorders have been reported less commonly.[11–44] However, in a 6-year prospective study, two-thirds of the patients diagnosed had an underlying affective disorder.[8] Other psychiatric diagnoses have included acute psychosis, atypical psychosis, brief reactive psychosis, schizophreniform psychosis, paranoia, character disorder and postpartum psychosis.[3,7–9a,11,43]

Finally, treatment with the combination of a neuroleptic and lithium may result in a more severe course in NMS.[12,32] Lithium by itself does not cause NMS. In the acute manic state of manic-depressive psychosis, neuroleptics are frequently utilized in combination with lithium. Since lithium requires 5 to 10 days to become effective, neuroleptics are given for immediate amelioration of symptoms.[32,33] In 1974, Cohen and Cohen[32] described a rare "severe encephalopathic syndrome" in four patients treated with lithium and haloperidol. Each patient experienced hyperpyrexia, mental status change, and parkinsonian signs and symptoms. The syndrome described by Delay and associates[1,2] was not mentioned in the paper but the descriptions were typical of NMS. In two cases, symptoms did not clear until lithium was discontinued. All patients suffered from long-term sequelae, most notably oral-buccal-lingual dyskinesia. It was concluded that a "sumative or synergistic effect" between the two drugs caused the syndrome. Spring and Frankel[33] reported a similar case caused by the same drug combination. They noted that the syndrome was identical to NMS except for the residual dyskinesia. These residual findings suggested that lithium may have enhanced the NMS. Since lithium can worsen drug-induced parkinsonism, cause a recurrence of tardive dyskinesia, and decrease central dopaminergic transmission,[44] it was felt that lithium must be playing some enhancing role in NMS.[33] In particular, it was felt that patients in the acute manic state were susceptible to NMS when treated with this drug combination.[33] Since haloperidol alone can cause NMS and tardive dyskinesia and since the lithium/haloperidol combination is commonly utilized without adverse effects, it is not surprising that this role for lithium has met with some resistance.[12,15,33] Currently, it is difficult to prove whether or not any relationship between lithium and NMS actually exists.

NMS has been described in normal individuals. A patient treated with haloperidol presurgically to induce sedation experienced NMS after a single dose.[45] A single dose of trimeprazine, a phenothiazine utilized for sedation and pruritis, resulted in fatal NMS in a normal child.[46] Metoclopramide, an antiemetic, drug has also been reported to cause NMS.[47,48]

NMS also occurs in nonpsychiatric patients with neurological disease. Breitbart et al.[49] reported three patients with AIDS dementia and NMS secondary to neuroleptic therapy. Burke et al.[4] reported NMS in a patient with Huntington's disease treated with tetrabenazine and alpha-methyl-tyrosine. In Parkinson's disease, NMS may occur in several situations. It may occur with sudden withdrawal of levodopa or with sudden withdrawal of levodopa and bromocriptine, as in a "drug holiday."[5,26,50–52] Withdrawal of antiparkinsonian medications including levodopa and amantadine in patients with Parkinson's disease and psychiatric disease treated with neuroleptics may result in NMS.[23,53] NMS may also occur during an "off" period in patients with "on/off" phenomenon.[54] An "off" period is pharmacologically similar to medication withdrawal. A NMS-like syndrome may also occur in parkinsonian patients treated with lithium for "on/off" phenomenon.[20,54]

Recently, NMS has been reported in association with cocaine abuse.[55] After cessation of acute intense cocaine abuse, seven people experienced a syndrome that resulted in rapid death. Clinical features included hyperthermia, delirium, and agitation followed by akinesia and various degrees of rigidity. In each case, respiratory failure and death ensued within hours. This syndrome most likely represents NMS.

Differential Diagnosis (Table 5)

NMS is a clinical diagnosis based on the presence of the proper historical setting and the characteristic constellation of signs. Levenson[9a] devised criteria as a guide to proper diagnosis. He considered fever, rigidity, and elevated serum CK as "major" criteria and tachycardia, abnormal blood pressure, tachypnea, altered consciousness, diaphoresis, and leukocytosis as "minor" features. NMS was diagnosed if all three major features or two major and four minor features were present. Although these criteria are not universally accepted,[11a] they are helpful in making a diagnosis. There are a number of illnesses and syndromes that are characterized by features seen in NMS. In the fully developed syndrome, these disorders can

Table 5

Differential Diagnosis of Neuroleptic Malignant Syndrome

Medical disorders:
  Infection (encephalitis, meningitis, meningoencephalitis)
  Postinfectious encephalomyelitis
  Tetanus
  Drug allergy
  Diabetic ketoacidosis
  Metabolic encephalopathy
  Tetany
  Strychnine poisoning
  Myocardial infarction

Malignant hyperthermia

Heat stroke (induced by phenothiazines)

Lethal catatonia

Other drug reactions:
  Central anticholinergic syndrome
  Monoamine oxidase inhibitor intoxication
  Monoamine oxidase inhibitor interactions with meperidine, dextromethorphan, tricyclic antidepressants
  Other neuroleptic-induced syndromes: parkinsonism, acute dystonic reactions, tardive dyskinesia/dystonia, mixed extrapyramidal syndromes

Polymyositis

Brain stem stroke (locked-in syndrome)

Wilson's disease (acute dystonic form)

be differentiated; however, in the early and very late stages, this may not be easy.[56] Since NMS is potentially fatal, any situation in which this diagnosis is considered warrants immediate treatment.

A diagnosis of NMS is further assured if other causes of febrile illness are ruled out. Most important in the differential diagnosis is *infection*. Any infection can result in elevation of temperature. Central nervous system infection such as encephalitis, meningitis, or meningoencephalitis can result in elevated temperature, mental status changes, increases in muscle tone and autonomic features.[8,9,15,18] Infection may be viral, bacterial, or fungal in origin. Lumbar puncture and CT scan are warranted in these patients. In many cases, antibiotics are often initiated as treatment for NMS is started. NMS and infection may coexist. NMS predisposes patients to infection because of dysphagia, respiratory complications, and immobility. Infection may increase the risk of NMS.[8] Other considerations related to infection include *postinfectious encephalomyelitis* and *tetanus*.[9] When NMS arises after starting a new neuroleptic, another possibility to consider is *drug allergy*.[4,8,23] In one study, 7 of 20 patients had a skin rash during development of NMS.[8] Absence of eosinophilia and lack of a consistent relationship between initiation of neuroleptics and onset of the rash make it unlikely that NMS is an allergic reaction.[8,23] In either case, withdrawal of the offending agent is necessary. Other medical illnesses to consider include *diabetic ketoacidosis, tetany, metabolic encephalopathies* (renal or hepatic), *myocardial infarction* (because of elevated CK), and *strychnine poisoning*.[57]

There are a number of disorders which have features very similar to NMS. They are usually differentiated by a clear history and knowledge of the situation in which the disorder arose. Most important of this group is *malignant hyperthermia* (MH).[4,8,9,15,23] MH is a myopathic disorder with varied inheritance (autosomal dominant and recessive forms are reported). This disorder generally occurs immediately after exposure to halogenated inhalation anesthesics and depolarizing muscle relaxants, such as succinylcholine. Within minutes of exposure, symptoms of hyperpyrexia, muscle rigidity, and changes in mentation occur. There is an associated elevation in CK and myoglobinurea. The disorder is felt to be the result of an abnormality of muscle membranes. In particular, there appears to be defective regulation of the transport of calcium in the sarcoplasmic reticulum in the presence of general anesthetic agents. MH occurs frequently in patients who have other myopathic disorders such as muscular dystrophy, myotonic dystrophy, and congenital myopathies. In addition, there is often a family history of anesthesia-associated MH and possibly death. In those at risk for MH, there usually is an elevation in resting CK. In addition, relatives may also have a high resting level of CK. MH is treated with dantrolene sodium, a muscle relaxant that may inhibit the release of calcium ions from the sarcoplasmic reticulum.[9] Because of similarities in clinical features of MH and NMS, a similar pathophysiological mechanism has been proposed.

Phenothiazines impair heat dissipation mechanisms by interrupting temperature regulation and inhibiting sweating, especially on hot humid days and in association with exercise or agitation. The resulting syndrome is *heat stroke*. This disorder manifests with hyperpyrexia, a depressed level of consciousness, and pallor. Muscle rigidity, profuse diaphoresis, and dyskinesias do not occur. The use of anticholinergic drugs in combination with neuroleptics may increase the risk of heat stroke, particularly in the elderly. This diagnosis should be considered in the differential diagnosis of NMS since the etiologic agents may be the same.[4,8,9,15,23] In either case, neuroleptics should be stopped and dehydration attended to.

NMS resembles the psychiatric disorder *lethal catatonia* (LC), a rare variant of catatonia. This disorder was described in the 19th century (long before neuroleptics became available) and has many names including Bell's mania, mortal catatonia, acute delirious mania, manic depressive exhaustion death, psychotic exhaustion syndrome, delirium acutum, and Scheid's cyanotic syndrome.[58,59] In 1934, Stauder[60] coined the term "lethal catatonia" when describing 27 cases. In 1987, Kalinowsky[61] felt a better term would be "pernicious catatonia" because it is not uniformly fatal. LC represents a syndrome that may occur in varying circumstances. It is most frequently seen in association with psychiatric disorders such as depression, mania, and psychosis (schizophrenia). In a small percentage (10–15%), it occurs in relation to organic illness including infection, cerebrovascular disorders, tumors, head injury, seizure disorders, and toxic-metabolic disorders.[58]

Clinical features of LC occur in three phases.[8,9,15,23,28,58] The prodromal phase, which lasts approximately 2 weeks, is characterized by a labile mood, insomnia, and anorexia. The hyperactive phase is most prominent. Intense motor excitement is characterized by violent destructive behavior, unprovoked assaultiveness, and suicide attempts. There is usually disorganization of thought, incoherent speech, hallucinations (visual and auditory), and bizarre delusions. Patients also demonstrate the classic features of catatonia and refuse nutrients. Autonomic features have been reported in this phase. These include tachycardia, diaphoresis, labile blood pressure, and cyanosis of extremities. Fever up to 110°F (43.3°C) also emerges in this phase which, lasts an average of 8 days but may continue for weeks. In the final phase, excitement gives way to exhaustion, electrolyte imbalance, extreme hyperthermia, stupor, coma, and cardiovascular collapse. In this phase, Stauder[60] described rigidity with bizarre posturing. This is not a common feature, and if rigidity is present, it is usually intermittent and alternates with flaccidity. The final phase lasts 36 hours to 4 days before death, which occurs in over 60%.

In the contemporary literature, this classic presentation is observed in approximately 70% of patients.[58] The other 30% present with a catatonic stupor without intense hyperactivity. In many of these patients, fever and rigidity occur after initiation of neuroleptics, suggesting that these may be cases of NMS in catatonic patients. Autopsy results in patients with LC have been unrevealing.[58] The pathophysiology of LC is hypothesized to be similar to NMS with abnormal dopaminergic transmission in mesolimbic/mesocortical pathways, resulting in catatonia and in the hypothalamus causing fever. This alteration occurs spontaneously and is not related to medications. Treatment of choice in LC is electroconvulsive therapy (ECT). Controversy surrounds the use or withdrawal of neuroleptics. Mann and associates[58] suggest that withdrawal of these medications is the best route to take. Finally, corticosteriods and ACTH have been utilized with some success.

Some authors claim that NMS and LC may be impossible to differentiate,[9,15] while others feel they may be the same disorder.[62] Mann and associates[58,63] suggest that NMS might be viewed as a "neuroleptic-induced toxic or iatrogenic form of organic lethal catonia." Similarities include fever, stupor, coma, rigidity, and response to ECT. Differences are more conspicuous and can allow for differentiation on a clinical basis.[59] LC does not occur in relation to neuroleptic therapy. When seen in the early stages, LC is easily distinguished from NMS since it is a syndrome of hyperactivity and resulting exhaustion and not a drug reaction. Although hyperactivity may be a risk factor in NMS, it is not as constant a feature and does not reach the extremes of that seen in LC. Some investigators[63] suggest using the time of onset of hyperpyrexia to differentiate "classic" LC from NMS. In NMS, fever does not occur during excitement but afterwards when the typical features emerge. In LC, hyperthermia starts in the excitement phase and progresses relentlessly. Rigidity and posturing are variable features of LC while extrapyramidal signs and symptoms are characteristic of NMS. Catatonia is always present in LC, but the classic features are notably absent in NMS. Treatment of the two syndromes is different. Although ECT may be useful in treating NMS, it is not the treatment of choice. Finally, death rates are substantially higher in LC than NMS. It is when LC is seen in its final stage, resembling any "near-death acute confusional state," without clear history, and in the presence of neuroleptic therapy, that differentiation from NMS is difficult.[59]

Adverse reactions to non-neuroleptic psychotropic medications may be similar to NMS. Differentiation of these syndromes may be impossible since patients are frequently treated with multiple drugs. Patients may also have combined syndromes when treated with multiple medications.[63a] A *central anticholinergic syndrome* often results in confusion, mild temperature elevation, dry flushed skin, dry mouth, dilated pupils, decreased bowel sounds, and urinary retention. Superficially this may appear similar to NMS; however, in NMS, there is diaphoresis and no change in pupillary function or dry mouth. In addition, anticholinergic toxicity does not result in rigidity or CK elevation.[8,15] *Monoamine oxidase (MAO) inhibitors* by themselves or in combination with other medications may result in adverse effects appearing similar to NMS. Overdose of monoamine oxidase inhibitors can result in agitation, delirium, hyperpyrexia, convulsions, and hypertension.[15,57] These toxic symptoms may take up to 12 hours to develop. The concurrent administration of meperidine or dextromethorphan and monoamine oxidase inhibitors results in agitation, delirium, hypotension, hyperpyrexia, and even death. Concurrent administration of tricyclic antidepressants with MAO inhibitors can result in a similar syndrome.[57] In none of these cases are patients rigid nor do they have elevation of CK.

Other syndromes inducing increased muscle tone, akinesia, dyskinesia, and elevations in CK can be differentiated from NMS on the basis of the history and physical findings. These include *neuroleptic induced parkinsonism, acute dystonic reactions, tardive dyskinesia/ dystonia,* and *combined drug-induced extrapyramidal syndromes.*[9a,64,65] *Polymyositis* and *brain stem infarction* resulting in a "locked in" syndrome might also be considered. Finally, the rare *acute dystonic form of Wilson's disease,* which occurs preterminally and is characterized by dystonia, rigidity, fever, and rapid emaciation should be considered. One case has been reported with elevated serum CK. This disorder may be difficult to differentiate from NMS, particularly if the diagnosis of Wilson's disease is not known.[66]

Epidemiology

The incidence of NMS is not actually known but it is rare. A number of publications (reviews, retrospective and prospective studies) have reported that the incidence ranges from 0.01% to greater than 2% in those treated with neuroleptics.[3,7,15,38,67–69] However, the three separate prospective evaluations since 1987 have reported frequencies below 1%.[38,67,69] Keck et al.[67] diagnosed six cases in an acute-care hospital setting from 679 patients treated with neuroleptics over an 18-month period. This suggests an incidence of 0.9% ($\pm$ 0.3%). Friedman and associates[38] diagnosed one case of NMS from 495 patients treated with neuroleptics in a state hospital over a 6-month period. This finding indicates a frequency of 0.2%. Finally, Gelenberg and associates[69] examined the incidence of NMS in a short-term psychiatric hospital over 1 year. Of 1470 patients treated with neuroleptics, NMS was diagnosed in one patient. This indicates an incidence of 0.07% (95% confidence interval 0.007%–0.4%). Reasons for a lower incidence in this hospital were thought to be related to the short stay of patients, use of modest doses of neuroleptics, and fewer false-positive diagnoses of NMS. Since prospective analyses lack the methodological flaws of retrospective studies, it would be likely that an incidence of <1% is accurate and supports the earlier notion that this syndrome is rare. In all studies, only psychiatric patients treated with neuroleptics were evaluated. The frequency of NMS in other at-risk groups has not yet been examined.

A number of reviews of case reports indicate that there may be a male predominance in this disorder, with a ratio of approximately 2:1 (male:female).[3,7,9a,11,14] It is unclear whether these findings suggest a true increased susceptibility in males. Alternatively, there may be a predominance of male subjects in populations treated with neuroleptics, or males may require treatment with higher doses of more potent neuroleptics more often than females. In one prospective study of 20 consecutive patients with this disorder seen over 6 years, the male to female ratio was the opposite, 1:2.[8] Although Caroff[3] initially reported a higher incidence in young patients, age of onset has been shown to vary from 1 to 92 years.[7,8,11,38]

Pathogenesis

The pathogenesis of NMS is not completely understood. It is generally accepted that alterations in dopaminergic transmission in the central nervous system associated with drug therapy is the most important mechanism. Abnormalities in muscle membrane function, changes in peripheral and central sympathetic outflow, and alterations in central serotonin metabolism have also been suggested. It is possible that all mechanisms simultaneously play a role in the pathogenesis of this disorder.

Central Dopaminergic Systems

That central dopaminergic mechanisms are important in the pathogenesis of NMS is strongly suggested by a number of clinical observations. These include the situations in which the disorder arises,[6] signs and symptoms,[37] and the response to dopamine replacement or dopamine agonist therapy. The treatment situations that result in NMS all have one feature in common: a decrease in central dopaminergic transmission. Neuroleptics, clozapine, and metoclopramide all act by blocking central dopamine receptors.[70] Those agents with the strongest ability to block dopamine receptors are most commonly associated with NMS, indicating that this feature is important.[15] Tetrabenazine and alpha methyltyrosine are central dopamine depletors that can cause NMS. Withdrawal of dopaminergic agents in Parkinson's disease and sudden "off" periods also result in a decrease in dopaminergic activity. Cocaine blocks dopamine reuptake in the synapse. As a result, there is an initial increase in dopaminergic activity in the synapse; however, continuous use ultimately leads to depletion of dopamine in the presynaptic neurons and secondary receptor changes. With a sudden cessation of cocaine use, a relative decrease in postsynaptic dopamine availability occurs.[55]

Many of the clinical features of NMS can be readily explained by central dopaminergic blockade.[27] Rigidity, akinesia, and dyskinesias are most probably the result of nigrostriatal dopamine pathway interruption.[10,12,23,26] Many of these features are seen in Parkinson's disease, which is a disease with known central dopamine deficiency. The role of dopamine in thermal regulation is well known.[71] These dopamine pathways are probably within the hypothalamus.[4,10,12,21,23,26] The preoptic hypothalamus is particularly concerned with thermal detection, and dopamine receptors have been located in this region.[55] The posterior hypothalamus is more involved with generation of effector signals.[23,26] Dopamine and dopamine agonists modulate hypothalamic temperature regulation while dopamine receptor antagonsists block this ability.[4,26] Hashimoto et al.[37] reported increased levels of prolactin in NMS which decreased as the serum neuroleptic levels did. Prolactin levels are regulated by hypothalamic-pituitary dopamine systems with a decrease in dopaminergic transmission resulting in increases in prolactin. Ansseau et al.[72] reported that apomorphine failed to elicit an adequate growth hormone response in a patient with NMS. These findings indicate that the hypothalamic dopamine system is altered in NMS. Interruption of the other central dopamine systems may explain mental status changes and autonomic dysfunction in NMS.[12] Further evidence that NMS is the result of a decrease in central dopaminergic activity derives from its response to dopaminergic agents. Bromocriptine, levodopa, and amantadine have all been found to be very useful in the treatment of NMS.

Cerebrospinal fluid studies of homovanillic acid (HVA) concentrations (the principle metabolite of dopamine) support the hypothesis that NMS is related to altered central dopaminergic transmission. Results of studies have varied, but the most common finding has been a decrease in HVA concentrations during NMS. These results suggest a decrease in dopamine metabolism during NMS. Nisijima and Ishiguro[73] reported these findings in eight patients who were compared to 10 normal controls. Verhoeven et al.[74] reported similar findings in a single case of NMS. They suggested that the decreased metabolism was due to abnormal sensitivity of presynaptic autoreceptors. Ansseau et al.[72] reported a slightly elevated HVA concentration in one patient while Granato and associates[75] reported normal HVA concentrations in one other case. The reasons for these discrepancies are unclear but may be related to timing of lumbar puncture, number of milliliters of fluid removed, and previous or concurrent therapy. One group[74] noted that HVA levels returned to normal with bromocriptine therapy. Another group[73] found that lower levels of HVA continued 14 to 121 days after recovery from NMS. The significance of these findings is not clear.

A definite pathological lesion has not been identified in NMS. In two reports, hypothalamic abnormalities were described. Jones et al.[76] described tiny parenchymal hemorrhages and perivascular hemorrhage within the hypothalamus. In addition, tiny foci of acute ischemia were described in the globus pallidus, internal capsule, and lateral corpus callosum. Horn et al.[77] found bilateral foci of pyknosis and disintegration of neurons and sponginess within the anterior and lateral hypothalamic areas and the tuberal nuclei. Less severe changes were seen in the ventral medial hypothalamic nucleus. Scattered petechial hemorrhages were also present in the periventricular gray matter of the anterior and posterior hypothalamus. The basal ganglia was not involved. Cerebral cortex had widespread small foci of nuclear pyknosis and increased cytoplasmic acidophilia, with vacuolation and disintegration of neurons. On the other hand, normal brain has been described,[29] and in patients with Parkinson's disease and NMS, autopsy findings have been typical of Parkinson's disease with no additional pathological changes.[51,54]

Muscle

NMS and MH share the clinical features of hyperthermia, muscle rigidity, and elevations in CK. It has been suggested that these two disorders may share pathophysiology as well.[76,78] The symptoms and signs of MH result from defective membrane regulation of the transport of calcium in the presence of particular general anesthetics. Therefore, MH is considered to be a primary disorder of muscle. Despite overwhelming evidence that NMS is the result of disruption of central nervous system dopaminergic pathways, muscle abnormalities similar to those seen in MH may exist.[10,76] In order to explore this possibility, muscle from patients with NMS has been studied by examining halothane- and caffeine-induced contraction of muscle fibers and by pathological evaluation. A screening procedure utilized for MH involves exposing muscle biopsy specimens to various concentrations of halothane and caffeine. Those at risk for MH have strong muscle contractions with small concentrations of these agents. The contractions are the result of changes in permeability and a sudden rise in intracellular calcium. Using muscle strips, Caroff et al.[78] found muscle from a patient with NMS to be as sensitive to halothane as muscle from MH would be. In single fiber studies, Araki et al.[79] observed that six of eight NMS patients had increased sensitivity to caffeine. It should be noted that neuroleptics can interfere with sarcoplasmic reticulum function in pharmacological concentrations by causing release of calcium in a manner similar to that of caffeine and halothane. Muscle strips from an NMS patient tested with fluphenazine demonstrated increased contraction and an increase in the release of calcium.[78] Muscle from patients with MH did not respond in the same manner. Muscle from patients with NMS and MH appear to be oversensitive to agents that cause muscle contraction.

Pathological studies have also supported the role of direct muscle involvement. In one study,[79] type IIB atrophy was seen in six cases of NMS. Electron microscopy showed glycogen particles accumulated in intermyofibrillar spaces in all examined muscles. Mitochondria were either disrupted or were shown to have inner membrane and cristae swelling. Another report[76] described increased muscle fiber size, which was "myopathic" in appearance, and acute disseminated segmental necrosis with regeneration and occasional multivacuolated fibers. However, normal muscle biopsy in NMS has also been described in a psychiatric patient,[29] one parkinsonian patient,[51] and a patient with Huntington's disease.[4] Despite clinical, pathophysiological, and pathological similarities, NMS and MH are distinct disorders. In NMS, many of the features are the result of abnormalities in the central nervous system while all features of MH are the result of peripheral myopathic disturbances. The situations resulting in MH and NMS are distinct. In addition, the clinical course of the two disorders differs. Following a short exposure to anesthetic agents, MH has an explosive onset reaching a plateau in hours. In NMS, onset can occur anywhere from hours to weeks after changes in neuroleptic medication, and may even occur at stable doses. NMS progresses less rapidly, reaching a plateau in about 3 days. The mortality rate of MH is approximately 70% while in NMS, early estimates were 20%.[3] In NMS, diazepam, curare, and pancurium result in muscle flaccidity while this does not occur in MH.[10,15,27,29] MH does not seem to occur in patients with a history of NMS or in their families.[4,31,80,81] It seems that some abnormality of muscle is present in NMS. Whether or not this abnormality causes some features of NMS or is the result of NMS is not clear.

Peripheral and Central Sympathetic Systems

Some features of NMS may be the result of interruption of the sympathoadrenomedullary system.[82] In one case, urinary and plasma catecholamines were increased during an episode of NMS. After the patient recovered, the catecholamine levels returned to normal. This abnormality may play an important role in autonomic dysfunction in this disorder. The reason for this increase in turnover of catecholamine in the adrenal medulla is unclear; however, dopamine receptors are present in the adrenal gland[83] and blockade of these receptors may be important. The significance of these abnormalities in the pathophysiology of NMS remains to be proven. There is also evidence suggesting that central sympathetic function is affected. In one report,[73] noradrenalin concentrations in CSF were increased during an episode of NMS and returned to normal with recovery. In addition, a clonidine challenge test, which assesses central alpha noradrenergic receptor sensitivity, failed to generate an adequate response.[72]

Central Serotonergic Systems

The concentration of 5-HIAA (the principle serotonin metabolite) was diminished in the CSF of eight patients during an NMS episode.[73] The significance of this finding is unclear.

Risk Factors

Decreased dopaminergic transmission is a necessary factor in NMS. However, there are other factors that may result in an increase in susceptibility. In a number of reports, physical exhaustion and dehydration were present in patients prior to the onset of NMS.[8,15,27,53] Evidence of the importance of dehydration is found in a description of four patients in whom NMS occurred despite stable doses of neuroleptics. Each of these patients became dehydrated just before the onset of the disorder.[8] Hyponatremia, hypokalemia,[84,85] thyrotoxicosis, and hypothyroidism[86] have also been considered as factors that might increase the risk of NMS. In a case control study, Keck et al.[86a] found that psychomotor agitation prior to NMS was important. In addition, those patients with higher total mean and maximal doses of neuroleptics, those with a greater number of IM injections, and those with increasing doses were all at significantly higher risk for NMS. The clinical situation that seems most likely to predispose to NMS appears to exist in a patient with significant psychomotor agitation, physical dehydration, exhaustion, and perhaps mild hyperthermia, who is then treated with large and rapidly escalating doses of IM (or oral) dopamine antagonist drugs. It has been suggested that in this situation, treatment with lower doses of neuroleptics and the use of diazepam, carbamazepine, verapamil, and electroconvulsive shock therapy might prevent the onset of this potentially fatal disorder.[86a]

In the original description of NMS,[1,2] it was thought that this disorder would "supervene selectively in brain-damaged subjects ..." Some evidence to support this concept has been presented.[3,8] Rosebush et al.[8] found that 42% of 20 consecutive patients with NMS had another form of brain pathology. Other reviews, however, have not indicated that this is an important risk factor.[7,11]

Treatment

NMS is a potentially fatal but treatable disorder. A high index of suspicion in appropriate situations and early recognition and intervention are the keys to patient survival.[87] If the diagnosis is suspected, treatment should be initiated immediately. In those patients on neuroleptics, initial supportive steps include stopping the offending agent, treatment of dehydration with IV fluids, ice packs and cooling blankets for fever, correction of metabolic abnormalities, and support for renal, pulmonary, or cardiovascular complications. In an early review,[3] a mortality rate of approximately 20% was reported. This rate was probably the result of late recognition and treatment with supportive measures only. Mortality is likely due to the prolonged duration of symptoms.[75] Further steps are needed to shorten the duration of the clinical course and improve survival.

Since 1982, a number of drugs have been used in addition to supportive measures to treat NMS with good success. There have been no controlled therapeutic trials. All data are based on case reports. The two most frequently used drugs are dantrolene sodium[24,88–90] and bromocriptine[25,74,91–93a] or a combination of the two.[25,40,75] In a review of 67 cases,[14] 56 were treated with dantrolene, bromocriptine or a combination and the mortality rate was only 5%. It appears that early treatment with these drugs can shorten the course of NMS compared to supportive care alone[14] and improve the outcome. Dantrolene sodium, a muscle relaxant, was first utilized in NMS because of therapeutic success in MH. It has the advantage of being available in a parenteral form. Suggested doses of intravenous dantrolene are 2–3 mg/kg three or four times a day for a total of approximately 10 mg/kg per day. Higher doses may result in hepatotoxicity. Oral doses of 50 to 600 mg per day have been recommended.[15,18,88] Bromocriptine, a direct dopamine receptor agonist, was utilized because of the apparent central dopaminergic abnormalities in NMS. First used successfully in 1983,[92] it is now considered the treatment of choice in those patients in whom oral medications can be administered. The initial dose should be 2.5 to 5 mg t.i.d. with increasing increments of 2.5 mg t.i.d. every 24 hours until a response is seen. Total daily dose as high as 60 mg per day has been administered.[75] Despite the ability of this drug to induce psychosis, in this situation, it appears that it is well tolerated in both psychiatric and nonpsychiatric patients. Return to the original psychiatric state is related to improvement of NMS and not treatment with bromocriptine.[93a] It has been recommended that in patients who cannot swallow, intravenous dantrolene should be started and bromocriptine could replace it as the patient improves.[18] Others have suggested using dantrolene and bromocriptine in combination since they address different pathophysiological aspects of the disorder.[25,40,75] It has been suggested that dantrolene would diminish CK levels and fever while bromocriptine would improve the extrapyramidal aspects and mental status changes. Dhib-Jalbut et al.[25] have pointed out that in those treated with only supportive measures, it may take 14 days for the CK to begin to drop, 4–17 days for fever to decrease, and perhaps weeks for improvement in rigidity, with the entire syndrome lasting several weeks. With bromocriptine or combined bromocriptine and dantrolene, the CK dropped in 48 hours, fever diminished in 24 hours, rigidity diminished in 48 hours to 4 days, and autonomic changes reversed in 24–72 hours. The whole episode may resolve in a week. If the syndrome is caused by orally administered neuroleptics, treatment should be continued for at least 10 days since recurrence may develop with early withdrawal from treatment. When depot neuroleptics are utilized, 2–3 weeks of therapy may be warranted since it may take this time for the neuroleptics to be cleared. It may be helpful to follow these patients with serial CK levels, serial myoglobin levels in the urine and blood, and close monitoring of clinical features.

Other therapies have been beneficial in a small number of patients. Amantadine (100 mg t.i.d.) has been useful because of its dopaminergic effects.[94] It has been suggested that patients with milder cases of NMS be treated with amantadine while dantrolene and bromocriptine would be used in more severe cases.[95] Since amantadine therapy has failed to improve signs of NMS in some cases,[75] starting bromocriptine from the outset would be a more sound strategy. Levodopa has also been examined as a treatment for NMS with some success.[13,96] However, only a few cases have been reported and although one would expect it to be as efficacious as bromocriptine, it is not uniformly successful.[29] This may be related to timing and dosage since unsuccessful trials of bromocriptine have also been reported.[39] A single patient responded to treatment with combined levodopa and subcutaneous lisuride, a D_2 receptor agonist. The lisuride was started because the patient could not tolerate bromocriptine or levodopa at higher doses (nausea and vomiting). Parenteral forms of dopaminergic drugs (e.g., lisuride, apomorphine) may be useful in patients with dysphagia.[97] Benzodiazepines such as diazepam and clonazepam have also been variably successful.[20,25] Again this success is not uniform and an inadequate number of patients has been examined to judge their usefulness. Anticholinergic drugs such as benztropine, trihexyphenidyl, and diphenhydramine have often been the first drugs given to patients when NMS arises because of their effectiveness in other extrapyramidal syndromes such as acute dystonic reactions and parkinsonism. These drugs have not been useful in NMS and should not be administered if NMS is suspected.[3,24,88,90,92] No decrease in mortality or duration of NMS has been reported with these drugs. In fact, some report that anticholinergics may actually be harmful in patients with NMS.[91] The symptoms of hyperthermia, autonomic dysfunction, and elevated CK should lead one to suspect NMS and not other extrapyramidal syndromes.

Finally, electroconvulsive therapy (ECT) has been utilized to treat NMS and coexisting psychosis.[81,100] When an acutely psychotic patient develops NMS after administration of neuroleptics, cessation of the drugs could lead to worsening of psychosis and NMS. These patients are difficult to manage and ECT is considered appropriate. ECT in some instances has been used to treat Parkinson's disease.[98,99] It is thought to act by increasing nigrostriatal dopaminergic transmission. Of 17 NMS cases treated with ECT reviewed by Addonizio and Susman,[81] a rapid therapeutic response was obtained in eight. Four patients experienced cardiac arrhythmias, including ventricular fibrillation and cardiac arrest, indicating that ECT is not without serious adverse effects. Others had no response. In four patients treated with ECT for persistent psychosis shortly after NMS cleared, no recurrences of NMS were seen despite reinstitution of neuroleptic therapy. The role, if any, of ECT as a treatment modality in NMS remains to be established.

In the case of Parkinson's disease where NMS occurs from withdrawal of antiparkinsonian medications, the usual supportive measures should be started and parkinsonian medications should be reinstituted immediately.[52] This situation is more likely to arise during a "drug holiday." The use of drug holidays is currently in question.[101] This therapeutic measure should not be utilized except under very specific circumstances and under the close supervision of a movement disorder specialist. The patient should be hospitalized in each case and vital signs monitored closely. The decrease in usage of this therapeutic measure will most likely result in less frequent occurrence of NMS. In addition, patients with Parkinson's disease should be instructed not to abruptly stop their medications but to taper them if required.

Since NMS occurs most frequently in psychiatric patients treated with neuroleptics, it is likely that a large percentage will require retreatment with these antipsychotic agents at some time. Obvious questions include whether these patients can be safely rechallenged with neuroleptics and what factors are important in reducing the risk of recurrence of NMS? It is clear that neuroleptics can eventually be reintroduced successfully in a majority of patients.[102,103] Recurrences have been described as mild and self-limited in some patients while fatalities have also been reported.[102,103] While recurrences have occurred both early and late,[84] the most important factor that might reduce the risk is the time from resolution of NMS to the reintroduction of antipsychotic agents. Studies have demonstrated that waiting 2 weeks or more (longer with depot drugs) allows for a much safer rechallenge[102,103] In situations where neuroleptics are started sooner, the occurrence of NMS may actually represent an exacerbation of the original episode. This may also occur with early withdrawal of the treatment for NMS. The dopamine-blocking potency of the drug used in the rechallenge of patients is another factor that may alter the risk of recurrence. Since NMS may be related to degree of dopamine receptor blockade, it seems likely that lower potency drugs, such as thioridazine, may result in fewer recurrences. This has been substantiated in a number of studies.[102,104] For the same reason, if patients are restarted on the same drug that originally caused NMS or one of similar potency, use of lower doses would also allow for safer rechallenge.[102,103] Other factors that may reduce the risk of recurrence include making sure the patient is well hydrated and that no metabolic imbalances exist. After reintroduction of the drug, the patient must be monitored carefully for any signs of recurrent NMS.

Future Considerations

Major strides have been made in understanding NMS in the past decade. However, a good portion of the information presented is based on case reports, retrospective reviews of case reports, and uncontrolled studies performed on small numbers of patients. As a result, conflicting results and conclusions exist in the literature and many unanswered questions remain. Future goals include a better understanding of the pathogenesis and risk factors so that NMS can be prevented, improved treatment for those cases that do occur, and careful evaluation of clinical and laboratory features so that precise acceptable diagnostic criteria can be formulated. The key to reaching these goals involves controlled prospective studies of NMS. Rosebush et al.[8] have shown how useful prospective analysis can be in describing clinical features. Similar studies of the situations leading to NMS, CSF, serum, and urine examinations of catecholamines and metabolites, pharmacological (and neuroendocrinological) studies, and examination of risk factors should give us more information on the pathogenesis of this disorder. This will assist in our ability to recognize those patients with increased risk. In addition, controlled drug trials are important. Use of placebo would be questionable in a potentially fatal disorder, but comparison of currently available medications would help delineate which treatment is safest and most effective.

Acknowledgments: The authors would like to thank William J. Weiner, M.D., for his thoughtful suggestions and support. We would also like to thank Faith Wood for her assistance in preparation of the manuscript.

References

1. Delay J, Pichot P, Lemperiere T, et al. Un neuroleptique majeur non-phenothiazinique et non-reserpinique, l'haloperidol, dans le traitment des psychosis. Annales medicopsychologiques 1960; 118:145–142.
2. Delay J, Denicker P. Drug induced extrapyramidal syndromes. In: Vinken PJ, Bruyn GW, eds. Handbook of Clinical Neurology Amsterdam, North Holland, 1968, pp 258–259.
3. Caroff SN. The neuroleptic malignant syndrome. J Clin Psychiatry 1980; 41:79–82.
4. Burke RE, Fahn S, Mayeux R, et al. Neuroleptic malignant syndrome caused by dopamine-depleting drugs in a patient with Huntington's disease. Neurology 1981; 31:1022–1026.
5. Toro M, Matsuda O, Mikizuchi K, Sugano K. Neuroleptic malignant syndrome-like state following withdrawal of antiparkinsonian drugs. J Nerv Ment Dis 1981; 169:324–327.
6. Genis D. Neuroleptic malignant syndrome: impaired dopaminergic systems? Neurology 1985; 35:1806.
7. Shalev A, Munitz H. The neuroleptic malignant syndrome: agent and host interaction. Acta Psychiatr Scand 1986; 73:337–347.
8. Rosebush P, Stewart T. A prospective analysis of 24 episodes of neuroleptic malignant syndrome. Am J Psychiatry 1989; 146:717–725.
9. Kurlan R, Hamill R, Shoulson I. Neuroleptic malignant syndrome. Clin Neuropharmacol 1984; 7:109–120.
9a. Levenson JL. Neuroleptic malignant syndrome. Am J Psychiatry 1985; 142:1137–1145.

10. Smego RA, Durack DT. The neuroleptic malignant syndrome. Arch Intern Med 1982; 142:1183–1185.
11. Addonizio G, Sussman VL, Roth SD. Neuroleptic malignant syndrome: review and analysis of 115 cases. Biol Psychiatry 1987; 22:1004–1020.
11a. Scrinvasan AV, Murugappan M, Kristamurty SG, Sayeed ZA. Neuroleptic malignant syndrome. J Neurol Neurosurg Psychiatry 1990; 53:514–516.
12. Szabadi E. Neuroleptic malignant syndrome. Br Med J 1984; 288:1399–1400.
13. Clarke CE, Shand D, Yuill GM, Green MHP. Clinical spectrum of neuroleptic malignant syndrome. Lancet 1988; 2:969–970.
14. Rosenberg MR, Green M. Neuroleptic malignant syndrome: review of response to therapy. Arch Intern Med 1989; 149:1927–1931.
15. Guze BH, Baxter LR. Neuroleptic malignant syndrome. N Engl J Med 1985; 313:163–166.
16. Cohen BM, Baldessarini RJ, Pope HG, Lipinski JF. Neuroleptic malignant syndrome. N Engl J Med 1985; 313:1293.
17. Adityanjee, Singh S, Singh G, Ong S. Spectrum concept of neuroleptic malignant syndrome. Br J Psychiatry 1988; 153:107–111.
18. Mueller PS. Diagnosis and treatment of neuroleptic malignant syndrome: a review. Neuroview 1987; 3:1–5.
19. Weinberg S, Twersky RS. Neuroleptic malignant syndrome. Anesth Analg 1983; 62:848–850.
20. Koehler PJ, Mirandolle JF. Neuroleptic malignant-like syndrome and lithium. Lancet 1988; 2:1499–1500.
21. Allan RN, White HC. Side effects of parenteral long-acting phenothiazines. Br Med J 1972; 1:221–222.
22. Lew TY, Tollefson G. Chlorpromazine-induced neuroleptic malignant syndrome and its response to diazepam. Biol Psychiatry 1983; 18:1441–1445.
23. Henderson VW, Wooten GF. Neuroleptic malignant syndrome: a pathogenetic role for dopamine receptor blockade? Neurology 1981; 31:132–137.
24. Coons DJ, Hillman FJ, Marshall RW. Treatment of neuroleptic malignant syndrome with dantrolene sodium: a case report. Am J Psychiatry 1982; 139:944–945.
25. Dhib-Jalbut, Hesselbrock R, Brott T, Silbergeld D. Treatment of neuroleptic malignant syndrome with bromocriptine. JAMA 1983; 250:484–485.
26. Figá-Talamanca L, Gualandi C, DiMeo L, et al. Hyperthermia after discontinuance of levodopa and bromocriptine therapy: impaired dopamine receptors a possible cause. Neurology 1985; 35:258–261.
27. Editorial. Neuroleptic malignant syndrome. Lancet 1984; 1:545–546.
28. Taylor MA. Catatonia: a review of a behavioral neurologic syndrome. Neuropsychiatry Neuropsychol Behav Neurol 1990; 3:48–72.
29. Morris HH, McCormick WF, Reinarz JA. Neuroleptic malignant syndrome. Arch Neurol 1980; 37:462–463.
30. Mezaki T, Ohtani SI, Abe K, et al. Benign type of malignant syndrome. Lancet 1989; 1:49.

31. Levenson JL, Fisher JG, Long term outcome after neuroleptic malignant syndrome. J Clin Psychiatry 1988; 49:154–156.
32. Cohen WJ, Cohen NH. Lithium carbonate, haloperidol and irreversible brain damage. JAMA 1974; 230:1283–1287.
33. Spring G, Frankel M. New data on lithium and haloperidol incompatability. Am J Psychiatry 1981; 138:818–821.
34. Anderson SA, Weinschank K. Peripheral neuropathy is a component of the neuroleptic malignant syndrome. Am J Med 1987; 82:169–170.
35. Lee S, Merriam A, Kim TS, Liebling M, Dickson DW, Moore GRW. Cerebellar degeneration in neuroleptic malignant syndrome: neuropathologic findings and review of the literature concerning heat related nervous system injury. J Neurol Neurosurg Psychiatry 1989; 52:387–391.
36. Muller T, Becker T, Fritze J. Neuroleptic malignant syndrome after clozapine plus carbamazepine. Lancet 1988; 2:1500.
37. Hashimoto F, Sherman CB, Jeffrey WH. Neuroleptic malignant syndrome and dopaminergic blockade. Arch Intern Med 1984; 144:629–630.
38. Friedman JH, Davis R, Wagner RL. Neuroleptic malignant syndrome: the results of a 6 month prospective study of incidence in a state psychiatric hospital. Clin Neuropharmacol 1988; 11:373–377.
39. Lazarus A. Neuroleptic malignant syndrome and amantadine withdrawal. Am J Psychiatry 1985; 142:142.
40. Rosse R, Ciolino C. Dopamine agonists and neuroleptic malignant syndrome. Am J Psychiatry 1985; 142:270–271.
41. Corrigan FM, Coulter F. Neuroleptic malignant syndrome, amitriptyline and thioridazine. Biol Psychiatry 1988; 23:320–321.
42. Spivak B, Weizman A, Wolovick L, et al. Neuroleptic malignant syndrome during abrupt reduction of neuroleptic treatment. Acta Psychiatr Scand 1990; 81:168–169.
43. Price DK, Turnbull GJ, Gregory RP, Stevens DG. Neuroleptic malignant syndrome in a case of post-partum psychosis. Br J Psychiatry 1989; 155:849–852.
44. Friedman E, Gershon S. Effect of lithium on brain dopamine. Nature 1973; 243:520–521.
45. Konikoff F, Kuritzky A, Jerushalmi Y, Theodor E. Neuroleptic malignant syndrome by a single injection of haloperidol. Br Med J 1984; 289:1228–1229.
46. Moyes DG. Malignant hyperpyrexia caused by trimeprazine. Br J Anaesth 1973; 45:1163–1164.
47. Robinson MB, Kennett RP, Harding AE, Legg NJ, Clarke B. Neuroleptic malignant syndrome associated with metoclopramide. J Neurol Neurosurg Psychiatry 1985; 40:1304.
48. Samie MR. Neuroleptic malignant-like syndrome induced by metoclopramide. Mov Disord 1987; 2:57–60.
49. Breitbart W, Marotta RF, Call P. AIDS and Neuroleptic malignant syndrome. Lancet 1988; 2:1488–1489.
50. Friedman JH, Feinberg SS, Feldman RG. A neuroleptic malignant-like syndrome due to L-dopa withdrawal. Ann Neurol 1984; 16:126–127.

51. Sechi GP, Tanda F, Mutani R. Fatal hyperpyrexia after withdrawal of levodopa. Neurology 1984; 34:249–251.
52. Hirschorn KA, Greenberg HS. Successful treatment of levodopa induced myoclonus and levodopa withdrawal-induced neuroleptic malignant syndrome: a case report. Clin Neuropharmacol 1988; 11:278–281.
53. Simpson DM, David GC. Case report of neuroleptic malignant syndrome associated with withdrawal from amantadine. Am J Psychiatry 1984; 141:796–797.
54. Pfeiffer RF, Sucha EL. "On-off"-induced lethal hyperthermia. Mov Disord 1989; 4:338–341.
55. Kosten TR, Kleber HD. Rapid death during cocaine abuse: a variant of neuroleptic malignant syndrome. Am J Drug Alcohol Abuse 1988; 14:335–346.
56. Friedman JH. Recognition and treatment of neuroleptic malignant syndrome. Curr Opinion Neurol Neurosurg 1988; 1:310–311.
57. Lazarus A. Neuroleptic malignant syndrome: detection and management. Psychiatr Ann 1985; 15:706–712.
58. Mann SC, Caroff SN, Bleier HR, et al. Lethal catatonia. Am J Psychiatry 1986; 143:1374–1381.
59. Castillo E, Robin RT, Holsboer-Trachler E. Clinical differentiation between lethal catatonia and neuroleptic malignant syndrome. Am J Psychiatry 1989; 146:324–328.
60. Stauder KH. Die toldliche katatonie. Arch Psychiatry Nervenkr 1934; 102:614–634.
61. Kalinowsky LB. Lethal catatonia and neuroleptic malignant syndrome. Am J Psychiatry 1987; 144:1106.
62. Kellam AMP. The neuroleptic malignant syndrome, so-called: a survey of the world literature. Br J Psychiatry 1987; 150:752–759.
63. Mann SC, Caroff SN. Lethal catatonia and neuroleptic malignant syndrome. Am J Psychiatry 1987; 144:1106–1107.
63a. Bennett DA. Combined neuroleptic malignant syndrome and central cholinergic syndrome. J Neurol Neurosurg Psychiatry 1990; 53:711.
64. Weiner WJ, Lang AE. Movement Disorders: A Comprehensive Survey, Mount Kisco, NY, Futura Publishing Co, 1989.
65. Factor SA, Matthews MK. Persistent dystonic-rigid syndrome caused by combined metoclopramide and prochlorperazine therapy. Southern Med J 1991; 84(5):626–628.
66. Denning TR, Berrios GE. Potential confusion of neuroleptic malignant syndrome and Wilson's disease. Lancet 1989; 2:43.
67. Keck PE, Pope HG, McElroy SL. Frequency and presentation of neuroleptic malignant syndrome: a prospective study. Am J Psychiatry 1987; 144:1344–1346.
68. Pope HG, Keck PE, McElroy SL. Frequency and presentation of neuroleptic malignant syndrome in a large psychiatric hospital. Am J Psychiatry 1986; 143:1227–1233.
69. Gelenberg AJ, Bellingham B, Wojcik JD, et al. A prospective survey of neuroleptic malignant syndrome in short-term psychiatric hospital. Am J Psychiatry 1988; 145:517–518.
70. Peringer E, Jenner P, Donaldson IM, Marsden CD, Miller R. Metoclo-

pramide and dopamine receptor blockade. Neuropharmacology 1976; 15:463–469.

71. Cox B, Dopamine. In: Lomax P, Schonbaum E (eds), Body Temperature, Regulation, Drug Effects and Therapeutic Implications, New York, Marcel Dekker, 1979, pp 234–255.

72. Ansseau M, Reynolds CF, Kupfer DJ, et al. Central dopaminergic and noradrenergic receptor blockade in a patient with neuroleptic malignant syndrome. J Clin Psychiatry 1986; 47:320–321.

73. Nisijima K, Ishiguro T. Neuroleptic malignant syndrome: a study of CSF monoamine metabolism. Biol Psychiatry 1990; 27:280–288.

74. Verhoeven WMA, Elderson A, Westenberg HGM. Neuroleptic malignant syndrome: successful treatment with bromocriptine. Biol Psychiatry 1985; 20:680–684.

75. Granato JE, Stern BJ, Ringel A, et al. Neuroleptic malignant syndrome: successful treatment with dantrolene and bromocriptine. Ann Neurol 1983; 14:89–90.

76. Jones EM, Dawson A. Neuroleptic malignant syndrome: a case report with post mortem brain and muscle pathology. J Neurol Neurosurg Psychiatry 1989; 52:1006–1009.

77. Horn E, Lach B, Lapierre Y, Hrdina P. Hypothalamic pathology in the neuroleptic malignant syndrome. Am J Psychiatry 1988; 145:617–620.

78. Caroff S, Rosenberg H, Gerber J. Neuroleptic malignant syndrome and malignant hyperthermia. Lancet 1983; 1:244.

79. Araki M, Takagi A, Higuchi I, Sugita H. Neuroleptic malignant syndrome: caffeine contracture of single muscle fibers and muscle pathology. Neurology 1988; 38:297–301.

80. Hermesh H, Aizenberg D, Lapidot M, Munitz H. Neuroleptic malignans. Neurology 1989; 39:1273.

81. Addonizio G, Susman VL. ECT as a treatment alternative for patients with symptoms of neuroleptic malignant syndrome. J Clin Psychiatry 1987; 48:102–105.

82. Feibel JH, Schiffer RB. Sympathoadenomedullary hyperactivity in neuroleptic malignant syndrome: a case report. Am J Psychiatry 1981; 138:1115–1116.

83. Bigornia L, Suozzo M, Ryan KA, Napp D, Schneider AS. Dopamine receptors on adrenal chromaffin cells modulate calcium uptake and catecholamine release. J Neurochem 1988; 51:999–1006.

84. Gibb WRG, Wedzicha JA, Hoffbrand BI. Recurrent neuroleptic malignant syndrome and hyponatremia. J Neurol Neurosurg Psychiatry 1986; 49:960–961.

85. Tomson CRV. Neuroleptic malignant syndrome associated with inappropriate antidiuresis and psychogenic polydipsia. Br Med J 1986; 292:171.

86. Moore AP, Macfarlane FA, Blumhardt LD. Neuroleptic malignant syndrome and hypothyroidism. J Neurol Neurosurg Psychiatry 1990; 53:517–518.

86a. Keck PE, Pope HG, Cohen BM et al. Risk factors for neuroleptic malignant syndrome: a case controlled study. Arch Gen Psychiatry 1989; 46:914–918.

87. Velamoor VR, Fernando MLD, Williamson P. Incipient neuroleptic malignant syndrome? Br J Psychiatry 1990; 156:581–584.

88. Goulon M, de Rohan-Chabot P, Elkharrat D, et al. Beneficial effects of dantrolene in the treatment of neuroleptic malignant syndrome: a report of two cases. Neurology 1983; 33:516–518.

89. May DC, Morris SW, Stewart RM, et al. Neuroleptic malignant syndrome: response to dantrolene sodium. Ann Intern Med 1983; 98:183–184.

90. Goekoop JG, Carbaat PA Th. Treatment of neuroleptic malignant syndrome with dantrolene. Lancet 1982; 2:49–50.

91. Dhib-Jalbut S, Hesselbrock R, Mouradian MM, Means ED. Bromocriptine treatment of neuroleptic malignant syndrome. J Clin Psychiatry 1987; 48:69–73.

92. Mueller PS, Vester JW, Fermaglich J. Neuroleptic malignant syndrome: successful treatment with bromocriptine. JAMA 1983; 249:386–388.

93. Zubenko G, Pope HG. Management of a case of neuroleptic malignant syndrome with bromocriptine. Am J Psychiatry 1983; 140:1619–1620.

93a. Adityanjee, Das P, Chawle HM. Neuroleptic malignant syndrome and psychotic illness. Br J Psychiatry 1989; 155:852–854.

94. McCarron MM, Boettger ML, Peck JJ. A case of neuroleptic malignant syndrome successfully treated with amantadine. J Clin Psychiatry 1982; 43:381–382.

95. Fogel BS, Goldberg RJ. Neuroleptic malignant syndrome. N Engl J Med 1985; 313:1292.

96. Harris M, Nora L, Tanner CM. Neuroleptic malignant syndrome responsive to carbidopa/levodopa: support for a dopaminergic pathogenesis. Clin Neuropharmacol 1987; 10:186–189.

97. Rodriguez ME, Luquin MR, Lera G, et al. Neuroleptic malignant syndrome treated with subcutaneous lisuride infusion. Mov Disord 1990; 5:170–172.

98. Fochtmann L. A mechanism for efficacy of ECT in Parkinson's disease. Convulsive Ther 1988; 4:321–327.

99. Douyon R, Serby M, Klutchko B, Rotrosen J. ECT and Parkinson's disease revisited: a "naturalistic" study. Am J Psychiatry 1989; 146:1451–1455.

100. Jessee SS, Anderson GF. ECT in the neuroleptic malignant syndrome: case report. J Clin Psychiatry 1983; 44:186–188.

101. Mayeux R, Stern Y, Mulvey K, Cote L. Reappraisal of temporary levodopa withdrawal ("drug holiday") in Parkinson's disease. N Engl J Med 1985; 313:724–728.

102. Rosebush PI, Stewart TD, Gelenberg AJ. Twenty neuroleptic rechallenges after neuroleptic malignant syndrome in 15 patients. J Clin Psychiatry 1989; 50:295–298.

103. Susman VL, Addonizio G. Recurrences of neuroleptic malignant syndrome. J Nerv Ment Dis 1988; 176:234–241.

104. Shalev A, Hermesh H, Aisenberg D, Munitz H. Neuroleptic malignant syndrome. N Engl J Med 1985; 313:1292–1294.

8

Antidepressant Therapy and Movement Disorders

David E. Riley, M.D.

Introduction

There are two important facets to the relationship between movement disorders and the treatment of depression: (1) movement disorders can be induced by drugs during the course of the treatment of depression, and (2) antidepressant therapies can affect pre-existing movement disorders. Both facets will be dealt with in this chapter.

A number of restrictions to the scope of this chapter must be cited. The discussion will be limited to therapies used mainly to treat the affective component of depressive illnesses (Table 1). Thus, drugs used for psychotic symptoms, specifically neuroleptics, will not be dealt with here (see Chapters 2–7). Similarly, anxiolytics, such as benzodiazepines, will not be covered (see Chapter 12). Drugs that have been dropped from production, such as nomifensine, will not be mentioned. The use of selegiline in Parkinson's disease will not be discussed, although this monoamine oxidase inhibitor was originally developed as an antidepressant. However, the area under review will be broadened by the inclusion of lithium, which is actually used

Lang AE, Weiner WJ (editors): *Drug-Induced Movement Disorders,* Mount Kisco, NY, © Futura Publishing Co., Inc., 1992.

Table 1

Antidepressant Therapies

---

1. Monoamine Reuptake Inhibitors
    Tricyclic
        imipramine (Tofranil, Janimine)
        desipramine (Norpramin, Pertofrane)
        trimipramine (Surmontil)
        clomipramine (Anafranil)
        amitriptyline (Elavil, Endep)
        nortriptyline (Pamelor, Aventyl)
        protriptyline (Vivactil, Triptil)
    A.   doxepin (Sinequan, Adapin)
    Tetracyclic
    B.   maprotiline (Ludiomil)
    Dibenzoxapine
    C.   amoxapine (Asendin)
    Triazolopyridine
    D.   trazodone (Desyrel)
    Aminoketone
    E.   bupropion (Wellbutrin)
    Phenyltolylpropylamine
    F.   fluoxetine (Prozac)

2. Monoamine Oxidase Inhibitors
    Hydrazine
        phenelzine (Nardil)
    A.   isocarboxazid (Marplan)
    Nonhydrazine
    B.   tranylcypromine (Parnate)

3. Electroconvulsive Therapy

4 Lithium

---

more for manic than depressive symptoms because of the clear association between mania and depressive disorders.

There are four major categories of therapy for affective disorders (Table 1), three are drugs and the other electroconvulsive therapy (ECT). The most commonly used pharmacological agents for depression may be collectively referred to as the monoamine reuptake (MARU) inhibitors. Acknowledging that inhibition of reuptake of catecholamines may not be the mechanism by which they exert their antidepressant effect,[1] this is nevertheless the shared biochemical property by which they are most readily identified. The original MARU inhibitor, imipramine, is a phenothiazine derivative that was relatively ineffective as an antipsychotic but was serendipitously found to have pronounced antidepressant effects. Many analogs were formulated and collectively came to be known as *tricyclic antidepressants* (Table 1) because of a common three-ring molecular structure. The tricyclics all share the ability to promote the effects of norepinephrine, serotonin, and, to a lesser extent, dopamine, by blocking their reuptake into presynaptic neurons, although their individual activities on each transmitter system vary (Table 2). In addition, many have pronounced anticholinergic effects. Nontricyclic MARU inhibitors are often lumped together as "atypical" antidepressants. Maprotiline has relatively conventional biochemical actions, but bupropion, fluoxetine, and trazodone are unusual in that they block reuptake of serotonin or dopamine more than norepinephrine. These relatively new agents with anomalous transmitter system preferences have the potential to be exploited for investigation

Table 2

Relative Potencies of Monoamine Reuptake Inhibitors on Major Monoamine Systems

Drug	Norepinephrine	Serotonin	Dopamine
amitriptyline	3*	3	5
amoxapine	2**	4	5
bupropion	5	6	4*
clomipramine	3	2*	5
desipramine	1**	4	5
doxepin	3*	4	5
fluoxetine	4	3*	5
imipramine	3*	3	5
maprotiline	2**	5	5
nortriptyline	2**	4	5
protriptyline	1**	4	5
trazodone	5	4*	6
trimipramine	4*	5	5

Numerical values reflect a descending potency from 1 to 6, as follows: the inhibitor constant for 1 = less than 1 nM, 2 = 1–10 nM, 3 = 10–100 nM, 4 = 100–1,000 nM, 5 = 1,000–10,000 nM, 6 = greater than 10,000 nM.
Based on data from reference 51.
* The drug's greatest potency for reuptake inhibition is on this neurotransmitter.
** The drug is highly selective for this neurotransmitter.

of the biochemical disturbances underlying movement disorders, as well as becoming useful therapeutic agents. Bupropion, for example, may prove to be the antidepressant of choice in Parkinson's disease because of its strong dopaminergic action, whereas fluoxetine may be more useful in some forms of serotonin-deficiency myoclonus. The antidopaminergic effect of amoxapine will be discussed.

Like MARU inhibitors, monoamine oxidase inhibitors also increase the efficacy of catecholamines released into the synapse, but they do so by suppressing their catabolism. The neurochemical actions of lithium on the brain show more experimental variability. The most consistent finding from clinical and animal studies is that lithium may enhance serotonergic activity.[2] It also appears to decrease cholinergic activity and block the development of dopamine supersensitivity, as measured by behavioral manifestations in animals.[2a] It is of interest that all three classes of drugs were first used for affective disorders in the late 1940s or early 1950s, and they lent a great deal of impetus to the rise of biological psychiatry as an accepted medical discipline.

The effects of ECT on neurochemical mechanisms are complex and include enhanced responsiveness of serotonin receptors, increased synthesis and release of norepinephrine, induction of dopamine receptor supersensitivity, and a modest down-regulation of muscarinic cholinergic receptors.[3] It is not clear whether any of these responses is related to the clinical efficacy of ECT.

Movement Disorders Induced by Antidepressant Therapy (Table 3)

To provide perspective regarding the epidemiologic importance of the disorders to be discussed, it should be stated that the frequency of movement disorders associated with antidepressant therapy does not approach that of disorders related to antidopaminergic drugs. Although antidepressants are widely used, the associations are often drawn from anecdotal evidence provided by individual case reports, with the notable exceptions of tremor and myoclonus (Table 3). Furthermore, the degree of familiarity with movement disorders appears to vary greatly from author to author, with consequently disparate terminology and ability to provide sufficient relevant descriptive detail. In short, the existence of many of these drug-

Table 3
Movement Disorders Caused by Antidepressants

Movement Disorder	Causative Agent	References
parkinsonism	fluoxetine	7, 8
	amoxapine	14
	phenelzine	23
	lithium	43, 44
tremor	MARU inhibitors	many (see text)
	MAO inhibitors	24*
	lithium	35, 36*
myoclonus	MARU inhibitors	20, 21*
	MAO inhibitors	25, 28*
	lithium	49, 50*
acute dystonic reaction	amitriptyline	10
	doxepin	10
	amoxapine	12
oculogyric crises	lithium	52
dystonia	trazodone	17
	tranylcypromine (?)	29
orofacial dyskinesias	trazodone	17
	amitriptyline	18
	ECT	30, 31
chorea	imipramine	19
	amitriptyline	19
	lithium	45–47
akathisia	amoxapine	13
tardive dyskinesia	amoxapine	15
tardive dystonia	amoxapine	11

* These are common side effects. References cited are selected from among many reports.
? = A particularly questionable association (see text).
MARU = Monoamine reuptake; MAO = monamine oxidase; ECT = electroconvulsive therapy.

movement disorder associations could be challenged on both clinical and epidemiological grounds.

Tricyclic Antidepressants

A rapid, low-amplitude action *tremor* can be found in up to 50% or more of patients receiving various tricyclics and represents one of the most common side effects in virtually all clinical trials of these drugs. It is thought to represent an "enhanced physiological tremor."[4] The mechanism of the enhancement is unknown, but the incidence is positively correlated with plasma drug concentrations.[5] The tremor may respond to propranolol.[6] It will disappear with dosage reduction or discontinuation of the drug.

Fluoxetine has produced *parkinsonism* in two patients, alone[7] or in conjunction with haloperidol.[8] Another patient developed reversible "severe, generalized muscular stiffness" on fluoxetine; examination findings were not recorded.[9]

An *acute dystonic reaction* has been reported in a patient treated with amitriptyline, and it recurred when she later received doxepin.[10]

There is a published report of a "dystonic reaction" to treatment with *amoxapine*.[11] However, the time course of evolution of the movement disorder and the brief worsening followed by resolution after discontinuation of the drug are more consistent with *tardive dystonia* than the acute dystonic reaction suggested by the author. In fact, amoxapine has been reported to induce *acute dystonia*,[12] *akathisia*,[13] *parkinsonism*,[14] and *tardive dyskinesia*.[15] Thus, amoxapine has been associated with virtually all of the major neurological syndromes produced by antipsychotic drugs. This is most likely related to the antidopaminergic effects exerted by the metabolite 7-hydroxyamoxapine, which has been shown to have a greater affinity for postsynaptic dopamine receptors than the antipsychotic loxapine.[16] Neither amoxapine itself nor its 8-hydroxy metabolite showed a similar binding property.

Trazodone has been linked to a reaction consisting of oromandibular and lingual dyskinesias, and dystonic posturing of the limbs.[17] The movement disorder began after 2 months of gradually increasing the dosage to 400 mg/day, and resolved 2 weeks after cessation of trazodone therapy. Treatment with amitriptyline has also been associated with reversible orofacial dyskinesias[18] in two patients. The authors interpreted these cases as examples of a tricyclic antidepressant causing "tardive dyskinesia," but there was no tardive relationship to the medication. They may represent a reaction to the anticholinergic properties of amitriptyline. Apart from amoxapine, as noted above, there are no convincing reports of tardive dyskinesia caused by antidepressant therapies.

Chorea is an extremely rare manifestation of acute MARU inhibitor poisoning, but has been well documented in two cases.[19] In each case, the chorea was temporarily relieved by intravenous physostigmine, suggesting that it resulted from the anticholinergic activity of the antidepressant drug.

Myoclonus is a common manifestation of acute toxicity of MARU inhibitors.[20] The association of myoclonus with tricyclic antidepressants in normal therapeutic doses has been studied carefully in a prospective fashion by Garvey and Tollefson.[21] They found that treatment with such agents led to "clinically significant" myoclonus in 9 of 98 patients. Four developed a peculiar sudden unsustained jaw closure that interfered with speech. In three patients, there was disabling upper limb myoclonus. The other two developed severe nocturnal myoclonus. All had stopped their medication or requested a change because of the myoclonus. All experienced a remission upon discontinuation of the offending agent, and the five who subsequently restarted the same drug all had a recurrence of the myoclonus. Less severe lower limb jerking was noted by 30 other patients, yielding an overall incidence of drug-induced myoclonus of 40%. MARU inhibitor-induced myoclonus has been associated with reversible increases in somatosensory evoked potential amplitudes, suggesting cortical excitation or disinhibition as a pathogenetic mechanism.[22] The neurochemical action of MARU inhibitors that can most readily be implicated in the production of myoclonus is the potentiation of serotonin.

Unilateral eye *tics* have been attributed to fluoxetine therapy in two patients.[22a] Although both clearly had abnormal involuntary contractions of the orbicularis oculi muscle, the classification of these movements as tics is questionable. In the better documented of the two cases, transient (10–20 seconds) episodes of ipsilateral subjective diminished hearing were also a feature. Both symptoms resolved after fluoxetine withdrawal but occurred again upon rechallenge.

Monoamine Oxidase (MAO) Inhibitors

A case of *parkinsonism* that resolved upon discontinuation was associated with a trial of phenelzine.[23]

Tremor is a common complication of treatment with MAO inhibitors. Evans and colleagues[24] prospectively analyzed side effects in 41 patients given phenelzine for depression. They found a 15% incidence of tremor, which was roughly comparable to the 21% incidence detected in another group treated with imipramine. The mechanism for the production of tremor is unknown.

Lieberman and colleagues[25] reviewed the subject of *myoclonus* induced by MAO inhibitors. They concluded that this was a common side effect that was chiefly manifested as twilight or nocturnal myoclonus, but daytime (i.e., during full alertness) myoclonus occurred as well. Myoclonus may be brought out by adding the serotonin precursor L-tryptophan to MAO inhibitor therapy.[26,27] However, this combination may also have antimyoclonic properties when given to patients with posthypoxic action myoclonus (see below). Further evidence of a role for serotonergic mechanisms in MAO inhibitor-induced myoclonus comes from a case report of relief by methysergide, a serotonin antagonist.[28]

Tranylcypromine was reported to produce truncal *dystonia* within 3 days of initiation of treatment in one patient.[29] The dystonia did not resolve with intramuscular benztropine, but did upon discontinuation of the MAO inhibitor. A rechallenge with tranylcypromine brought out the same dystonia. However, the same patient had a truncal dystonic reaction to propranolol, and so the specificity of the response to MAO inhibition must be questioned.

ECT

ECT was associated with the development of persistent tardive dyskinesia in three patients with ongoing or recent neuroleptic use.[30] In three patients with little, no, or only remote exposure to antidopaminergic drugs, ECT brought out orofacial dyskinesias that spontaneously resolved in 2 weeks to 6 months.[31] ECT has been purported to be a risk factor for tardive dystonia,[32] but this association was based on particularly meager data. ECT used as adjunctive therapy for schizophrenia has actually been associated with a lower prevalence of tardive dyskinesia, possibly by sparing patients from higher doses of neuroleptics.[33]

Brief post-ECT asterixis in one patient led to a search for metabolic disorders and an eventual diagnosis of primary hyperparathyroidism.[34] Given their relative rarity, post-ECT movement disorders should prompt a careful review of the preanesthetic and anesthetic drugs employed.

Lithium

Like the *tremor* induced by tricyclic antidepressants, that associated with lithium use is thought to represent an enhancement of physiological tremor. Its occurrence rate and severity increase with higher serum levels of lithium. Estimates of its incidence vary because of differing doses used or because of co-administration of other tremor-producing drugs, but generally fall in the range of 33% to 65%.[35] The mechanism of tremor amplification may involve β_2-adrenergic hyperactivity, as suggested by the greater response of the tremor to metoprolol given at nonselective doses, and to propranolol, than to metoprolol given at β_1 receptor-selective doses.[36] Lithium-induced tremor may improve in response to a variety of beta-blockers or from dosage reduction.

No better example of the confusion generated by reports of side effects of therapy for depression exists than the claim of a high frequency of "cogwheel rigidity" among patients chronically treated with lithium. The authors of one paper[37] perpetuated the misconception that "cogwheel rigidity" is a form of extrapyramidal disorder, whereas it actually represents a fusion of two distinct findings—cogwheeling and rigidity. The latter certainly is a manifestation of basal ganglia disease, but the cogwheel phenomenon is a sign associated with the presence of an action tremor.[38,39] It is commonly found in patients with essential tremor[40] who have no abnormalities of muscle tone. What the above authors most likely found was simply a cogwheel phenomenon in patients with lithium-induced tremor, superimposed upon normal tone or poor relaxation. The conclusion that lithium caused extrapyramidal side effects[37] was probably erroneous. This view is supported by the knowledge that the "cogwheel rigidity" failed to respond to anticholinergic medication[37] and that subsequent authors could not confirm the finding of rigidity in patients treated with lithium.[41]

Two patients reported to develop an "extrapyramidal syndrome" (parkinsonism) on lithium[42] can be dismissed on separate grounds. The first patient developed parkinsonism that was not affected by lithium administration or withdrawal, thus no association can be drawn. The second patient's manifestations were limited to tremor and "cogwheel rigidity." However, in a third patient, parkinsonism documented while taking lithium resolved upon drug withdrawal and recurred with subsequent exposures.[43] Another patient with lithium-induced parkinsonism also demonstrated orofacial and hand dyskinesias and foot dystonia. After 4 years, his movement disorders all stopped within days of cessation of the lithium.[44]

Chorea has been reported as a side effect of lithium in a small number of patients, possibly as a result of anticholinergic activity. In one case, the movement disorder recurred with haloperidol treatment.[45] In another case, the patient had been treated with antidopaminergic drugs intermittently for 6 years, and the chorea persisted for 3 months after lithium was stopped.[46] Thus, there is some question whether lithium directly caused the chorea or precipitated the emergence of a tardive dyskinesia. The latter conclusion conflicts with experimental evidence suggesting a protective effect of lithium versus tardive dyskinesia.[2,2a] Chorea was reported in one patient with no psychiatric history who became toxic from lithium sulfate taken as a sodium-free salt substitute.[47] Two cases of lithium poisoning[48] were interpreted elsewhere[46] as examples of chorea associated with lithium. However, the descriptions are limited to "twitches of the small muscles of the hands and face" that were accompanied by jerking of the whole limbs. There is no reason to have segregated these two cases from the other four in the report, all of whom evidently had myoclonus.

Lithium frequently causes *myoclonus* as a toxic manifestation or, at times, with therapeutic serum levels.[49] This is likely related to enhancement of serotonergic activity. The myoclonus reported to occur in one patient as a result of combined treatment with tricyclics and lithium[50] was clearly related to the initiation of lithium, and its cessation was just as clearly related to discontinuation of the drug. The authors' contention that the abolition of myoclonus was prompted by a switch in tricyclics ignores the prolonged excretion time of lithium (10–14 days) which was stopped 3 days earlier. Their assertion that desipramine is "a less potent serotonin reuptake blocker" than nortriptyline is not supported by published data showing that these two agents have virtually identical serotonergic potencies.[51]

Oculogyric crises were noted in a patient who was taking lithium in addition to a longstanding regimen of haloperidol and amitriptyline.[52] The ocular *dystonia* resolved upon discontinuation of the lithium. Lithium has not been reported to cause dystonia of any kind when used as monotherapy. Finally, as discussed in Chapter 7, it has been suggested that concomitant lithium therapy may be a contributing factor in patients developing the neuroleptic malignant syndrome due to antipsychotic agents.

Effect of Antidepressant Therapy on Movement Disorders

Depression is a common feature of a number of basal ganglia disorders, particularly Parkinson's disease and Huntington's disease. For the most part, the management of the depression is identical to that used for patients with pure affective disorders. One important exception is the use of nonselective MAO inhibitors in Parkinson's disease. Although these drugs have been used in hopes of improving parkinsonism in the past, the strong potential for hypertensive crises absolutely contraindicates their application to patients treated with other dopaminergic agents. This section will not deal directly with this use of antidepressants. Instead, it will focus on those instances where antidepressant treatments have altered movement disorders (parkinsonism or dyskinesias) or have shown no effect where one was previously reported (Table 4).

As with the literature concerning antidepressant-induced movement disorders, a note of caution is in order. There is a wide range of neurological sophistication among authors of case reports reviewed in this section. There has also been a recurrent failure to suspect alternative explanations for the observed clinical changes, such as the natural variability of Gilles de la Tourette syndrome, or the simultaneous introduction or discontinuation of other therapies. These difficulties are typified by the case of a man with a 35-year history of manic-depressive disorder,[53] treated with lithium and neuroleptics. He was described as having nonprogressive parkinsonism, and "choreoathetoid dyskinetic movements of his hands and feet" for 7 years. He was inexplicably said to have Parkinson's disease, which the authors defended by saying it was "diagnosed by neurologists," although they did not state why none of them thought of treating the patient for this condition. He was given unilateral electroconvulsive therapy for acute mania. In a telling statement from the authors, it is said "the clinical condition of the patient did not improve. However, his bradykinesia, festinating gait, tremor, and rigidity improved markedly." Following bilateral ECT, the mania resolved completely and the parkinsonism almost so; however, the patient developed orolingual dyskinesias. The authors concluded that "ECT was associated with recovery from a manic episode, improvement of coexistent parkinsonism, and a marked change in

Table 4
Treatment of Movement Disorders with Antidepressants

Treatment	Movement Disorder	Results	References
MARU inhibitors	parkinsonism	improved	54–56
	PSP	improved	57, 58
		mixed	59
	tics	mixed	89–92
	dystonia	rare benefit	102
trazodone	essential tremor	improved	83
		no effect	84, 85
MAO inhibitors	postanoxic action myoclonus	improved	86–88
	chorea	improved	126
ECT	Parkinson's disease	improved	many (see text)
	drug-induced parkinsonism	improved	64–68
	tics	none or improved	96–98
	tardive dyskinesia	mixed	65, 66, 112–116
	tardive dystonia	improved	103, 104
lithium	parkinsonism	mixed	76–82
	tics	mixed	99–101
	dystonia	mixed	102, 105–111
	chorea	none or improved	120, 127–130
	tardive dyskinesia	mixed	117–125

MARU = Monoamine reuptake; MAO = monoamine oxidase; ECT = electroconvulsive therapy; PSP = progressive supranuclear palsy.
See ref. 60a for review.

the anatomic distribution of dyskinetic movements." This would be exciting news indeed if one didn't notice that at the time of initiation of ECT, the patient was withdrawn from haloperidol, which may have led to resolution of drug-induced parkinsonism and an exacerbation of tardive dyskinesia.

This article is not to be singled out for criticism. This is the caliber of reporting found in many publications related to the topic of this chapter, some of which are referenced here. _Caveat lector_.

Parkinsonism

Largely because of their known anticholinergic effects, it was not long after their introduction that *MARU inhibitors* were thought to be potentially useful for Parkinson's disease. Relief of parkinsonism by imipramine was first reported in a 1959 open-label study.[54] There were numerous confirmatory case reports, and the findings were substantiated by the results of a 1965 double-blind trial in which 63% of patients receiving imipramine improved versus 16% of placebo-treated patients.[55] The population studied included post-encephalitic and "arteriosclerotic" patients, as well as those with idiopathic parkinsonism, and there was no therapeutic difference among the groups. Response to imipramine was independent of the response to depression. Desipramine was also found to have significant symptomatic benefit for Parkinson's disease patients in a double-blind placebo-controlled study.[56] It was not stated how many of the 10 of 16 who improved were depressed.

Amitriptyline has been reported to improve many of the manifestations of progressive supranuclear palsy in two patients.[57,58] In a double-blind, double-crossover, placebo-controlled study of four patients, amitriptyline produced modest but statistically significant improvement in performance of daily activities and disability; desipramine conferred a lesser benefit.[58] A retrospective review of drug trials for progressive supranuclear palsy showed that imipramine, amitriptyline and fluoxetine each produced improvement or worsening in approximately equal numbers of patients.[59]

Since early reports in the 1940s and 1950s, *ECT* has repeatedly been shown to improve the motor manifestations of Parkinson's disease. This benefit has stood up to double-blind random scrutiny.[60] Older patients appear to experience a significantly greater degree of benefit. All of the manifestations of Parkinson's disease, including tremor, appear to share equally in the effects of ECT. Levodopa-related fluctuations may be eliminated.[60,61] In some patients, the improvement appears to be transient while in others it may last for 6 months or more.[61,62] An abstract report of four patients with complete eradication of parkinsonism for many years without treatment[63] probably represents alleviation of depression-related motor disturbances rather than true Parkinson's disease. ECT may also relieve drug-induced parkinsonism, whether administered therapeutically[64–67] or prophylactically.[68] The prophylactic benefit of ECT was independent of neuroleptic dosage, indicating that this was not simply due to a "sparing" effect, in contrast to the possible protective role of ECT in tardive dyskinesia mentioned earlier.

As with the effect of MARU inhibitors, there is some controversy as to whether the benefit of ECT in Parkinson's disease is a direct result of the treatment or a secondary effect of treating the depression. Some authors have pointed out that depression may worsen parkinsonism and its treatment may thus produce relief from its manifestations.[69,70] As noted, differentiation between parkinsonism and the psychomotor retardation of depression may cause diagnostic confusion, yet there are several reasons to believe that ECT has a direct effect on true parkinsonism. In depressed patients with Parkinson's disease, there is often a dissociation between the effects on motor manifestations and mood. Parkinsonism may improve before the depression, or there may be a clear motor response in the absence of detectable affective benefit. ECT also works in Parkinson's disease patients who are not depressed.[60,61] Manic Parkinson's disease patients treated with ECT have also shown improvement in their parkinsonian symptoms and signs.[53,71] Finally, ECT may provoke dyskinesias that resolve with reduction of antiparkinsonian medication.[60,62] This supports a direct action on dopaminergic systems rather than an indirect effect of mood elevation.

The effect of ECT on Parkinson's disease may be related to enhanced dopamine receptor sensitivity.[72] An alternative (or coexisting) mechanism might be greater penetration of medications into the central nervous system because of increased permeability of the blood-brain barrier.[73] However, this latter theory would not account for patients whose Parkinson's disease improved with ECT when not taking antiparkinsonian medication.[74,75,75a]

Although occasionally a cause of parkinsonism, *lithium* was reported to reduce "off" periods by greater than 60% in four of five patients with levodopa-related fluctuations.[76] Three of these suffered increased dyskinesias. A previous case report had also noted significant benefit from lithium on "off" periods.[77] However, a trial of lithium in 12 patients with fluctuations produced improvement in only three, and this was transient.[78] Lithium was found to increase akinesia and decrease dyskinesias in two other patients.[79] A similar trial failed to show a reduction in dyskinesias.[80] In the largest group studied to date, 21 patients showed no significant change in their parkinsonism or dyskinesias.[81] Lithium has been reported to decrease painful "off"-period dystonia, verified by a double-blind placebo-controlled trial in seven patients.[82]

Tremor

A report of two patients whose essential tremor improved with *trazodone*[83] prompted Koller to investigate this effect in a double-blind placebo-controlled study.[84] Ten patients experienced no significant subjective or objective amelioration of either the postural or kinetic components of their tremor. It was concluded that a serotonergic deficit probably does not play a role in the pathogenesis of essential tremor. Another group of 25 patients given intravenous infusions of trazodone failed to show any response.[85]

Myoclonus

MAO inhibitors have been used successfully to treat postanoxic action myoclonus, a condition strongly associated with serotonin deficiency. Iproniazid was reported to produce significant improvement in one case, although not as much as L-5-hydroxytryptophan.[86] Phenelzine has also been of benefit in one case.[87] Isocarboxazid given alone showed slight or no effect in four patients with action myoclonus, but potentiated improvement when combined with tryptophan.[88] A fifth patient with strictly spontaneous myoclonus showed no benefit from either or both drugs.

Tics

Tricyclic antidepressants usually exacerbate tics in Gilles de la Tourette syndrome (GTS),[89] perhaps by potentiation of dopamine. However, occasional patients are reported to show improvement.[90,91] As usual, the characteristic fluctuating course of GTS makes assessment of these reports difficult. When studied with a double-blind crossover approach, there was no apparent effect of desipramine or clomipramine, except in one patient who worsened on the latter.[92] More recently, imipramine[93] and fluoxetine[94] have been used to treat attention deficit disorder and obsessive-compulsive disorder, respectively, associated with GTS; however, they do not appear to have a consistent effect on the frequency or severity of tics. One exceptional case was reported to show a "dramatic" response of both GTS and attention deficit disorder manifestations with eventual complete resolution on desipramine alone.[95]

ECT had no effect on GTS in two patients,[96,97] but one patient who developed a disabling complex motor tic at age 59 in association with severe depression experienced a complete resolution of both conditions following four bilateral and six unilateral treatments.[98]

Lithium has had mixed effects on the manifestations of GTS, producing improvement in some cases[99,100] but worsening in others.[101]

Dystonia

In a retrospective study of patients with dystonia, only one of 25 patients was found to have a "good response" to treatment with tricyclic *MARU inhibitors*.[102]

ECT was reported to induce a complete remission in a patient with tardive dystonia,[103] and a marked, though transient, improvement in another.[104]

Individual cases of improvement of spasmodic torticollis or segmental dystonia with *lithium* have been reported.[105–107] However, in an unselected group of nine patients, there was no objective improvement.[108] A patient with generalized dystonia also failed to improve on lithium. In a group of 14 dystonia (not further qualified) patients, only one enjoyed a "good response."[102] By contrast, lithium was found to show marked (persistent for greater than 3 months) improvement in 9 of 34 patients with cranial-cervical dystonia so treated; an unsustained benefit was noted in a further 17 patients.[109] The same group has found that lithium enhances the response of cranial-cervical dystonia to tetrabenazine.[110] A double-blind placebo-controlled study of six patients with various forms of dystonia found no benefit in any patient.[111]

Choreoathetosis

Tardive Dyskinesia

ECT worsened tardive dyskinesia in a patient with parkinsonism receiving haloperidol for depression.[65] Both the parkinsonism and depression improved. In seven other patients with tardive dyskinesia, ECT had little or no effect.[112,113] However, seven patients have experienced relief of tardive dyskinesia when treated with ECT.[66,114–116]

Lithium given to patients with tardive dyskinesia has been reported to aggravate the dyskinesias[117] and attenuate the salutary effects of reserpine.[118] More often, it has been found to have a beneficial effect that may be mild[119] or marked.[120-122] However, a double-blind, placebo-controlled study of 11 patients showed no effect of lithium on tardive dyskinesia.[123] Sixteen of 18 patients with tardive dyskinesia who were pretreated with amitriptyline (or imipramine) improved on lithium to a variable degree.[124] In the largest study reported to date, lithium administered to 23 patients in a double-blind placebo-controlled crossover fashion produced no overall significant change.[125] However, when individual responses were considered, two patients had complete eradication of their tardive dyskinesia, three others enjoyed an "important improvement," and two experienced a noticeable worsening.

Huntington's Disease

MAO inhibitors were reported to reduce the severity of chorea in two patients with Huntington's disease, simultaneously with an improvement in their affective state.[126] The observed benefit on chorea was contrary to the expected result of using agents known to increase brain dopamine levels, and it was attributed to "a consequence of mental well-being" rather than a direct effect of the drugs.

Lithium has been used to treat the chorea of Huntington's disease. In one study,[120] there was a "striking reduction of hyperkinetic symptoms" in three of six patients. In another report,[127] treatment with lithium produced a 40–50% improvement in chorea, as measured by a "brachio-kinesio-meter," in three of four patients with Huntington's disease. However, when examined in a double-blind, placebo-controlled fashion, lithium has not produced improvement of chorea.[128-130] A patient with hemichorea also failed to improve on lithium.[108]

Conclusion

Antidepressant agents can be implicated as causes of certain movement disorders. MARU inhibitors, MAO inhibitors, and lithium all cause tremor and myoclonus with a sufficiently high frequency that these can be regarded as common side effects. Clinicians should also be aware that amoxapine, through one of its metabolites, blocks dopamine receptors sufficiently to cause all side effects associated with neuroleptics, including tardive dyskinesias. Other movement disorder-antidepressant associations are largely anecdotal and their pathophysiology is poorly understood. With a few well-documented exceptions, these should be considered tenuous relationships.

The lack of definitive treatment for many movement disorders has led to numerous trials with a variety of neuropsychiatric agents, and antidepressants are no exception. By far the most consistent benefit has been shown in the treatment of Parkinson's disease with ECT. Treatment of Parkinson's disease with other antidepressants has yielded mixed results. For other movement disorders, treatment with antidepressant agents has also produced variable effects, and conclusions are difficult to draw because of the small numbers of patients usually involved. Double-blind studies have often failed to confirm the findings of open-label trials.

The often conflicting reports of the effects of medications underscore the complex biochemical factors underlying movement disorders and the variety of neurotransmitter changes that can be brought about by a single drug. This is especially true of lithium, which may cause or aggravate parkinsonism, tardive dyskinesia, or tics in some patients while ameliorating them in others. They also emphasize that we must consider that multiple pathophysiologies underlie the expression of many movement disorders.

The advent of MARU inhibitors which are more selective for serotonin or dopamine than norepinephrine pathways, may herald a new era of improved ability to treat a variety of neurological conditions, including movement disorders, and provide keys to understanding their neurochemical nature.

References

1. Heninger GR, Charney DS. Mechanism of action of antidepressant treatments: implications for the etiology and treatment of depressive disorders. In: Meltzer H (ed), Psychopharmacology: The Third Generation of Progress, New York, Raven, 1987, pp 535–544.
2. Bunney WE, Garland-Bunney BL. Mechanisms of action of lithium in

affective illness: basic and clinical implications. In: Meltzer H (ed), Psychopharmacology: The Third Generation of Progress, New York, Raven, 1987, pp 553–565.

2a. Klawans HL, Weiner WJ, Nausieda PA. The effect of lithium on an animal model of tardive dyskinesia. Progr Neuropsychol Pharmacol 1977; 1:53–60.

3. Lerer B. Neurochemical and other neurobiological consequences of ECT: implications for the pathogenesis and treatment of affective disorders. In: Meltzer H (ed), Psychopharmacology: The Third Generation of Progress, New York, Raven, 1987, pp 577–588.

4. Young RR. Physiological and enhanced physiological tremor. In: Findley LJ, Capildeo R (eds), Movement Disorders: Tremor, New York, Oxford University Press, 1984, pp 127–134.

5. Nelson JC, Jatlow PI, Quinlan DM. Subjective complaints during desipramine treatment. Arch Gen Psychiatry 1984; 41:55–59.

6. Kronfol Z, Greden JF, Zis AP. Imipramine-induced tremor: effects of a beta-adrenergic blocking agent. J Clin Psychiatry 1983; 44:225–226.

7. Bouchard RH, Pourcher E, Vincent P. Fluoxetine and extrapyramidal side effects. Am J Psychiatry 1989; 146:1352–1353.

8. Tate JL. Extrapyramidal symptoms in a patient taking haloperidol and fluoxetine. Am J Psychiatry 1989; 146:399–400.

9. Brod TM. Fluoxetine and extrapyramidal side effects. Am J Psychiatry 1989; 146:1353.

10. Lee HK. Dystonic reactions to amitriptyline and doxepin. Am J Psychiatry 1988; 145:649.

11. Gardos G. Undiagnosed dystonic reaction secondary to amoxapine. Psychosomatics 1984; 25:66–69.

12. Lydiard RB, Galenberg AJ. Amoxapine: an antidepressant with some neuroleptic properties? A review of its chemistry, animal pharmacology and toxicology, human pharmacology and clinical efficacy. Pharmacotherapy 1981; 1:163–175.

13. Barton JL. Amoxapine-induced agitation among bipolar depressed patients. Am J Psychiatry 1982; 139:387.

14. Gammon GD, Hansen C. A case of akinesia induced by amoxapine. Am J Psychiatry 1984; 141:283–284.

15. Lapierre YD, Anderson K. Dyskinesia associated with amoxapine antidepressant therapy: a case report. Am J Psychiatry 1983; 140:493–494.

16. Coupet J, Rauh CE, Szues-Myers VA, Yunger LM. Amoxapine, an antidepressant with antipsychotic properties: a possible role for 7-hydroxyamoxapine. Biochem Pharmacol 1979; 28:2514–2515.

17. Kramer MS, Marcus DJ, Di Ferdinando J, et al. Atypical acute dystonia associated with trazodone treatment. J Clin Psychopharmacol 1986; 6:117–118.

18. Fann WE, Sullivan JL, Richman BW. Dyskinesias associated with tricyclic antidepressants. Br J Psychiatry 1976; 128:490–493.

19. Burks JS, Walker JE, Rumack BH, Ott JE. Tricyclic antidepressant poisoning. Reversal of coma, choreoathetosis, and myoclonus by physostigmine. JAMA 1974; 230:1405–1407.

20. Noble J, Matthew H. Acute poisoning by tricyclic antidepressants:

clinical features and management of 100 patients. Clin Toxicol 1969; 2:403–407.

21. Garvey MJ, Tollefson GD. Occurrence of myoclonus in patients treated with cyclic antidepressants. Arch Gen Psychiatry 1987; 44:269–272.

22. Forstl H, Pohlmann-Eden B. Amplitudes of somatosensory evoked potentials reflect cortical hyperexcitability in antidepressant-induced myoclonus. Neurology 1990; 40:924–926.

22a. Cunningham M, Cunningham K, Lydiard BR. Eye tics and subjective hearing impairment during fluoxetine therapy. Am J Psychiatry 1990; 147:947–948.

23. Teusink JP, Alexopoulos GS, Shamoian CA. Parkinsonian side effects induced by a monoamine oxidase inhibitor. Am J Psychiatry 1984; 141:118–119.

24. Evans DL, Davidson J, Raft D. Early and late side effects of phenelzine. J Clin Psychopharmacol 1982; 2:208–210.

25. Lieberman JA, Kane JM, Reife R. Neuromuscular effects of monoamine oxidase inhibitors. Adv Neurol 1986; 43:231–249.

26. Baloh RW, Dietz J, Spooner JW. Myoclonus and ocular oscillations induced by L-tryptophan. Ann Neurol 1982; 11:95–97.

27. Pope HG, Jonas JM, Hudson JI, Kafka MP. Toxic reactions to the combination of monoamine oxidase inhibitors and tryptophan. Am J Psychiatry 1985; 142:491–492.

28. Askenasy JJ, Yahr MD. Is monoamine oxidase inhibitor induced myoclonus serotoninergically mediated? J Neural Transm 1988; 72:67–76.

29. Pande AC, Max P. A dystonic reaction occurring during treatment with tranylcypromine. J Clin Psychopharmacol 1989; 9:229–230.

30. Uhrbrand L, Faurbye A. Reversible and irreversible dyskinesia after treatment with perphenazine, chlorpromazine, reserpine and electroconvulsive therapy. Psychopharmacologia 1960; 1:408–418.

31. Flaherty JA, Naidu J, Dysken M. ECT, emergent dyskinesia, and depression. Am J Psychiatry 1984; 141:808–809.

32. Friedman JH, Kucharski LT, Wagner RL. Tardive dystonia in a psychiatric hospital. J Neurol Neurosurg Psychiatry 1987; 50:801–803.

33. Gardos G, Samu I, Kallos M, Cole JO. Absence of severe tardive dyskinesia in Hungarian schizophrenic out-patients. Psychopharmacology 1980; 71:29–34.

34. Dysken MW, Halaris AE. Post-ECT asterixis associated with primary hyperparathyroidism. Am J Psychiatry 1978; 135:1237–1238.

35. Vestergaard P. Clinically important side effects of long-term lithium treatment: a review. Acta Psychiatr Scand 1983; 67(suppl):11–36.

36. Zubenko GS, Cohen BM, Lipinski JF. Comparison of metoprolol and propranolol in the treatment of lithium tremor. Psychiatry Res 1984; 11:163–164.

37. Shopsin B, Gershon S. Cogwheel rigidity related to lithium maintenance. Am J Psychiatry 1975; 132:536–538.

38. Lance JW, Schwab RS, Peterson EA. Action tremor and the cogwheel phenomenon in Parkinson's disease. Brain 1963; 86:95–110.

39. Findley LJ, Gresty MA, Halmagyi GM. Tremor, the cogwheel phenomenon and clonus in Parkinson's disease. J Neurol Neurosurg Psychiatry 1981; 44:534–546.

40. Cleeves L, Findley LJ, Koller W. Lack of association between essential tremor and Parkinson's disease. Ann Neurol 1988; 24:23–26.

41. Branchey MH, Charles J, Simpson GM. Extrapyramidal side effects in lithium maintenance therapy. Am J Psychiatry 1976; 133:444–445.

42. Tyrer P Alexander MS, Regan A, Lee I. An extrapyramidal syndrome after lithium therapy. Br J Psychiatry 1980; 136:191–194.

43. Lang AE. Lithium and parkinsonism. Ann Neurol 1984; 15:214.

44. Reches A, Teitler J, Lavy S. Parkinsonism due to lithium carbonate poisoning. Arch Neurol 1981; 38:471.

45. Shopsin B, Johnson G, Gershon S. Neurotoxicity with lithium: differential drug responsiveness. Int Pharmacopsychiatry 1970; 5:170–182.

46. Zorumski CF, Bakris GL. Choreoathetosis associated with lithium: case report and literature review. Am J Psychiatry 1983; 140:1621–1622.

47. Peters HA. Lithium intoxication producing chorea athetosis with recovery. Wis Med J 1949; 48:1075–1076.

48. Coats DA, Trautner EM, Gershon S. The treatment of lithium poisoning. Australia Ann Med 1957; 6:11–15.

49. Rosen PB, Stevens R. Action myoclonus in lithium toxicity. Ann Neurol 1983; 13:221–222.

50. Devanand DP, Sackeim HA, Brown RP. Myoclonus during combined tricyclic antidepressant and lithium treatment. J Clin Psychopharmacol 1988; 8:446–447.

51. Richelson E, Pfenning M. Blockade by antidepressants and related compounds of biogenic amine uptake into rat brain synaptosomes: most antidepressants selectively block norepinephrine uptake. Eur J Pharmacol 1984; 104:277–286.

52. Sandyk R. Oculogyric crises induced by lithium carbonate. Eur Neurol 1984; 23:92–94.

53. Roth SD, Mukherjee S, Sackeim HA. Electroconvulsive therapy in a patient with mania, parkinsonism, and tardive dyskinesia. Convulsive Ther 1988; 4:92–97.

54. Sigwald J, Bouttier D, Raymondeaud C, Marquez, Gal JC. Etude de l'action sur l'akinesie parkinsonienne de deux derives de l'iminodibenzyle. Presse Med 1959; 67:1697–1698.

55. Strang RR. Imipramine in treatment of parkinsonism: a double-blind placebo study. Br Med J 1965; 2:33–34.

56. Laitinen L. Desipramine in treatment of Parkinson's disease. Acta Neurol Scand 1969; 45:109–113.

57. Kvale JN. Amitriptyline in the management of progressive supranuclear palsy. Arch Neurol 1982; 39:387–388.

58. Newman GC. Treatment of progressive supranuclear palsy with tricyclic antidepressants. Neurology 1985; 35:1189–1193.

59. Golbe LI, Sage JI, Duvoisin RC. Drug treatment of 83 patients with progressive supranuclear palsy. Neurology 1990; 40(Suppl 1):438.

60. Andersen K, Balldin J, Gottfries CG, et al. A double-blind evaluation of electroconvulsive therapy in Parkinson's disease with "on-off" phenomena. Acta Neurol Scand 1987; 76:191–199.

60a. Faber R, Trimble MR. Electroconvulsive therapy in Parkinson's disease and other movement disorders. Mov Disord 1991; 6:293–303.

61. Balldin J, Granerus AK, Lindstedt G, Modigh K, Walinder J. Predictors of improvement after electroconvulsive therapy in parkinsonian patients with on-off symptoms. J Neural Transm 1981; 52:199–211.
62. Douyon R, Serby M, Klutchko B, Rotrosen J. ECT and Parkinson's disease revisited: a "naturalistic" study. Am J Psychiatry 1989; 146:1451–1455.
63. Baruch P, Jouvent R, Vindreu C, Drowillon C, Widlocker D, Agid Y. Improvement of parkinsonism in ECT-treated depressed patients: Parkinson's disease or depression related extrapyramidal disorder? In: Abstracts of the IVth World Congress of Biological Psychiatry, Philadelphia, 1985.
64. Ananth J, Samra D, Kolivakis T. Amelioration of drug-induced parkinsonism by ECT. Am J Psychiatry 1979; 136:1094.
65. Holcomb HH, Sternberg DE, Heninger G. Efficacy of electroconvulsive therapy on mood, parkinsonism and tardive dyskinesia in a depressed patient: ECT and dopamine system. Biol Psychiatry 1983; 18:865–873.
66. Chacko RC, Root L. ECT and tardive dyskinesia: two cases and a review. J Clin Psychiatry 1983; 44:265–266.
67. Goswani U, Dutta S, Kuruvilla K, Papp E, Perenyi A. Electroconvulsive therapy in neuroleptic-induced parkinsonism. Biol Psychiatry 1989; 26:234–238.
68. Gangadhar BN, Choudhary JR, Channabasavanna SM. ECT and drug-induced parkinsonism. Indian J Psychiatry 1983; 25:212–213.
69. Wilder J. Parkinsonism, depression and ECT. Am J Psychiatry 1975; 132:1083–1084.
70. Ward L, Stern GM, Pratt RT, McKenna P. Electroconvulsive therapy in parkinsonian patients with the "on-off" syndrome. J Neural Transm 1980; 49:133–135.
71. Atre-Vaidya N, Jampala VC. Electroconvulsive therapy in parkinsonism with affective disorder. Br J Psychiatry 1988; 152:55–58.
72. Balldin J, Eden S, Granerus AK, et al. Electroconvulsive therapy in Parkinson's syndrome with "on-off" phenomenon. J Neural Transm 1980; 47:11–21.
73. Bolwig TG, Hertz MM, Paulson OB, Spotoft H, Rafaelsen OJ. The permeability of the blood brain barrier during electrically induced seizures in man. Eur J Clin Invest 1977; 7:87–93.
74. Asnis G. Parkinson's disease, depression and ECT: a review and case study. Am J Psychiatry 1977; 134:191–195.
75. Yudofsky SC. Parkinson's disease, depression, and electroconvulsive therapy: a clinical and neurobiologic synthesis. Compr Psychiatry 1979; 20:579–581.
75a. Stern MB. Electroconvulsive therapy in untreated Parkinson's disease. Mov Disord 1991; 6:265.
76. Coffey CE, Ross RD, Ferren EL. The effect of lithium on the "on-off" phenomenon in parkinsonism. Adv Neurol 1983; 37:61–73.
77. Ross DE. "On-off" syndrome treated with lithium carbonate: a case report. Am J Psychiatry 1981; 138:1626–1627.
78. Lieberman A, Gopinathan G. Treatment of "on-off" phenomena with lithium. Ann Neurol 1982; 12:402.

79. Dalen P, Steg G. Lithium and L-dopa in parkinsonism. Lancet 1973; 1:936–937.
80. van Woert MH, Ambani LM. Lithium and L-dopa in parkinsonism. Lancet 1973; 1:1390–1391.
81. McCaul JA, Stern GM. Lithium in Parkinson's disease. Lancet 1974; 1:1117.
82. Quinn N, Marsden CD. Lithium for painful dystonia in Parkinson's disease. Lancet 1986; 1:1377.
83. McLeod NA, White LE. Trazodone in essential tremor. JAMA 1986; 256:2675–2676.
84. Koller W. Tradozone (sic) in essential tremor: probe of serotoninergic mechanisms. Clin Neuropharmacol 1989; 12:134–137.
85. Caccia MR, Osio M, Galimberti V, Cataldi G, Mangoni A. Propranolol, clonidine, urapidil and trazodone infusion in essential tremor: a double-blind crossover trial. Acta Neurol Scand 1989; 79:379–383.
86. Lhermitte F, Marteau R, Degos CF. Analyse pharmacologique d'un nouveau cas de myoclonies d'intention et d'action post-anoxiques. Rev Neurol 1972; 126:107–114.
87. De Lean J, Richardson JC, Hornykiewicz O. Beneficial effects of serotonin precursors in postanoxic action myoclonus. Neurology 1976; 26:863–868.
88. Chadwick D, Hallett M, Harris R, et al. Clinical, biochemical, and physiological factors distinguishing myoclonus responsive to 5-hydroxytryptophan, tryptophan plus a monoamine oxidase inhibitor, and clonazepam. Brain 1977; 100:455–487.
89. Fras I. Gilles de la Tourette's syndrome: effects of tricyclic antidepressants. NY State J Med 1978; 78:1230–1232.
90. Messiha FS, Knopp W. A study of endogenous dopamine metabolism in Gilles de la Tourette's disease. Dis Nerv Syst 1976; 37:470–473.
91. Yaryura-Tobias JA, Neziroglu FA. Gilles de la Tourette syndrome: a new clinico-therapeutic approach. Prog Neuropsychopharmacol 1977; 1:335–338.
92. Caine ED, Polinsky RJ, Ebert MH, Rapoport JL, Mikkelsen EJ. Trial of chlorimipramine and desipramine for Gilles de la Tourette syndrome. Ann Neurol 1979; 5:305–306.
93. Dillon DC, Salzman IJ, Schulsinger DA. The use of imipramine in Tourette's syndrome and attention deficit disorder: case report. J Clin Psychiatry 1985; 46:348–349.
94. Riddle MA, Hardin MT, King R, Scahill L, Woolston JL. Fluoxetine treatment of children and adolescents with Tourette's and obsessive compulsive disorders: preliminary clinical experience. J Am Acad Child Adolesc Psychiatry 1990; 29:45–48.
95. Hoge SK, Biederman J. A case of Tourette's syndrome with symptoms of attention deficit disorder treated with desipramine. J Clin Psychiatry 1986; 47:478–479.
96. Araneta E, Magen J, Musci MN, Singer P, Vann CR. Gilles de la Tourette's syndrome; symptom onset at age 35. Child Psychiatry Hum Dev 1975; 5:224–230.
97. Guttmacher LB, Cretella H. Electroconvulsive therapy in one child and three adolescents. J Clin Psychiatry 1988; 49:20–23.

98. Swerdlow NR, Gierz M, Berkowitz A, Nemiroff R, Lohr J. Electroconvulsive therapy in a patient with severe tic and major depressive episode. J Clin Psychiatry 1990; 51:34–35.

99. Erickson HM, Goggins JE, Messiha FS. Comparison of lithium and haloperidol therapy in Gilles de la Tourette syndrome. Adv Exp Med Biol 1976; 90:197–205.

100. Hamra BJ, Dunner FH, Larson C. Remission of tics with lithium therapy: case report. J Clin Psychiatry 1983; 44:73–74.

101. Borison RL, Ang L, Hamilton WJ, Diamond BI, Davis JM. New pharmacological approaches in the treatment of Tourette syndrome. Adv Neurol 1982; 35:377–382.

102. Greene P, Shale H, Fahn S. Experience with high dosages of anticholinergic and other drugs in the treatment of torsion dystonia. Adv Neurol 1988; 50:547–556.

103. Kwentus JA, Schulz SC, Hart RP. Tardive dystonia, catatonia, and electroconvulsive therapy. J Nerv Ment Dis 1984; 172: 171–173.

104. Adityanjee, Jayaswal SK, Chan TM, Subramaniam M. Temporary remission of tardive dystonia following electroconvulsive therapy. Br J Psychiatry 1990; 156:433–435.

105. Couper-Smartt J. Lithium in spasmodic torticollis. Lancet 1973; 2:741–742.

106. Marti-Masso JF, Obeso JA, Carrera N, Astudillo W, Martinez Lage JM. Lithium therapy in torsion dystonia. Ann Neurol 1982; 11:106–107.

107. Lippmann S, Kareus J. Lithium for spasmodic torticollis. Am J Psychiatry 1983; 140:946.

108. McCaul JA, Stern GM. Lithium and haloperidol in movement disorders. Lancet 1974; 1:1058.

109. Jankovic J, Ford J. Blepharospasm and orofacial-cervical dystonia: clinical and pharmacological findings in 100 patients. Ann Neurol 1983; 13:402–411.

110. Jankovic J, Orman J. Tetrabenazine therapy of dystonia, chorea, tics, and other dyskinesias. Neurology 1988; 38:391–394.

111. Koller WC, Biary N. Lithium ineffective in dystonia. Ann Neurol 1983; 13:579–580.

112. Rosenbaum AH, Niven RG, Hanson NP, Swanson DW. Tardive dyskinesia: Relationship with a primary affective disorder. Dis Nerv Syst 1977; 38:423–427.

113. Asnis GM, Leopold MA. A single-blind study of ECT in patients with tardive dyskinesia. Am J Psychiatry 1978; 135:1235–1238.

114. Price TR, Levin R. The effect of electroconvulsive therapy on tardive dyskinesia. Am J Psychiatry 1978; 135:991–993.

115. Gosek E, Weller RA. Improvement of tardive dyskinesia associated with electroconvulsive therapy. J Nerv Mental Dis 1988; 176:120–122.

116. Webb M. Effects of electroconvulsive therapy and depression on tardive dyskinesia. Ann Neurol 1988; 23:181.

117. Crews EL, Carpenter AE. Lithium-induced aggravation of tardive dyskinesia. Am J Psychiatry 1977; 134:933.

118. Reches A, Hassan MN, Jackson V, Fahn S. Lithium interferes with reserpine-induced dopamine depletion. Ann Neurol 1983; 13:671–673.

119. Reda FA, Escobar JI, Scanlan JM. Lithium carbonate in the treatment of tardive dyskinesia. Am J Psychiatry 1975; 132:560–562.
120. Dalen P. Lithium therapy in Huntington's chorea and tardive dyskinesia. Lancet 1973; 1:107–108.
121. Prange AJ, Wilson IC, Morris CE, Hall CD. Preliminary experience with tryptophan and lithium in the treatment of tardive dyskinesia. Psychopharmacol Bull 1973; 9:36–37.
122. Ehrensing RH. Lithium and melanocyte-stimulating-hormone releasing-inhibiting hormone in tardive dyskinesia. Lancet 1974; 2:1459–1460.
123. Mackay A, Sheppard G. Failure of lithium treatment in established tardive dyskinesia. Psychol Med 1980; 10:583–587.
124. Rosenbaum AH, Maruta T, Duane DD, Auger RG, Martin DK, Brenengen EE. Tardive dyskinesia in depressed patients: successful therapy with antidepressants and lithium. Psychosomatics 1980; 21:715–719.
125. Jus A, Villeneuve A, Gautier J, et al. Deanol, lithium and placebo in the treatment of tardive dyskinesia. Neuropsychobiol 1978; 4:140–149.
126. Ford MF. Treatment of depression in Huntington's disease with monoamine oxidase inhibitors. Br J Psychiatry 1986; 149:654–656.
127. Mattsson B. Huntington's chorea and lithium therapy. Lancet 1973; 1:718–719.
128. Aminoff MJ, Marshall J. Treatment of Huntington's chorea with lithium carbonate: a double-blind trial. Lancet 1974; 1:107.
129. Carman JS, Shoulson I, Chase TN. Huntington's chorea treated with lithium carbonate. Lancet 1974; 1:811.
130. Vestergaard P, Baastrup PC, Petersson H. Lithium treatment of Huntington's chorea: a placebo-controlled clinical trial. Acta Psychiatr Scand 1977; 56:183–188.

9

Spontaneous Movement Disorders in Psychiatric Patients

Roger Kurlan, M.D., Christopher O'Brien, M.D.

Introduction

There are a variety of movement disorders that may accompany neuropsychiatric conditions and that must be differentiated from those induced by drugs. For example, the characteristic chorea or dystonia of Huntington's disease may be difficult to distinguish from tardive dyskinesias caused by neuroleptic drugs used to treat psychiatric symptoms of the illness. These classic movement disorders, including chorea, dystonia, athetosis, myoclonus, tics, tremor, and parkinsonism, may also be seen in psychiatric patients as part of a conversion disorder, malingering, or Munchausen's syndrome.[1-3] They will not be discussed further. Rather, we will concentrate on a different group of disorders of excessive or reduced movement that have generally been considered to fall within the realm of psychiatric patient populations. The hyperkinetic disorders of this group consist of a variety of complex repetitive movements and include habits, mannerisms, stereotypies, and compulsions. Specific examples of

Lang AE, Weiner WJ (editors): *Drug-Induced Movement Disorders*, Mount Kisco, NY, © Futura Publishing Co., Inc., 1992.

each of these disorders, such as tapping, touching, or posturing, may appear identical and may be impossible to differentiate by observation from each other or from the more classic types of movement disorders such as tics or dystonia. *Categorization of the movements is largely based on the setting in which they occur.* For example, repetitive foot tapping might be considered a habit for a normal person, a mannerism for a schizophrenic patient, a stereotypy for a severely retarded individual, a compulsion when performed in response to an obsessive thought pattern, or a complex motor tic for an individual with Tourette's syndrome. The hypokinetic conditions, including bradykinesia, catatonia, rigidity, catalepsy, negativism, and mutism, must generally be distinguished from various forms of drug-induced parkinsonism.

Hyperkinetic Disorders

Habits

Habits are repetitive, coordinated movements that are commonly seen in otherwise normal individuals, particularly during times of anxiety, self-consciousness, boredom, or fatigue. Common examples of habits are shown in Table 1. Depending on their circumstance, identical actions might be classified as compulsions or complex motor tics. A variety of habits are seen in normal children, but they tend to disappear over time as they are learned to be socially inappropriate. Some habits, such as nose picking, may be socially offensive. Chain smoking and gum or tobacco chewing could be considered to fall within this group.

Some habits are particularly common in the course of normal development.[4] Finger (usually thumb) sucking, or substituted sucking of a pacifier, blanket, or other objects, is regarded as a normal habit in early childhood. It has been estimated to occur in 80% of all infants and usually disappears by the age of 3 or 4. Occasional finger sucking, however, persists in up to 30% of 12-year-olds. If finger sucking persists in severe form much beyond the age of 9 years, it tends to be associated with general emotional immaturity. The cause of finger sucking is unknown, but incompleteness of the sucking phase of feeding is a theory supported by the observation that if feeding of some domestic animals is interrupted prior to satiety,

---

Table 1

Common Habits

Eyes
Eye rubbing

Ears
Ear rubbing, pulling, and picking

Nose
Nose picking, scratching, and rubbing

Mouth
Thumb and finger sucking, nail biting, picking at teeth, chewing tongue

Hair
Hair, mustache, or beard pulling, rubbing, and twirling

Head
Head or chin scratching or rubbing

Hands
Fist clenching, popping finger joints, nail picking, twiddling thumbs, finger tapping and drumming, manipulation of clothing, eyeglasses, or jewelry

Genitals
Manipulation of genitals, thigh rubbing

Legs
Foot tapping, abduction-adduction of legs

---

licking or sucking behaviors may appear. There is ongoing debate concerning the relationship between inadequate breast feeding and the later development of finger sucking.

Nail biting is a habit that usually appears between ages 4 and 6 years and is reported in 40–55% of adolescents. After puberty, its frequency declines rapidly so that only 20% of young adults continue to bite their nails. Whereas finger sucking is usually seen when the child is unoccupied or getting ready for bed, nail biting is associated with times of anxiety or stress. Pencil or pen biting and chewing gum may represent substituted behaviors for nail biting.

Mannerisms

A mannerism is a peculiar or unusual characteristic mode of performing a normal activity, such as eating or walking.[4] The term is applied to odd, idiosyncratic, or bizarre variations of normal human behavior. Many normal people possess a mannerism or two that may be regarded as no more than a slight eccentricity. Mannerisms may be used to attract attention, particularly in individuals who are insecure and wish to appear more confident than they actually are. Schizophrenic patients display an astonishing number of odd, senseless variations in normal activities for which the term "mannerism" has been applied. Some examples include bizarre gaits (e.g., lifting legs like a stork), unnatural, affective flourishes incorporated into eating behavior, imitating a famous person's behavior or speech, and a variety of distorted expressive gestures. Mannerisms may remain constant for years or may be altered constantly. Some mannerisms may be so extreme as to actually interfere with the underlying action. Schizophrenic speech may also be associated with manneristic qualities, such as speaking in rhyme, telegrammatic jargon, or adding "ism" to the end of every word.

Stereotypies

A stereotypy is a coordinated, repetitive, rhythmic, and patterned movement, posture or vocalization that is carried out virtually the same way during each repetition and is observed in an individual with defective mentation or deprived of visual or auditory sensory input. The movements are stereotypic in that their form, body distribution, amplitude, and timing are predictable. Stereotypies may include simple (e.g., body rocking, smiling) or more complex (e.g., walking in circles, sitting down and arising from a chair) movements (Table 2). While the movements are usually uniform, at times incomplete forms of a given stereotypy may be seen. For example, instead of rocking the body back and forth, a patient may merely nod the head. Stereotypies are generally considered to be involuntary and non-goal-directed. However, as these movements are characteristically seen in individuals with severe cognitive impairment

---

Table 2

Common Stereotypies

Mouth
Bruxism, lip movements, biting, grimacing, smiling, frowning, vocalizations (e.g., snorting, blowing, groaning, hissing, singing,
screaming)

Head
Banging, nodding, shaking, weaving, bizarre posturing

Arms and Hands
Finger waving and flicking before the eyes, holding hand at arm's
length and watching the fingers move, finger drumming or pill-
rolling movements, hand rubbing, fist pounding, hand to face,
mouth, or ear movements, touching or stroking parts of the body,
fragments of common actions (e.g., smoking, combing hair)

Trunk
Body rocking, twirling, and circling, pelvic swaying and thrusting,
sitting and arising

Legs
Jumping, hopping, lotus position, walking in circles or back and
forth

Self-Injurious Behavior
Lip manipulation, hand biting, eye poking and gouging, scratching,
self-beating

---

whose motivation cannot be assessed, the true intentional quality of
these behaviors remains to be clarified. Indeed, it has been suggested
that stereotypies may be purposeful in that they serve as a form of
self-stimulation. When not accompanied by severe cognitive deficit,
stereotypies can be temporarily suppressed. Although patients usually have little control over stereotypies, the movements often decrease when the patients engage in activities such as counting or
drawing. Conditions in which stereotypies occur are listed in Table
3.

Mental retardation and autistic disorders are characteristically
associated with stereotypies.[5] In one study of 102 institutionalized
mentally retarded adults, 34% demonstrated at least one type of

---

Table 3

Conditions Associated with Stereotypic Behavior

Mental retardation
Autism
Pervasive developmental disorder of children
Rett syndrome
Neuroacanthocytosis
Childhood encephalopathies
    Viral encephalitis
    Ceroid lipofuscinosis
    Phenylketonuria
Schizophrenia
Severe agitated depression
Tardive stereotypies (stereotyped orofacial dyskinesia and stereotypies
    of tardive akathisia)
Akathisia (acute or tardive)
Congenital blindness
Congenital deafness
Developmental stereotypies

---

stereotypy, including rhythmic movements (26%), bizarre posturing (13%), and object manipulation (7%).[6] Stereotypies, including self-stimulatory behavior, often constitute the most recognizable features of children and adults with autism of any cause.[7-9] Rett syndrome is an autistic disorder reported only in girls that is characterized by stereotypic movements and other movement disorders.[10] The most common stereotypies include hand wringing, washing, clapping, clenching, patting, and rubbing. In addition, other stereotypic behaviors may be seen, such as body rocking, shifting of weight from one leg to the other, bruxism, and ocular deviations. In patients with mental retardation and autism, stereotypic self-injurious behavior may be observed. This seems particularly evident for patients with body rocking, a stereotypy most often associated with self-hitting.[11] While head banging and other self-injurious behavior may occur in normal children, this type of behavior is usually abnormal.[12]

Childhood onset pervasive developmental disorder, a condition that is similar to autism but has a later age at onset and does not present with the complete clinical picture of autism, is also associated with stereotypic behavior. Children with encephalopathy caused by phenylketonuria, infantile ceroid lipofuscinosis (hand "knitting" stereotypies),[13] or a prenatal viral infection such as rubella or cytomegalovirus, may develop an autistic syndrome with stereotypies.

A variety of stereotypic behaviors were described in schizophrenic patients long prior to the introduction of neuroleptic drug therapy. Stereotypies are particularly characteristic of the catatonic variety.[14] Stereotypic maintenance of unusual postures, shifting position, repetitively moving mouth and jaw, tapping or touching objects, and repetitive verbalizations are typical motor features of the catatonic state. When catatonia is associated with stereotypic behavior, the diagnosis of mania should be considered.[15] Particularly strange and excessive stereotypic behavior may be seen in catatonic and other severe psychiatric disorders for which the terms "parakinesia,"[16] "bizarrery," or "grotesquery"[17] have been applied.

Children with congenital deafness and blindness may also exhibit a variety of stereotypic behaviors.[18] Stereotypies are generally much more bizarre and highly repetitive in autistic children than in those with a disordered special sensory system. The stereotypies of visually disturbed children, however, may at times strongly resemble those of autism. The stereotypies of deaf children are accompanied by noises, whereas those of blind children are not. It has been suggested that severe mental retardation or autism may represent forms of sensory deprivation, analogous to congenital deafness or blindness, in that external stimuli are not processed in a cognitively appropriate fashion.

The term "stereotypy" is often employed to describe patterned and repetitive movements in other settings, although we prefer usage that is restricted to patients with severely defective mentation or severe congenital hearing or visual loss. No clear, generally accepted definition of this movement disorder has been formulated. At least some stereotyped activities, such as sucking and clasping behaviors, are associated with normal neonatal motor patterns that function to maintain close contact with the mother and that have generally been considered reflexive. With further development, other stereotypic behaviors may appear, including body rocking, bruxism, and head banging, the latter seen in up to 15% of normal children. One might consider these behaviors to represent a form of "physiological" or "developmental" stereotypy, representing a process similar to the recognized developmental chorea and dystonia of infancy and childhood.[19] Stereotypies are also commonly observed in otherwise normal children during times of emotional excitement.

The most typical form of tardive dyskinesia, the orofacial-lingual-masticatory movement, has often been classified as a choreic disorder. However, as the movements are less random and more predictable than classic chorea, it has been labeled by some as "rhythmic" chorea or stereotypy.[5] Since all known types of involuntary movement disorders can result from the use of neuroleptic drugs, it would not be unexpected that drug-induced stereotypies may occur as well. The repetitive restless movements of patients with akathisia, such as crossing and uncrossing of legs, arising and sitting down, marching in place, and picking at clothes, have also been called stereotypic.[5]

Stereotypic behavior is common in animals, particularly those housed in restraining environments with low stimulation.[5,20] With the development of stereotypies, there is a reduction in the spectrum of behaviors normally displayed by unrestrained animals. Therefore, stereotypy has been viewed as either a self-generating sensory stimulus or a motor expression of underlying tension and anxiety.[5] Unfortunately, such animal stereotypic behavior as repetitive biting, turning, and circling are not clearly related to similar behaviors in man.[21]

Developmental and behavioral theories have been proposed to explain the origin of stereotypies in man.[22] It has been suggested that social isolation may convert normal developmental stereotypic behavior into autistic stereotypies such as thumb sucking or self-clasping, a concept that has been confirmed for primates and other animals that are isolated in development.[22] The appearance of stereotypic behavior in mentally retarded children may be related to a tendency for these children to be physically isolated or for them to be effectively isolated by their mental dysfunction. Alternatively, it has been proposed that stereotypies in these children may represent an attempt to decrease what is interpreted as an overstimulating environment.[24] Others have suggested that stereotypies are an attempt to increase self-stimulation to a predetermined level.[25] One behavioral theory suggests that stereotypies arise from essentially normal behaviors that are further shaped and reinforced by a process of operant conditioning.[25]

Most studies of stereotypic behavior in experimental animals have emphasized the role of dopaminergic systems in the basal ganglia and limbic structures.[5,22] Intrastriatal injection of dopamine and systemic administration of dopaminergic drugs, such as amphetamine or apomorphine, in rats produces dose-related stereotypic behavior.[26–29] These stereotypies can be prevented by pretreatment with dopamine receptor antagonist drugs.[26] Recent studies indicate that the D_2 dopamine receptor subtype mediates stereotypic behavior in animals and that activation of D_1 receptors potentiates these D_2-mediated effects.[27–29] A correlation between amphetamine-induced stereotypic behavior and striatal extracellular release of dopamine and serotonin has been demonstrated using the technique of in vivo microdialysis in freely moving rats.[30] Brain neuropeptides, such as cholecystokinin, neurotensin, and opioids, particularly in limbic sites, may play an important role in the pathogenesis of stereotypic behavior.[31] The relevance of the stereotypic behaviors seen in animals to those seen in man remains unclear. Furthermore, stereotypies appear differently in different species and the term "stereotypy" is often used in the scientific literature of animal research to describe activities that are not clearly stereotyped.[21]

Compulsions

Compulsions are repetitive and seemingly purposeful behaviors that are often performed according to certain rules (i.e., are ritualistic) and are often carried out in order to ward off anticipated future harm or a dreaded event. For example, repetitive hand washing is done to prevent contamination or disease, or an individual may believe that repetitive counting of objects will prevent harm from coming to a loved one. In this respect, compulsions occur in response to an obsessive thought pattern. Obsessions are defined as recurrent, persistent ideas, thoughts, images, or impulses that are not experienced as voluntarily produced but rather as thoughts that invade consciousness and are experienced as senseless or repugnant. Attempts are made to ignore or suppress them. Obsessions are usually unpleasant and may be frightening or violent. Examples of common compulsions and obsessions are shown in Tables 4 and 5.[32]

A pervasive pattern of compulsive perfectionism and inflexibility, including excessive devotion to work, indecisiveness, restricted expression of affection, and lack of generosity, is referred to as obsessive-compulsive personality disorder. For individuals in whom obsessions and/or compulsions interfere with normal daily functioning, the diagnosis of obsessive-compulsive disorder (OCD) is made. OCD

Table 4

Common Compulsions

Excessive or ritualistic handwashing, showering, bathing, toothbrushing, or grooming

Repeated rituals (going in/out door, up/down from chair, etc.)

Checking (doors, locks, stove, appliances, emergency brake on car, etc.)

Rituals to remove contact with contaminants

Touching

Measures to prevent harm to self or others

Ordering, arranging

Counting

Hoarding, collecting

Cleaning household or inanimate objects

From reference 32.

is classified as an anxiety disorder since obsessive thought patterns are associated with the development of anxiety, which may in turn be relieved by performance of compulsions. Interference with the patient's ability to carry out compulsive behavior is also anxiety-provoking. First symptoms of OCD usually occur by the early 20's, may begin suddenly or slowly, and often have an episodic course. Obsessive-compulsive symptoms are common in other psychiatric illnesses as well. About 20% of patients with major depression have obsessive symptoms and schizophrenics may manifest a variety of bizarre obsessions. The development of obsessive-compulsive symptoms in later life may indicate emergence of a dementia.

Approximately 50% of patients with Tourette's syndrome will show evidence of obsessive-compulsive symptoms.[33,34] Although compulsions may at times be difficult to differentiate from complex motor tics, certain characteristics of compulsions are helpful in making this distinction. Compulsions are often associated with obsessions and/or performed in response to an obsessive thought. Furthermore, compulsions are performed according to certain rules while tics are not. The presence of such rules indicates a ritualistic disorder, and examples include performance of an action a specified number of times, in a specified order, or at a specified time of day (e.g., bedtime rituals). Thus, a patient who must tap the floor in multiples

Table 5

Common Obesessions

Concern with dirt, germs, environmental toxins
Something terrible happening (fire, death/illness of self or loved one)
Symmetry, order, exactness
Scrupulosity (religious)
Concern or disgust with bodily wastes or secretions (urine, stool, saliva)
Lucky or unlucky numbers
Forbidden, aggressive, or perverse sexual thoughts, images, or impulses
Fear might harm others, self
Intrusive nonsense sounds, words, or music

From reference 32.

of three prior to rising from a chair is likely experiencing compulsive tapping, while patients who tap with no specified rule may be showing tapping tics. Compulsions may be performed to ward off some feared consequence, although this history is usually absent in Tourette's patients with OCD. Finally, while tics usually respond favorably to neuroleptic medications, compulsions do not, but rather often they improve following treatment with antidepressant medications that preferentially block serotonin reuptake.

In addition to Tourette's syndrome, obsessive-compulsive symptoms are associated with a variety of other basal ganglia disorders, including Sydenham's chorea, Huntington's disease, and postencephalitic parkinsonism.[35] This clinical observation has suggested that disordered basal ganglia function may underlie the development of obsessive-compulsive symptoms. Individual cases with discrete lesions of the basal ganglia and obsessive-compulsive features have also been reported.[35] Indeed, a decreased volume of the caudate nuclei by computed tomography and increased caudate and lateral orbito-frontal cortical metabolic rates by positron emission tomography have been described in patients with OCD.[35,36] Disruption of basal ganglia-frontal lobe connections with psychosurgical procedures (particularly anterior capsulotomy and cingulotomy) have been used therapeutically to treat patients with disabling OCD.[35,37] Taken together, these observations are consistent with a pathogenetic model of OCD involving dysfunction of basal ganglia and frontal lobe-basal ganglia interactions.

Recent studies have pointed out the importance of genetic factors for OCD. In Tourette's syndrome, an autosomal dominant disorder with incomplete penetrance and variable expression, it appears that particularly in females, the genetic trait may be expressed by obsessive-compulsive symptoms alone.[38] Large families in which primary OCD is segregating have been described as well.

Significant interest in the diagnosis of OCD has been aroused by the recent availability of effective medications. Clomipramine (Anafranil) and fluoxetine (Prozac) are recently introduced antidepressant medications that are potent inhibitors of serotonin reuptake. Both medications have proven benefit for patients with OCD, including those in association with Tourette's syndrome.[39,40] A role for disturbance of central serotonin systems in the pathogenesis of the disorder has thereby been implicated.

Hypokinetic Disorders

Motor disturbances characterized by slowness or paucity of movement are commonly encountered in psychiatric populations. Historically, patients with such hypokinetic conditions have been classified under a variety of headings. Catatonia, stupor, negativism, and catalepsy are terms that have been used, at times interchangeably.[22,41–43]

One can conceptually divide the hypokinetic disorders into active and passive types. Active immobility is brought about by increased muscle tone or effort, such as maintaining a bizarre posture against gravity. In contrast, passive immobility is related to reduced muscle tone or activation. The limp and inactive posture of a depressed person serves as an example. Active and passive immobility appear to have distinct pathophysiological correlates and therefore require different therapeutic considerations.

Most studies of hypokinesia in neurological and psychiatric populations have emphasized the role of the basal ganglia in this type of movement disorder.[22,43] In particular, neuropharmacological manipulation of the dopaminergic system has produced the most consistent effects on hypokinesia in humans and in animal models. In general, dopaminergic stimulation ameliorates passive immobility whereas dopamine antagonism reverses active immobility. Data from animal models support the concept that passive and active immobility reflect distinct neural substrates, the former associated with dopamine underactivity, the latter overactivity.[44] The ability of dopamine receptor antagonists to produce immobile states in animals corresponds very closely to the drug's affinity for nigrostriatal dopamine receptors.[45] For example, neuroleptics with little influence on the nigrostriatal dopamine system, such as clozapine, have little effect in this model system.[46] There also appear to be important differences in the effects on D_1 and D_2 receptor subtypes, as blockade of D_2 receptors results in fixed postures in some animal species and this response is modulated by D_1 stimulation or blockade.[41] Much study is needed to clarify the neuropharmacological basis of these phenomena.

As our knowledge of pathogenesis has improved, a number of distinct etiologies of hypokinesis have been identified (e.g., tertiary syphilis) and accordingly removed from the purely psychiatric realm. Although forms of hypokinesia in psychiatric patients may be induced by medications (e.g., drug-induced parkinsonism), a variety of hypokinetic conditions may also be observed in those who are not medicated. These will be the focus of this section (Fig. 1).

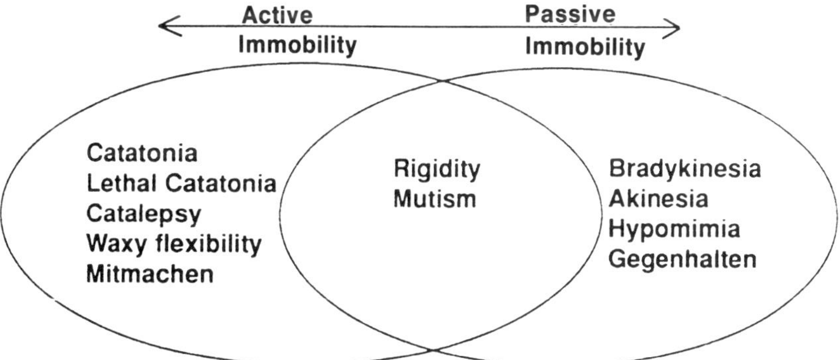

Figure 1: Immobility observed in patients with spontaneous hypokinesia can be viewed across a continuum ranging between active and passive types.

Bradykinesia, Akinesia, and Hypomimia

Although usually associated with neurological parkinsonian conditions, these terms refer to perhaps the most common form of hypokinesia observed in nonmedicated psychiatric patients, particularly those with depression or schizophrenia. Bradykinesia describes diminished velocity of normal movement and akinesia describes poverty of all movement. These two phenomena may be seen independently of each other and each may occur in the absence of rigidity. Diminished facial expression with a decreased rate of blinking is termed "hypomimia," a feature that is most often encountered in parkinsonian conditions and is essentially akinesia of the face. As such, hypomimia may be found, like generalized bradykinesia or akinesia, in a wide spectrum of psychiatric patients. In contrast to depressed or withdrawn patients, the hypomimic state in Parkinson's disease often does not correspond to the patient's reported emotional state.

Bradykinesia, akinesia, and hypomimia are frequently seen in psychiatric patients prior to drug therapy. Most often, slow movement and easy fatiguability are encountered in patients with depression but these features have also been reported in other affective disorders, schizophrenia, and developmental disturbances. Signs of parkinsonism, when prominent, may be virtually indistinguishable from those of idiopathic Parkinson's disease except by the clinical context in which they occur. Parkinsonian features in the setting of affective disturbance have been termed "pseudo-parkinsonism" and the treatment and course are quite different from the idiopathic degenerative disorder. Pseudo-parkinsonism responds best to antidepressant therapy, is attended by recognizable widespread affective disturbance, and tends not to progress inexorably. In contrast, idiopathic Parkinson's disease responds best to dopaminergic agents, demonstrates specific patterns of cognitive impairment, and progresses to disabling neurological dysfunction over 5–15 years.[47] Associated systemic illness (e.g., hypothyroidism, arthritis) must be excluded as a cause of bradykinesia or akinesia in psychiatric patients.

The pathophysiological basis for these bradykinetic phenomena in psychiatric patients is not clear. Abnormalities in several neurotransmitter systems have been implicated, particularly dopamine (DA) and norepinephrine (NE).[43] Opioid, cholinergic, serotonergic, GABAergic, and other systems have been suggested as secondary mediators.[44] Low levels of DA and its major metabolite, homovanillic acid (HVA), are found in cerebrospinal fluid (CSF) and brains of patients with bradykinesia in the setting of Parkinson's disease.[47] In schizophrenics, the so-called "negative" symptoms (e.g., withdrawal, hypokinesia) correlate with reduced HVA levels in CSF as well.[43] In concert with the hypothesis that central dopamine deficiency is important pathogenetically, negative symptoms in schizophrenics are not generally improved by dopamine antagonist medications. This is in contrast to positive symptoms (e.g., hallucinations, delusions) that have been attributed to DA hyperactivity. Low CSF HVA levels have also been reported in depressed patients with psychomotor retardation. The studies of other neurotransmitters in schizophrenic and affective disorders are inconclusive as to the relationship between hypokinesia and serotonin, NE, GABA, opioid, and neuropeptide concentrations.[43]

Attempts to pharmacologically manipulate central neurotransmitter systems have shown some therapeutic benefit for psychiatric patients with bradykinesia and akinesia. Norepinephrine re-uptake blockade with tricyclic antidepressants, anticholinergic therapy, and dopaminergic activation with a variety of antiparkinsonian agents may increase the frequency and velocity of movements in such patients (Table 6). It is unclear, however, whether the antide-

---

Table 6

Pharmacological Treatment of Bradykinesia

Antidepressants
    Protriptyline
    Nortriptyline

Dopaminergic Agents
    Levodopa/Carbidopa
    Amantadine
    Bromocriptine
    Pergolide

Stimulants
    Methylphenidate
    Pemoline

pressant effects are independent of the influences on motor function. Finally, the extent to which parkinsonism in depression might be due to specific nigrostriatal dysfunction remains unknown.

The complex and heterogeneous nature of these neurobehavioral phenomena is evident from the observation that akinesia or varieties of bradykinetic movements may be abolished in psychotic patients following treatment with antipsychotic medication.[22,43] In this setting, the disordered movement responds to dopamine antagonist treatment, consistent with an active immobility model of hypokinesia. In such patients, hypokinesia would thereby not be considered to represent part of a parkinsonian syndrome.

Catatonia

Over the past 150 years, the term "catatonia" has been applied to nearly all of the movement abnormalities observed in psychiatric patients. As currently conceived, catatonia describes a constellation of altered motor and mental activity most often including abnormalities of posture, muscle tone, and movement frequency, accompanied by withdrawal, agitation, or psychosis. A continuum of motor abnormalities exists, ranging from a markedly inhibited, immobile state to a highly agitated state with increased motor activity and hyperkinetic features. The described clinical entities of rigidity, mutism, and catalepsy can be considered to fall within this catatonic motor spectrum. Thus, both excess movements and hypokinesias, including active and passive forms, may be part of the catatonic syndrome.

Three individuals are historically recognized for their careful study of motor abnormalities in psychiatric patients. Karl Ludwig Kahlbaum defined catatonia in 1868 as a condition with multiple "symptom-complexes" emerging at different times during disease progression.[42] These symptom-complexes were described as clusters of abnormal thought processes (e.g., disorientation) and motor dysfuntion (e.g., increased tone). It is not clear whether catatonia was felt by Kahlbaum to be a distinct disease, as he emphasized the association of catatonia with depression, mania, epilepsy, generalized paresis, and other conditions. Periods of excitation and hyperkinesia as well as stupor and hypokinesia were also described. Catatonia was not felt to be a degenerative condition since good recovery was at times observed. Kahlbaum's concepts were later modified and incorporated into the theories of Kraeplin and later Bleuler within the nosologic entity of schizophrenia.[48,49]

The current *Diagnostic and Statistical Manual of Psychiatry* (DSM-III-R) defines catatonia as "a demonstration of generalized inhibition manifest by stupor, mutism, negativism, or waxy flexibility," and catatonia is included as a subtype of schizophrenia.[50] Examples of other motor disturbances commonly reported in catatonia include both hypokinetic (bradykinesia, mutism, rigidity, posturing, catalepsy) and hyperkinetic (mannerisms, stereotypies, and echopraxia) forms. Similar motor disturbances occur, however, in all types of schizophrenia and range from subtle clumsiness or postural stiffness at one extreme to bizarre gait or rigid immobility at the other.[22,43]

Limited information about the prevalence or natural history of motor disturbances in schizophrenics is available. Prior to the availability of neuroleptic drugs, abnormalities of motor function were frequently noted.[41,43] However, interpretation of past prevalence surveys is difficult as definitions were inconsistent and many diagnosed "psychiatric" conditions would now carry a specific neurological diagnosis. Over the last decade, it has been estimated that 30–50% of schizophrenics show signs of catatonia, although the prevalence of this motor disturbance among all psychiatric patients has been decreasing over the last century.[22,43] It is likely that many cases of catatonic schizophrenia reported early in this century were "symptomatic" with the majority due to postencephalitic states. Obviously, incidence and prevalence data are dependent upon precise definition of diagnostic terms, a goal not yet achieved. In his concise 1976 review, Gelenberg states "catatonia is not a rare phenomena, does not automatically imply a functional disorder, and certainly does not always indicate schizophrenia".[41] Several recent prevalence studies are reviewed by Manschreck, who concludes that "disturbances of voluntary motor behavior (i.e., those that were not attributable to drug effects or known neurological disorder) occur in virtually all cases of conservatively defined schizophrenic disorder".[43] He also notes that these motor phenomena may frequently be overlooked and that patients should be observed for extended periods of time.

In summary, the catatonic syndrome represents a continuum of altered motor activity accompanied by disordered affect and thought processes. The motor abnormalities may include both hyperkinesia and hypokinesia and appear to reflect disruptions of central neurotransmission in the basal ganglia. Although considered as a subset of schizophrenia, catatonia deserves recognition within a broader neuropsychiatric context. Patients with catatonia as part of an affective disorder are no different in demographic characteristics or treatment response than affectively disturbed patients without catatonia.[51] From a practical point of view, the individual signs of the catatonic syndrome (i.e., stupor, mutism, negativism, and waxy flexibility) are best considered separately as this may afford greater diagnostic precision and, in turn, more efficacious treatment. Moreover, each of these individual features has overlapping but not identical differential diagnoses, many outside the sphere of schizophrenia.[41]

Cyclic and Familial Catatonia

Patients with single or multiple episodes of catatonia without obvious predisposing neurological or psychiatric cause (e.g., bipolar affective disorder) and often occurring in a familial pattern have been described.[52] While some members of these families had seizures, treatment with anticonvulsants in no way altered the occurrence of catatonia. Electroconvulsive therapy (ECT) produced the best response and long-term benefit. The pathogenesis of this disorder remains unknown.

Lethal Catatonia

A description of a clinical syndrome characterized by extreme physical excitement and exhaustion was provided by Stauder in 1934.[53] These patients, all young adults, progressed from agitation to fixed postures and ultimately death. Acrocyanosis, tachycardia, and fever were usually present and autopsy revealed no obvious cause of death. The syndrome shares some clinical similarity with neuroleptic malignant syndrome (NMS), but several important differences exist.[54,55] NMS occurs with rapid onset, often without excitatory prodrome, and is usually secondary to drug-induced dopamine receptor blockade. Lethal catatonia, on the other hand, was described long prior to the introduction of antipsychotic medications and often includes an excitatory prodrome. Differentiation of these two conditions is critical since very different treatment approaches are employed. Lethal catatonia is best treated with antipsychotics, benzodiazepines, and supportive care, while NMS requires immediate cessation of such drugs and treatment with dopaminergic agents and dantrolene (see Chapter 7). The true incidence of lethal catatonia, while low, remains unknown. As the early treatment of psychosis may prevent the full expression of this condition, in the current era of readily available antipsychotic therapy, NMS has become a much more common concern.

Rigidity

Three types of abnormal muscle tone have been described in psychiatric patients unexposed to psychotropic medications. *Waxy flexibility* is said to be present when a posture or limb position is maintained for an extended period of time after positioning by another individual. Many unusual postures or positions have been described over the years, some with such frequency that they have earned their own names. The "psychological pillow," for example, describes a reclining patient with head held without support just above the bed surface. While these motor disturbances may still be seen in patients with affective and schizophrenic disorders, the prevalence of this phenomena has apparently decreased over this past century for unknown reasons. Waxy flexibility is categorized as a form of active immobility since treatment with neuroleptics is the most effective therapy. ECT also has alleviated this disturbance.

Two other alterations of muscle tone may be mistaken for waxy flexibility. *Mitmachen* describes an immediate return to a resting or initial limb position after manipulation by the examiner. For example, a hand turned palm up by the examiner is returned to its prior pronated position. This sign is not specific to any psychiatric syndrome, although it is most commonly seen in schizophrenia. *Gegenhalten* (counter holding) refers to variable resistance to all passive movement. Now termed "paratonia," this sign reflects bihemispheric dysfunction and can be found in a wide range of conditions such as Alzheimer's disease, multi-infarct dementia, and metabolic encephalopathy.

Catalepsy

Most simply, catalepsy can be considered a synonym for waxy flexibility as it refers to the maintenance of an abnormal posture for prolonged periods of time following positioning by another. However, some authors use the term "waxy flexibility" in reference to a "plastic resistance" to movement and reserve "catalepsy" specifically for prolonged maintenance of an abnormal posture. In catalepsy, muscle tone is variable, ranging from marked resistance to near hypotonia. In the past, the term "catalepsy" was also employed to describe altered mental states and other motor disturbances, such as tonic seizures. Catalepsy has now, however, been placed conceptually within the spectrum of catatonia. Psychiatric patients may maintain abnormal cataleptic postures without exposure to psychotropic medications. Limbs may be held above the head, the trunk may be twisted, extended, or flexed, and the ball of one foot might support a large man for hours. Patients seem surprisingly undisturbed by these uncomfortable postures in contrast to patients with a focal dystonia, such as spasmodic torticollis, in which discomfort is often a primary feature. Catalepsy may be seen in patients with affective disturbances, both psychotic and nonpsychotic, as well as schizophrenic disorders. The true incidence of catalepsy in unmedicated patients is not known.

The term "catalepsy" is also employed frequently in the behavioral neuroscience literature in reference to animal models used to evaluate central neurochemical systems.[56] In order to assess the impact of drugs on DA, opioid, and other neurotransmitter systems, animals are placed in an unusual posture, for example, limbs on elevated bars or pegs, and the time taken to correct to normal posture is recorded. This form of catalepsy is most often induced by neuroleptic or opiate medications. A similarity between human and animal catalepsy has been inferred on the basis of neuropharmacological response, although this relationship remains speculative.

Negativism

A vaguely defined term, negativism has been applied to both observable behavior and inferred "internal" mental processes.[4,22] As a movement disorder, negativism describes a motor activity or inactivity contrary to the intended goal. This may appear, for example, in a schizophrenic patient as an inability to shake hands due to limb withdrawal despite repeated attempts at initiating the gesture. Similar actions have also been termed motor "blocking" or "ambitendency."[4] As a concept, negativism appears to have little diagnostic, phenomenologic, or therapeutic utility. When "negative" motor activity is observed clinically, consideration should be given to more precisely defined movement disorders or thought disturbances. For example, a patient with complex motor tics or obsessive-compulsive disorder may be similarly unable to carry out skilled actions.

Mutism

Absence of sound production in unmedicated psychiatric patients may occur without evidence for aphasia, laryngeal, or labial dysfunction. Mutism in a psychiatric patient capable of phonation is suggestive of psychosis or severe depression, but absence of sound production accompanied by akinesia raises the possibility of structural damage within the brain. Akinetic mutism has been associated with lesions of the third ventricle, thalamic nuclei, and cingulate gyrus.[57] Traumatic closed-head injury may result in a similar clinical pattern, perhaps due to the torque-induced shearing of axons in the regions surrounding the midbrain and corpus callosum. Dopaminergic medications such as bromocriptine, levodopa/carbidopa, and amantadine may have beneficial effect in some akinetic mute patients with or without identifiable structural abnormalities.[58,59]

References

1. Marsden CD. Hysteria-a neurologist's view. Psychol Med 1986; 16:277–288.
2. Fahn S, Williams DT. Psychogenic dystonia. Adv Neurol 1988; 50:431–455.
3. Ranawaya R, Riley D, Lang A. Psychogenic dyskinesias in patients with organic movement disorders. Mov Disord 1990; 5:127–133.
4. Lee AJ (ed). Tics and Related Disorders, Edinburgh, Churchill Livingstone, 1985, pp 104–124.
5. Jankovic J. Stereotypies. Presented at the annual meeting of the American Academy of Neurology, Miami, 1990.
6. Dura JR, Mullick JA, Rasnake LK. Prevalence of stereotypy among institutionalized nonambulatory profoundly mentally retarded people. Am J Mental Deficiency 1987; 91:548–9.
7. Allen DA. Autistic spectrum disorders: clinical presentation in preschool children. J Child Neurol 1988; 3(Suppl):S48-S56.
8. Schreibman L. Diagnostic features of autism. J Child Neurol 1988; 3(Suppl):S57-S64.
9. Wing L, Attwood A. Syndromes of autism and atypical development. In: Cohen DJ, Donnelan AM, Paul R (eds), Handbook of Autism and

Pervasive Developmental Disorders, New York, John Wiley and Sons, 1987, pp 3–19.

10. Fitzgerald PM, Jankovic J, Percy AK. Rett syndrome and associated movement disorders. Mov Disord 1990; 5:195–202.

11. Rojahn J. Self-injurious and stereotypic behavior of noninstitutionalized mentally retarded people: prevalence and classification. Am J Mental Deficiency 1986; 91:268–276.

12. Jankovic J. Orofacial and other self-mutilations. In: Jankovic J, Tolosa E (eds), Facial Dyskinesias, Advances in Neurology, Vol 49, New York, Raven Press, 1988, pp 365–381.

13. Santavuori P, Haltia J, Raitta C. Infantile type of so-called neuronal ceroid lipofuscinosis. I. A clinical study of 15 cases. J Neurol Sci 1973; 18:257.

14. Rogers D, Hymas N. Sporadic facial stereotypies in patients with schizophrenia and compulsive disorders. In: Jankovic J, Tolosa E (eds), Facial Dyskinesias, Advances in Neurology, Vol 49, New York, Raven Press, 1988, pp 383–394.

15. Abrams R, Taylor MA, Stolurow KA. Catatonia and mania: patterns of cerebral dysfunction. Biol Psychiatry 1979; 14:111–117.

16. Leonhard K. In: Robins E (ed), Berman R (trans), The Classification of Endogenous Psychoses, New York, Halsted Press, 1979.

17. Fish FJ. In: Hamilton M (ed), Fish's Clinical Psychopathology: Signs and Symptoms in Psychiatry, Bristol, Wright, 1974.

18. Sakuma M. A comparative study by the behavioral observation for stereotypy in exceptional children. Folia Psychiatr Neurol Jpn 1975; 29:371–391.

19. Shoulson I, Rothfield K, McBride M, Kurlan R. Physiologic chorea and dystonia of infancy. Neurology 1987; 37(Suppl):99.

20. Dantzer R. Behavioral, physiological and functional aspects of stereotyped behavior: a review and re-interpretation. J Animal Sci 1986; 62:1776–1786.

21. Randrup A. Munkvad I. Stereotyped activities produced by amphetamine in several animal species and man. Psychopharmacologia 1967; 11:300–310.

22. Lohr JB, Wisniewski AA (eds). Movement Disorders: A Neuropsychiatric Approach, New York, Guilford Press, 1987, pp 91–108.

23. Berkson G. Abnormal stereotyped motor acts. In: Zubin J, Hunt HF (eds), Comparative Psychopathology: Animal and Human, New York, Grune and Stratton, 1967, pp 76–94.

24. Hutt SJ, Hutt C, Lee D, et al. A behavior and electroencephalographic study of autistic children. J Psychiat Res 1965; 3:181–197.

25. Baumeister AA, Forehand R. Stereotyped acts. In: Ellis NR (ed), International Review of Research in Mental Retardation. Vol 6, Academic Press, New York, 1973, pp 53–96.

26. Tschanz JT, Rebec GV. Atypical antipsychotic drugs block selective components of amphetamine-induced stereotypy. Pharmacol Biochem Behav 1988; 31:519–522.

27. Koller WC, Herbster G. D_1 and D_2 dopamine receptor mechanisms in dopaminergic behaviors. Clin Neuropharmacol 1988; 11:221–231.

28. Chipkin RE, McQuade RD, Iorio LC. D_1 and D_2 dopamine binding site upregulation and apomorphine-induced stereotypy. Pharmacol Biochem Behav 1987; 28:477–482.
29. Costall B, Marsden CD, Naylor RJ, Pycock CJ. Stereotyped behavior patterns and hyperactivity induced by amphetamine and apomorphine after discrete 6 hydroxydopamine lesions of extrapyramidal and mesolimbic nuclei. Brain Res 1977; 123:89–111.
30. Kuczenski R, Segal D. Concomitant characterization of behavioral and neurotransmitter response to amphetamine using in vivo microdialysis. J Neurosci 1989; 9:2051–2065.
31. Blumstein LK, Crawley JN, Davis LG, Baldino F. Neuropeptide modulation of apomorphine-induced stereotyped behavior. Brain Res 1987; 404:293–300.
32. Swedo SE, Rapoport J. Phenomenology and differential diagnosis of obsessive-compulsive disorder in children and adolescents. In: Rapoport JL (ed), Obsessive-Compulsive Disorders in Children and Adolescents, Washington, DC, American Psychiatric Press, 1989, pp 13–32.
33. Frankel M, Cummings JL, Robertson MM, Trimble MR, Hill MA, Benson DF. Obsessions and compulsions in Gilles de la Tourette's syndrome. Neurology 1986; 36:378–382.
34. Pitman RK, Green RC, Jenike MA, Mesulam MM. Clinical comparison of Tourette's disorder and obsessive-compulsive disorder. Am J Psychiatry 1987; 144:1166–1171.
35. Wise SP, Rapoport JL. Obsessive-compulsive disorders: is it basal ganglia dysfunction? In: Rapoport JL (ed), Obsessive-Compulsive Disorder in Children and Adolescents, Washington, DC, American Psychiatric Press, 1989, pp 327–344.
36. Baxter L, Phelps M, Mazziotta J, et al. Local cerebral glucose metabolic rates of obsessive-compulsive disorder compared to unipolar depression and normal controls. Arch Gen Psychiatry 1987; 44:211–218.
37. Kurlan R, Kersun J, Ballantine HT, Caine ED. Neurosurgical treatment of severe obsessive-compulsive disorder associated with Tourette's syndrome. Mov Disord 1990; 5:152.
38. Pauls DL, Leckman JF. The inheritance of Gilles de la Tourette's syndrome and associated behaviors: evidence for autosomal dominant transmission. N Engl J Med 1986; 315:993–997.
39. Leonard HL. Drug treatment of obsessive-compulsive disorder. In: Rapoport JL (ed), Obsessive-Compulsive Disorder in Children and Adolescents, Washington, DC, American Psychiatric Press, 1989, pp 217–236.
40. Como PG, Kurlan R. An open-label trial of fluoxetine for obsessivecompulsive disorder in Tourette's syndrome. Neurology 41(6):872–874.
41. Gelenberg AJ. The catatonic syndrome. Lancet 1976; i:1339–1341.
42. Barnes MP, Saunders M, Walls TJ, Saunders I, Kirk CA. The syndrome of Karl Ludwig Kahlbaum. J Neurol Neurosurg Psychiatry 1986; 49:991–996.
43. Manschreck TC. Motor abnormalities in schizophrenia. In: Nasrallah HA, Weinberger DR (eds), Handbook of Schizophrenia, Vol 1, 1986, pp 65–96.
44. Klemm WR. Drug effects on active immobility responses: what they

tell us about neurotransmitter systems and motor fluctuations. Progr Neurobiol 1989; 32:403–422.

45. Campbell A, Herschel M, Cohen BM, Baldessarini RJ. Tissue levels of haloperidol by radioreceptor assay and behavioral effects of haloperidol in the rat. Life Sci 1980; 27:633–640.

46. Honma T, Fukushima H. Correlation between catalepsy and dopamine decrease in the rat striatum induced by neuroleptics. Neuropharmacology 1976; 15:601–607.

47. Weiner WJ, Lang AE. Parkinson's disease. In: Weiner WJ, Lang AE (eds), Movement Disorders: A Comprehensive Survey, Mount Kisco, NY, Futura Publishing Co, 1989, pp 23–115.

48. Kraepelin E. Dementia Praecox and Paraphrenia (Barclay RM, trans), Huntington, NY, Robert E Krieger, 1971 (facsimile 1919 edition).

49. Bleuler E. Dementia praecox or the group of schizophrenias. (Zinkin J, trans), New York, International Universities Press, 1950.

50. American Psychiatric Association, Diagnostic and Statistical Manual of Mental Disorders, third edition, revised, Washington, DC, American Psychaitric Association Press, 1987.

51. Taylor MA, Abrams R. Catatonia: prevalence and importance in the manic phase of manic-depressive illness. Arch Gen Psychiatry 1977; 34:1223–1225.

52. Gjessing LR. A review of periodic catatonia. Biol Psychiatry 1974; 8:23–45.

53. Stauder KH: Die todliche katatonie. Arch Psychiatr Nervenkr 1934; 102:614–634.

54. Mann SC, Caroff SN, Bleier HR, Welz WKR, Kling MA, Hayashida M. Lethal catatonia. Am J Psychiatry 1986; 143:1374–1381.

55. Castillo E, Rubin RT, Holsboer-Trachsler E. Clinical differentiation between lethal catatonia and neuroleptic malignant syndrome. Am J Psychiatry 1989; 146:324–328.

56. Sanberg PR, Bunsey MD, Giordano M, Norman AB. The catalepsy test: its ups and downs. Behavioral Neurosci 1988; 5:748–759.

57. Plum F, Posner JB. The Diagnosis of Stupor and Coma, third edition, Philadelphia, F.A. Davis Co., 1980.

58. Ross ED, Stewart RM. Akinetic mutism from hypothalamic damage: successful treatment with dopamine agonists. Neurology 1981; 31(11):1435–1439.

59. Guidice MA, et al. Improvement in motor functioning with levodopa and bromocriptine following closed head injury. Neurology 1986; 36(1)198–199.

10

Dyskinesia Induced by Levodopa and Dopamine Agonists in Patients with Parkinson's Disease

John G. Nutt, M.D.

History

The seminal report of Cotzias, Van Woert, and Schiffer, published in 1967, which stated that orally administered D,L-dopa ameliorated the signs and symptoms of Parkinson's disease, included the observation that athetoid movements were induced in some patients by the drug.[1] This was an unexpected side effect of the drug because the earlier report from Birkmeyer and Hornykiewicz on the acute effects of D,L-dopa administered intravenously to patients with parkinsonism had not described production of involuntary movements.[2] A subsequent report from Cotzias et al. in 1969 indicated the magnitude of the problem; 50% of the patients receiving D,L-dopa or L-dopa developed dyskinesia.[3] The rapid acceptance of levodopa as the

Supported in part by grant RO1-NS21062 from the National Institute of Disease and Stroke.

Lang AE, Weiner WJ (editors): *Drug-Induced Movement Disorders,* Mount Kisco, NY, © Futura Publishing Co., Inc., 1992.

therapy of choice for parkinsonism resulted in a number of clinical reports in the early 1970s, many of which emphasized the high prevalence of levodopa-induced dyskinesia.[4-6] In the mid- to late 1970s, distinctive patterns of dyskinesia were recognized, including "peak dose" dyskinesia, "dysphasic dyskinesia," and "off" dystonia.[7-11]

Apomorphine was the first dopamine agonist to be tried in Parkinson's disease, the first investigations antedating the introduction of levodopa. Schwab, Amador, and Lettvin found that small subcutaneous or oral doses produced modest improvement in the parkinsonism and no dyskinesia.[12] The interest in apomorphine was revived by Cotzias, who noted a more dramatic effect of the drug on parkinsonism as well as the fact that it would induce dyskinesia in some patients in whom dyskinesia had appeared during chronic levodopa therapy.[13] Chronic oral administration of aporphines were shown by Cotzias et al. to produce dyskinesia that was very similar to that induced in the patients by levodopa.[14]

Bromocriptine, introduced by Calne et al. in 1974, was also found to induce dyskinesia in patients who had developed dyskinesia on levodopa.[15] Other orally effective direct-acting dopamine agonists (pergolide, lisuride, PHNO, mesulergine) also induce dyskinesia. However, patients treated only with bromocriptine from the initiation of dopaminergic therapy, unexposed to levodopa, rarely develop dyskinesia.[16,17] This has focused interest on the factors important for the induction of dyskinesia in Parkinson's disease.

Another important development in the history of levodopa and dopamine agonist-induced dyskinesia was the introduction of the MPTP-treated monkey as a model of parkinsonism.[18] Physiological and pharmacological investigations of this model have yielded insight into the physiology and pharmacology of drug-induced dyskinesia in parkinsonian patients and allowed separation of drug- and disease-related factors.

Clinical Features

Forms of Levodopa-Induced Involuntary Movements

Choreoathetosis

Choreoathetosis is the most common pattern of involuntary movement induced by levodopa and dopamine agonists. This form of dyskinesia often begins with very subtle rocking movements of the trunk, nodding movements of the head, or sinuous movements of the fingers, ankles, or toes. The choreoathetosis may become very severe and may affect any skeletal muscle group. This levodopa-induced dyskinesia may be indistinguishable from the movements of Huntington's disease or tardive dyskinesia. Choreoathetosis may be as disabling as the parkinsonism, but in most patients, it produces little disability and most prefer choreoathetosis to the parkinsonian state.

Dystonia

Dystonia is the second most common pattern for levodopa-induced dyskinesia. Dystonia in patients with parkinsonism need not be related to use of dopaminergic drugs. Some patients have dystonia, particularly of the foot, as an early manifestation of their parkinsonism and well before any drug therapy is started.[19] Most commonly, dystonia is related to the use of dopaminergic drugs. The dystonia is often brought out by movement or use of the affected muscle group. It may affect any part of the body. Dystonia affecting the cranial musculature may interfere with speech and swallowing. A patient with this type of dystonia may appear relatively normal when sitting quietly although the corners of the mouth may be excessively retracted. On attempting to speak, involuntary contractures of facial, lingual, and masticatory muscles become apparent and may disrupt speech, chewing, and swallowing. Dystonic posturing of the ankle and toes, often accompanied with pain, is another distinct pattern in patients receiving levodopa chronically.

Dystonia often coexists with choreoathetosis in the same patient. Both may appear concurrently, with the dyskinesia being a mixture of choreic and dystonic movements, or there may be dystonic movements at one time and choreoathetotic movements at another time.

Ballism

Levodopa-induced involuntary movements can be extremely severe in some patients, producing wild, flinging, ballistic movements of the limbs that are very disabling and may result in injury.

Stereotyped Movements

Stereotyped movements may occur with chronic levodopa therapy. These may take the form of stepping or kicking movements of the legs, particularly as the patient passes from "off" to "on." Peculiar patterns of gait may be seen, most commonly a tendency to lift one leg too high to give the patient a gait sometimes characterized as a "hemi-goose-step march." Occasionally, stereotyped movements could be characterized as tics, but it is rare for tics to be the only manifestation of levodopa-induced involuntary movements with an absence of other choreoathetotic movements.

Myoclonus

Myoclonus may be seen in parkinsonian patients treated chronically with levodopa.[20] This almost always occurs in the setting of cognitive impairment and psychiatric symptoms. It may thus be a sign of a metabolic encephalopathy. It is uncommon that the myoclonus is so severe as to produce disability itself or to require treatment.

Tremor

Tremor is, of course, part of the parkinsonism tetrad. However, it is worth noting that the tremor of Parkinson's disease may be augmented by levodopa. This tends to be a transitory phenomenon during each dose cycle. The tremor tends to be of lower amplitude when the patient is more severly "off" and to become more pronounced just as the patient begins to turn "on" and even be transiently mixed with choreoathetotic dyskinesia. The tremor may also be exaggerated as the patient turns "off."

Akathisia

Akathisia is the subjective sensation of the need to move not caused by other sensory complaints or anxiety (see Chapters 4 and 6). It is generally manifested by restlessness and fidgety movements. Restlessness is a rather nonspecific symptom. In the absence of the compulsion to move, this should probably not be considered akathisia. Akathisia may be seen in untreated Parkinson's disease but more commonly occurs in patients receiving dopaminergic drugs. A relationship to the dopaminergic drug cycle may be present in some patients; in some, the drugs appear to relieve the symptoms and, in others, they appear to induce them.[21]

Temporal Patterns of Dyskinesia

Peak Dose Dyskinesia

Peak dose dyskinesia is dyskinesia occurring when the effects of levodopa on the parkinsonism are most apparent.[22] For this reason, it is sometimes called "on" dyskinesia. Although termed "peak dose" dyskinesia, the dyskinesia often does not directly relate to plasma peaks of levodopa, as is also true for the improvement in parkinsonism.[23] The dyskinesia is most conmonly choreoathetotic but may be dystonic, ballistic, or stereotyped. This form of dyskinesia tends to be present throughout the period of time the patient is experiencing a reduction in the parkinsonian symptomatology (sometimes referred to as a "square-wave" response).[24] This is the most commonly observed pattern of levodopa-induced dyskinesia.

Diphasic Dyskinesia

Diphasic dyskinesia refers to choreoathetotic, dystonic, stereotyped, or ballistic movements that appear as the levodopa begins to take effect and as the drug effects wane.[7-9,22] Thus, the patient may have bursts of dyskinesia as the drug begins to produce an antiparkinsonism effect succeeded by another burst of dyskinesia as the drug effects wear off. In between these periods of exaggerated dyskinesia, there may be good antiparkinsonian effects with minimal chorea. This diphasic exacerbation of dyskinesia is not always apparent with each dose cycle and may be noticeable only at the end of some dose cycles. Diphasic dyskinesias can be extremely severe with ballistic movements accompanied by marked sweating, hypertension, and tachycardia. Sudden death has occurred during these episodes, presumably related to cardiac arrythmias.[22] This severe form of diphasic dyskinesia is, luckily, uncommon.

Diphasic dyskinesia, however, in a lesser form may be extremely common. Many patients will have an exacerbation of their tremor just before they begin to turn on, immediately followed by dyskinesia. The dyskinesia and tremor may even be mixed or alternate for several minutes. The dyskinesia may then partially remit and the patient is left with a milder degree of dyskinesia but good control of the parkinsonism until the effects of the medicine begin to wear off when the sequence is again repeated. A diphasic pattern of dyskinesia has also been seen in monkeys with MPTP-induced parkinsonism treated with levodopa or apomorphine.[25]

"Off" Dystonia

Dystonia, generally affecting the legs and frequently painful, occurs when dopaminergic drug levels are low, such as when the patients have been without medicine overnight or as the effects of a dose wear off.[10,11,22] Because of the predisposition for it to occur in the morning, it also is termed "early morning dystonia."[10] Commonly, the dystonia produces flexion or extension of the toes, inversion, or plantar flexion of the ankles, and internal rotation of the leg. However, dystonia may affect the trunk and arms, although this is less conon. Cramping pain is almost always present with "off" dystonia. As implied by the term "off," dystonia is present when the parkinsonism is more apparent, i.e., when the drug is not working or the patient is "off." The dystonia is frequently precipitated when the patient attempts to walk or becomes anxious. "Off" dystonia can generally be clinically differentiated from "peak dose" or "diphasic" dystonic dyskinesias by the timing of the dyskinesia in relation to the dose cycle and by the presence of crampy pain.

Spatial Patterns of Dyskinesia

Dyskinesia is Worse on the Side Most Affected by Parkinsonism

Idiopathic parkinsonism is often asymmetrical, the tremor, rigidity, and bradykinesia appearing in one arm or leg first and spreading over months to years to involve the other limbs. The asymmetry in severity at presentation may persist throughout the course of the disease. Peak dose dyskinesia as well as "off" dystonia are generally first apparent on this most affected side of the body and may be more severe on the most affected side throughout the course of the illness.[27]

Thalamotomy Reduces Contralateral Dyskinesia

Stereotaxic lesions of the ventrolateral nucleus of the thalamus reduce contralateral tremor and rigidity. In addition, they will reduce contralateral levodopa-induced limb dyskinesia.[6,28,29] Occasionally, thalamotomies are used in patients with severe levodopa-induced dyskinesia to make it possible for the patient to obtain the therapeutic benefits of the drug.[28]

Somatic Musculature Affected by Dyskinesia

Peak dose and diphasic dyskinesia commonly affect cranial, trunk, and limb musculature. Extraocular muscles are spared as is smooth muscle. Patients with Parkinson's disease and levodopa-induced fluctuations in motor function may have respiratory complaints, particularly dyspnea. Sometimes dyspnea is associated with dyskinetic movements of the respiratory muscles.[31] However, dopaminergic drugs may induce dyspnea without obvious dyskinesia of chest or abdominal musculature. It has been postulated that dyskinesia of the diaphragm or upper airway musculature may be responsible or that there is a direct effect on medullary respiratory centers.[30,31] Dyspnea may also be an "off" symptom, perhaps related to chest wall rigidity[32] or involuntary movements of the upper airway.[33]

Parkinsonism and Dyskinesia Present Concurrently

When dyskinesia develops in a patient after a dose of levodopa, it need not appear in all body parts simultaneously. Some patients will note that dyskinesia appears in the arms while the legs are still very parkinsonian. Alternatively, the legs may develop dyskinesia while a typical parkinsonian rest tremor persists in the arms. This often appears to be a transient state when presumably striatal dopamine is near a critical level. With higher doses, only dyskinesia is present, and when the drug is withheld for several hours, only parkinsonian bradykinesia and tremor are present. It is less common to see a marked side to side dissociation with, for example, one arm dyskinetic and the other tremorous. Similarly, mixtures of parkinsonism and dyskinesia occur simultaneously in some neuroleptic-treated patients.[34]

Severity of Dyskinesia

Effects of Duration of Treatment

Levodopa-induced dyskinesia is rarely present upon initiation of therapy but appears after weeks, months, or years of chronic therapy, suggesting that its emergence is somehow induced by a drug action on the dopaminergically denervated striatum. The dyskinesias first appear as very subtle, fidgety movements that gradually increase in severity over months or years. Likewise, "off" dystonia appears with chronic therapy and at first is infrequent and minor but may increase in severity to dominate the patient's complaints. Peak dose dyskinesia, diphasic dyskinesia, and "off" dystonia disappear if dopaminergic agents are withdrawn.

Dose Responsiveness of Dyskinesia

Peak dose dyskinesia is generally considered to be dose-responsive, i.e., dyskinesia is more severe with larger doses of drug.[22] It is also assumed that, at least initially, there is a therapeutic window and that more drug is required to produce dyskinesia than to produce the antiparkinsonian effects.[22,35,36] It is for these reasons, i.e., to keep the plasma concentrations within the therapeutic window, that many physicians reduce the dose of levodopa and increase the frequency of dosing when dyskinesia appears.

A contrary view suggests that the severity of dyskinesia is not very dose-related, although the duration of the dyskinesia is related to the size of the dose or the peak plasma levodopa levels.[23,37] If the patient has dyskinesia, it is generally either present or absent without a gradient of severity.[24] The diphasic pattern of dyskinesia exhibited by many patients and the effects of stress and activity may confuse any relation between dose and severity of dyskinesia that does exist. Finally, these later studies[23,24,37] have not found a consistent therapeutic window where the antiparkinsonian effects can be obtained without dyskinesia.

Role of Emotion and Stress

The severity of dyskinesia waxes and wanes throughout the day and even during a single dose cycle. One clear contributing factor to this is the emotional state of the patient. Stress will often exacerbate the dyskinesia.[24] However, stress may sometimes completely abolish the dyskinesia and concomitantly turn the patient "off." Both effects may be seen in the same patient and presumably the effects of stress depend on whether the brain dopamine levels are well above threshold (stress then increasing dyskinesia) or close to threshold (stress turning the patient "off").

Role of Activity

Dyskinesia lessens when the patient is sitting or lying quietly and disappears or is greatly reduced if the patient is asleep. Conversely, dyskinesia is often brought out by motor activity.[24] To some extent, this increase in dyskinesia resembles mirror movements or "motor overflow." For example, when the patient begins to use one hand in a motor task, dyskinesia will appear in the other limbs.

Relation of Dyskinesia to Therapeutic Response

The original report describing the therapeutic efficacy of oral levodopa for Parkinson's disease noted that dyskinesia tended to occur in the patients who had an impressive therapeutic benefit from the drug.[1] This observation has been verified by many subsequent investigators.[5,6] Conversely, patients who receive little or no therapeutic benefit from levodopa generally have little or no dyskinesia.

Natural History

Appearance of Dyskinesia

Dyskinesia is not apparent with the first doses of levodopa or dopamine agonists. However, dyskinesia may appear during the first month of chronic treatment with levodopa and successively more patients develop it over the ensuing months.[4–6] The appearance of dyskinesia, however, is delayed for years in some patients. Likewise, in monkeys with MPTP-induced parkinsonism, the first doses of dopaminergic drugs do not induce dyskinesia, but repeated administration over days to weeks is required.[25,38–40] "Off" dystonia is generally seen in patients treated for years rather than months.[10,11,26]

The relationship of development of dyskinesia to the appearance of the fluctuating response ("wearing off" and "on-off") is problematic. There is evidence that a short-duration response (a motor fluctuation) to levodopa may be seen with the first doses of the drug but that these fluctuations are so subtle as to escape the patient's and physician's notice under most circumstances.[37,41] The appearance of dyskinesia intermittently throughout the day may therefore offer the first evidence, recognized by patient and physician, that motor function varies during the day.

When dyskinesia first appears, it is often very subtle and difficult to distinguish from restlessness or fidgetiness. With time, the severity of the dyskinesia increases and the movement is more clearly choreic, dystonic, or stereotyped. However, the severity of the dyskinesia eventually tends to plateau and remain at a constant level for many years. Initially, dyskinesia may be present only in the most affected limb or affect the face, neck, or trunk. With continued therapy, the dyskinesia may spread to involve other body parts or it may remain localized. The same pattern of increase in severity of dyskinesia and gradual involvement of more muscle groups is seen in parkinsonian monkeys treated with levodopa.[25,38-40]

Dose-to-Dose Pattern

The patient's dyskinesia is generally related to the dose cycle. This pattern may not be identical with each dose, perhaps because of the interdose variability in absorption and blood-to-brain transport of levodopa. Many patients notice that the control of the parkinsonism is not as good in the afternoon, and often the afternoons may be associated with more dyskinesia. This may be due to poorer absorption of levodopa in the afternoon and increasing plasma amino acid concentrations.[42]

Withdrawal of Dopaminergic Agents

Withdrawal of levodopa or dopamine agonists will cause an immediate disappearance of peak dose and diphasic dyskinesia. The "off" dystonia will also disappear within 24 hours or so.[26] The consequence, of course, is that the patient is left in a state of parkinsonism.

Epidemiology

Definitions

Prevalence studies of levodopa-induced dyskinesias generally lack rigor. First, the criteria for diagnosis of levodopa-induced dyskinesia are not explicitly defined. Dyskinesia appears gradually, making it difficult to draw the line between vague fidgety movements and definite dyskinesia. Second, rarely are "on" dyskinesia, diphasic dyskinesia, and "off" dystonia differentiated. Finally, most studies describing prevalence of dyskinesia do not indicate whether the presence of dyskinesia is based on direct observation or on the patient's history. Patients' histories are notoriously unreliable because patients often cannot differentiate tremor, dyskinesia, and cramps. The chances of the physician observing and characterizing dyskinesia depend upon whether the patient is seen throughout one or more dose cycles and whether the patient is put through activating procedures such as carrying out motor and mental tasks. These considerations become particularly important when dyskinesia is an important end-point, such as in studies comparing the effects of various treatment regimens in previously untreated patients.

Prevalence of Dyskinesia in Levodopa-Treated Patients

The prevalence of dyskinesia reported by various investigators is remarkably similar. Barbeau et al.[4] reported that 49% of their series of 100 patients exhibited dyskinesia at 3 months. The percentage rose during the ensuing 2 years, but this was partially because of dropout of nonresponding patients as well as increase in the percent of treated patients with dyskinesia. Five of the six patients treated for 21 months had dyskinesia. Markham[5] found that 21% of 100 patients had chorea at 3 months and 38% at 1 year. In the same group of patients, 68% showed 50% or more improvement in the parkinsonism at 1 year. Mones et al.[6] reported that 3 or more months of levodopa improved 74% of the patients and induced dyskinesia in 44% of these improved patients. Dyskinesia was noted in only one of the nonresponding patients. Lesser et al.[43] found dyskinesia in 43% of levodopa-treated patients with idiopathic parkinsonism attending a movement disorder clinic. Quinn et al.[43a] found that dyskinesias were particularly common in patients with young-onset Parkinson's disease (onset between ages 21 and 40 years). Of their 51 patients, 15.7% had developed dyskinesias within 1 week of beginning levodopa. At 1 year, 3 years, and 6 years of treatment, the percentages of patients with dyskinesias were 54.9%, 74.5%, and 100%, respectively.

The prevalence of dyskinesia may plateau with continuation of levodopa therapy. Sweet and McDowell[44] noted that prevalence peaked in their patient series at 57% after 3 years of treatment and fell to 49% after 5 years of treatment. Barbeau[45] reported on prevalence of dyskinesia in a series of 80 patients in whom dyskinesia was present in 66% of the patients after 1 year of treatment, in 55% after 6 years, and 33% after 11 years. Again, the percentage of patients with dyskinesia in these series with longer follow-up may represent: (1) a dropout of the patients with poor or no response to the drug or patients who rarely develop dyskinesia, (2) loss of patients from other causes, and (3) changes in treatment strategies.

Risk Factors

Association with Age and Sex

It is a widely held clinical impression, bolstered by clinical series, that individuals with younger age of onset of Parkinson's disease have a higher prevalence of levodopa-induced dyskinesia.[43,46,47] However, age alone may not be responsible for this difference. Young onset individuals have a good response to levodopa, tolerate higher doses, and are treated for a longer time. These variables rather than age itself, may be responsible for younger onset patients having a greater frequency and severity of levodopa-induced dyskinesia. Estrogens may affect basal ganglia function and parkinsonian symptomatology,[48] and one might expect that the sex of the patient could be a risk factor for developing dyskinesia. However, no studies have indicated that levodopa-induced dyskinesia occurs more frequently in one sex than the other.

Relation to Pathological Substrate of Parkinsonism

Levodopa-induced dyskinesia appears almost exclusively in Parkinson's disease. Markham[5] and Mones et al.[6] reported that levodopa did not induce dyskinesia in normals nor in patients with dystonia, Huntington's disease, torticollis, or other miscellaneous diseases. Likewise, Chase et al. found no dyskinesia in patients with motor neuron disease treated with levodopa.[49] Barbeau, however, did note that it could augment the dyskinesias of dystonia musculorum deformans, Huntington's disease, Wilson's disease, and induce it in progressive supernuclear palsy.[4] Levodopa-induced dyskinesia and motor fluctuations occur in patients with MPTP-induced parkinsonism[50] and in parkinsonism secondary to obstructive hydrocephalus.[51] Goodwin et al. reported a single depressed patient who developed dyskinesia (without further description) while taking high doses of levodopa.[52] Dyskinesias as well as other features of motor fluctuations occasionally do occur in patients with multiple system atrophy, including oliovpontocerebellar atrophy[52a] and striatonigral degerneration.[52b] Nevertheless, the vast majority of patients with the parkinsonism plus syndromes such as progressive supranuclear palsy, multiple systems atrophy, or cortical-basal ganglionic degeneration receive little therapeutic benefit from dopaminergic agents and, likewise, very rarely develop dyskinesia. Induction of dyskinesia by levodopa is generally a reliable indication that the patient has idiopathic parkinsonism and not a parkinsonism plus syndrome.

These observations in patients are consistent with studies in nonhuman primates. Levodopa will induce hyperactivity and stereotyped movements in normal monkeys, but these motor patterns are different from the choreoathetosis and dystonia induced in the MPTP-induced parkinsonian monkey.[53–57]

Relation to Severity of Parkinsonism

Mones et al. noted a tendency for levodopa-induced dyskinesia to appear in patients more severly affected with parkinsonism.[6] Furthermore, Langston and Ballard found that dyskinesia appeared very early in the severely parkinsonian individuals who developed the syndrome after taking MPTP.[50] Although the evidence from various clinical series is not overwhelming that disease severity is a major risk factor for the development of dyskinesia, the fact that it almost always occurs first on the side most severely affected by the parkinsonism argues for severity of disease as an important risk factor for the development of dyskinesia.[27] In the monkey with MPTP-induced parkinsonism, levodopa induces dyskinesia only in the monkeys with more severe depletion of striatal dopamine,[40] supporting the importance of disease severity.

Relation to Levodopa Responsiveness

Cotzias et al.[1] and many subsequent investigators[5,6] have noted that dyskinesia appears in those patients who enjoy the most improvement in motor function with levodopa. Conversely, patients who receive little therapeutic benefit from levodopa are at low risk to develop dyskinesia, regardless of the severity of the parkinsonism. Many of these individuals have an alterative diagnosis found at autopsy.

Drug Exposure

Drug-induced dyskinesia in parkinsonism is almost exclusively found in patients treated with levodopa. Although nondopaminergic agents have been occasionally reported to produce dyskinesia (see chapter 12), this is decidedly rare. The dopamine agonist, bromocriptine, infrequently induces dyskinesia in patients who have never received levodopa,[16,17] although bromocriptine will induce dyskinesia in patients in whom dyskinesia has previously been induced by chronic levodopa therapy. The same is true in nonhuman primates with MPTP-induced parkinsonism. Bromocriptine will relieve the parkinsonism but will not induce dyskinesia unless the monkey has been previously treated with levodopa.[39] Although there is less experience with the other dopamine agonists such as pergolide and lisuride, they appear to have a low propensity to induce dyskinesia de novo as well. It should be noted, however, that the dopamine agonists are also less efficacious against parkinsonian disability than is levodopa and therefore the ability to induce dyskinesia may be proportional to antiparkinsonian efficacy.

There is a general impression that emergence of dyskinesia in levodopa-treated patients is related to the total daily dose or cumulative exposure.[4,43,46] This has been invoked as a reason to delay initiating levodopa and to keep levodopa doses as low as possible.[58] Indeed, Poewe, Lees, and Stern found that patients treated for 6 years with the maximum tolerated dose of levodopa had a prevalence of dyskinesia of 88% versus 54% in a group treated with low-dose levodopa.[59] However, the observation that dyskinesia can occur in a significant portion of patients within the first 3 months of therapy[4-6] makes the cumulative dose unlikely to be a major risk factor in the development of dyskinesia. The size of individual doses may, however, be important. The concomitant use of anticholinergics, antihistiminics, or amantadine has not been linked with increased risk to develop dyskinesia in patients treated with levodopa.

Summary of Risk Factors

Young, more severely affected patients with Parkinson's disease, who have a good therapeutic response to levodopa, are at high risk for developing dyskinesia. Patients with other neurological diseases or with parkinsonism that is not responsive to levodopa are at low risk. Patients treated only with dopamine agonists, anticholinergics, or amantadine rarely develop dyskinesia.

Pathophysiology

Model of Basal Ganglia Function and Dysfunction

Studies of the anatomical and neurotransmitter interconnections among the basal ganglia, their alterations in various disease states, and physiological studies in monkeys with MPTP-induced parkinsonism have produced a working hypothesis for the pathophysiology of parkinsonism and involuntary movements.[60–63] The major pathways and their neurotransmitters are indicated in Figure 1. Parkinsonism appears to be related to increased firing of the principal output projections of the basal ganglia to the thalamus from the globus pallidus interna (GPi) and the substantia nigra reticulata (SNr). Involuntary movements such as chorea, dystonia, and ballism result from a decreased firing of GPi and SNr. The rate of firing of the GPi and SNr is controlled by the balance between a direct putaminal-pallidal pathway utilizing neurons with GABA and substance P as neurotransmitters and an indirect pathway from putamen to the globus pallidus externa (GPe), thence to the subthalamic nucleus (STN) and then to the GPi and SNr. The loss of the dopaminergic nigrostriatal pathway in parkinsonism increases the activity in the indirect pathway from putamen to GPi via STN and reduces the activity in the direct pathway (Fig. 2). In support of this explanation is the recent observation that lesions of the STN will reverse many of the signs of parkinsonism in monkeys with MPTP-induced parkinsonism.[64] In hyperkinetic disorders, there appears to be a preponderance of the direct pathway effects and reduced activity in the indirect pathway, which in turn leads to reduced output from the GPi and SNr (Fig. 3). The subthalamic nucleus lesion, which abolishes

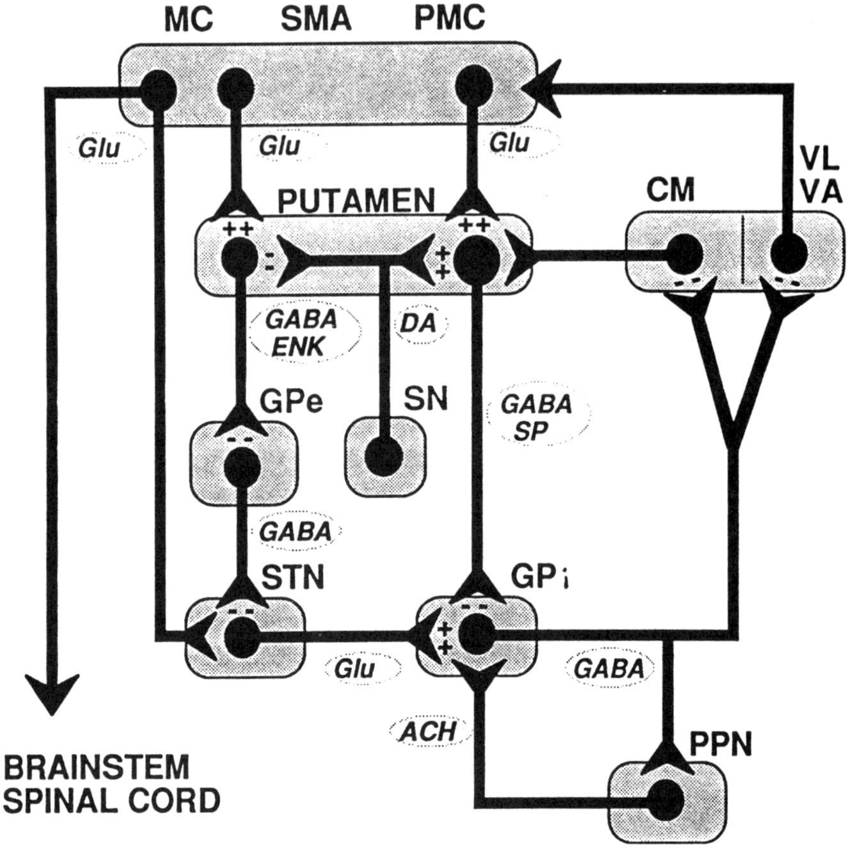

Figure 1: Current concept of neuronal connections and their neurotransmitters of basal ganglia, thalamus, and motor cortex. The cortical-subthalamic nucleus pathway and loops through the pedunculopontine nucleus and through the centromedian nucleus of thalamus are pathways of unknown function in motor control which are omitted in Figures 2 and 3. CM = nucleus centromedian, GPe = globus pallidus externa, GPi = globus pallidus interna, MC = motor cortex, PMC = premotor cortex, PPN = pedunculopontine nucleus, SMA = supplementary motor cortex, SN = substantia nigra, STN = subthalamic nucleus, VA and VL = nucleus ventral anterior and ventral lateral. The shaded letters represent neurotransmitters; ACH = acetylcholine, DA = dopamine, ENK = enkephalin, GLU = glutamic acid, SP = substance P. Adapted from DeLong and Crutcher[63] and Alexander.[62]

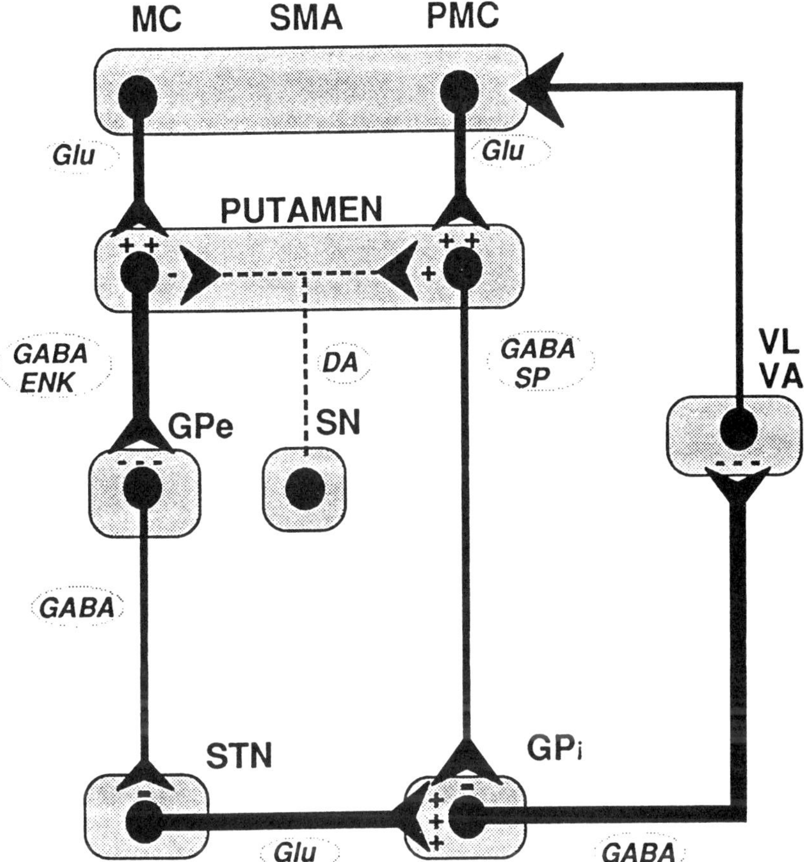

Figure 2: Model of basal ganglia function producing parkinsonism. Reduced dopaminergic input to the putamen results in a predominance of excitatory input to GPi from subthalamic nucleus. Abbreviations are the same as Figure 1. Adapted from DeLong.[63]

parkinsonism of MPTP-treated monkeys, produces dyskinesia by shifting the balance of afferent input to the GPi from the indirect putaminal-pallidal pathway to the direct connection.[65]

Upon initiation of levodopa, few patients have a dramatic improvement in their parkinsonism symptoms, and it is only with days to months of therapy that the drug begins to markedly reduce the parkinsonian signs. Likewise, dyskinesia does not immediately appear with initiation of levodopa. Thus, levodopa treatment may pro-

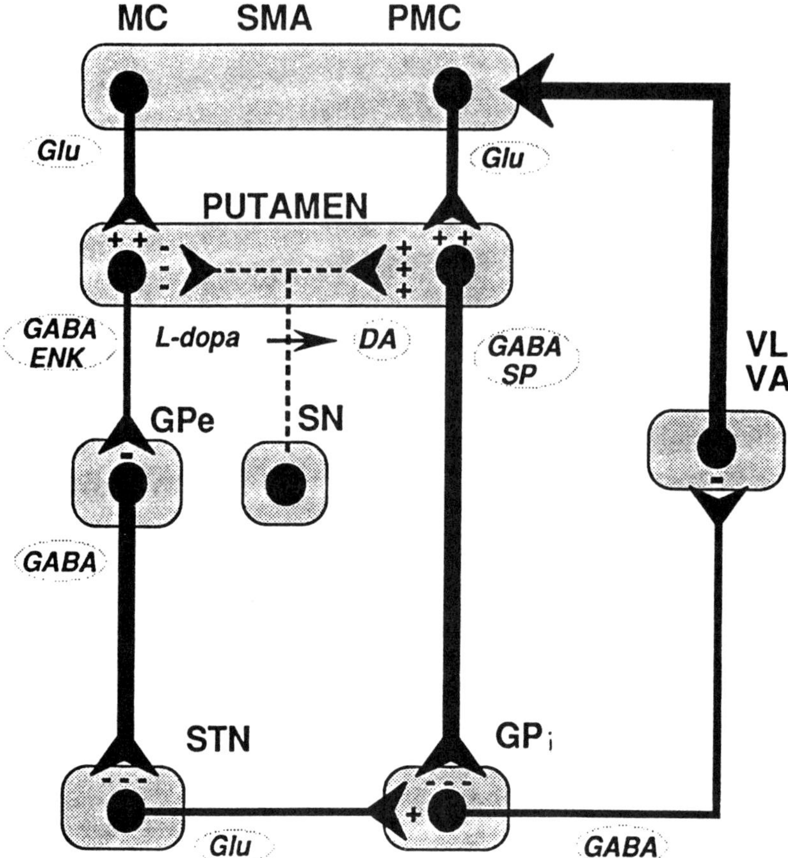

Figure 3: Model of basal ganglia function producing levodopa-induced dyskinesia in a parkinsonian subject. Levodopa, converted to dopamine in the putamen, reverses the balance of excitation and inhibition in the GPi by augmenting the direct inhibitory input while reducing the indirect excitatory input. This reduces or abolishes the parkinsonism but concomitantly induces dyskinesia. Abbreviations as in Figure 1. Adapted from DeLong.[63]

gressively shift the preponderance of input to the globus pallidus interna from the indirect pathway mediated through the subthalamic nucleus to the direct pathway, clinically manifest by increasing improvement of parkinsonism accompanied by dyskinesia. In patients whose parkinsonism does not respond to levodopa, striatal or pallidal pathology limits the ability of the drug to reduce activity in the indirect pathway, resulting in no clinical improvement but also no dyskinesia. An obvious but unanswered question is whether lesions or pharmacological manipulation of the STN would improve these patients with striatal pathology.

Pharmacological Mechanisms

Dopaminergic Denervation Required

Levodopa and the dopamine agonists very rarely induce dyskinesia in patients who do not have parkinsonism. This suggests that dopaminergic denervation is necessary for levodopa-induced dyskinesias. Studies in monkeys reinforce this concept. Extremely large doses of levodopa can produce hyperactivity and stereotyped movements in normal primates but requires doses that are often associated with toxicity including death.[53–57] These movements appear to be qualitatively different from the choreiform and dystonic dyskinesia that occurs in monkeys with MPTP-induced parkinsonism.[57,61]

This is not an "all or nothing" phenomenon; the extent of dopaminergic denervation is also an important variable in the susceptibility to levodopa-induced dyskinesia, as discussed earlier.

Induced by Levodopa

Repeated Dosing Necessary

Dyskinesia does not appear with the initial administration of levodopa in patients or in monkeys with MPTP-induced parkinsonism. Repeated dosing is necessary. Thus, dyskinesia is not explicable by dopaminergic stimulation of a dopaminergically denervated, supersensitive striatum. Some alteration of the drug response is induced by repeated dosing with levodopa. Potentially important drug-induced neurochemical changes include alterations in dopamine D_1 or D_2 receptor numbers,[39,65,66] adenylate cyclase activity,[65] or striatal GAD activity.[66]

Role of D_1 and D_2 Effects

Bromocriptine, a drug with D_2 agonist and D_1 antagonist properties, will only rarely induce dyskinesia in patients who have not been previously or are not concurrently treated with levodopa. This could be explained by the fact that bromocriptine rarely produces the antiparkinsonian effects that can be achieved with levodopa.[16,17] However, in the monkey with MPTP-induced parkinsonism, doses of bromocriptine that produce as much improvement in the signs of parkinsonism as does levodopa, still do not induce dyskinesia.[39] This has suggested that drug effects mediated by the D_1 receptor may be particularly critical to the development of dyskinesia. However, once patients or MPTP-treated monkeys develop dyskinesia with levodopa, then either D_1- or D_2-selective dopamine agonists can elicit dyskinesia.[25,67,68] Studies in rodents also suggest differences in the sensitization induced by D_1 and D_2 receptor agonists.[69,70] The newly described D_3 receptor[71] awaits pharmacological characterization.

Temporal Pattern of Drug Administration in Rodents

The temporal pattern of drug administration is important in determining whether the animals will demonstrate tolerance or sensitization to subsequent drug administration. Continuous administration of dopaminergic agents tends to reduce the response to subsequent doses.[72–75] Intermittent administration, which may be closer to the clinical situation in humans, results in sensitization.[66,70,72–74] Thus, the manner in which levodopa is administered may be critical to the development of dyskinesia in humans and increases the interest in new delivery systems for the drug.[76]

Biphasic Effects

Many neurally active drugs exhibit biphasic effects, one effect predominating at low doses and an entirely different effect predominating at high doses. For example, dopamine agonists and levodopa reduce motility in animals at low doses and increase motility at high doses.[77–79] The drug effect at any given time is a summation of these two (or more) separate effects. This biphasic drug effect is postulated to be mediated by different dopamine receptors, the difference perhaps reflecting dopamine receptor subtypes, the transduction process to which the receptors are coupled or the neuronal location of the receptors. This pharmacological phenomenon could explain the different types of levodopa-induced dyskinesia, peak dose, and diphasic dyskinesia resulting from sensitization of receptors and/or systems responsive to high concentrations of dopamine agonists and "off" dystonia resulting from sensitization of a different dopamine receptor subpopulation responsive to lower concentrations of dopamine agonists.

Treatment

Determining Pattern of Dyskinesia

To treat dyskinesia, one obviously needs to know what pattern of dyskinesia the patient experiences. This information is often very difficult to obtain from the patient because the patient has difficulty differentiating tremor, "off" dystonia, "on" dystonia, and choreoathetosis. In addition, patients with dyskinesia are, by definition, having fluctuations in motor response. It is important to understand the fluctuations in control of parkinsonism symptoms (wearing off, on-off) because any changes in medical regimen will effect this as well as the dyskinesia. If the history is not perfectly clear, and the physician has not observed the dyskinesia described by the patient, it is worthwhile having the patient stay in the clinic through one or two dose cycles so that the various forms of dyskinesia as well as the fluctuation in the parkinsonism can be observed. Monitoring the plasma levels of levodopa during this time may help delineate the relationship between plasma levels of drug and clinical responses.[80] However, it is important to recall that clinical response and plasma levels do not directly correlate; striatal dopamine concentrations are the important parameter and not plasma dopa. The relationships among plasma levodopa levels and levodopa-induced rise in dopamine concentration in the vicinity of the striatal dopamine receptors and clinical response remain unclear. For plasma levodopa levels to be of assistance in managing a patient, plasma levels and clinical ratings at 30- to 60-minute intervals through one or more dose cycles are necessary.

Peak Dose ("On") Dyskinesia

Therapeutic Window

The relationship between the dose or plasma levels of levodopa that produce dyskinesia and those that reduce parkinsonism are controversial. There is some evidence that initially the threshold for inducing dyskinesia is much higher than the threshold for inducing the improvement in parkinsonism.[3,35,36] This would suggest that when dyskinesia appears, smaller doses of the drug could be administered to produce the antiparkinsonian effects without eliciting dyskinesia. In practice, this therapeutic window is elusive, if it exists at all.

Other investigators have felt that once dyskinesia appears, it is generally present when the antiparkinsonian effect is apparent.[23,24,37] This implies that there is no therapeutic window and full therapeutic efficacy of levodopa will be accompanied by dyskinesia in those patients in whom dyskinesia has developed. This formulation suggests that reducing the dose of levodopa will not separate the antiparkinsonian effects and dyskinetic effects of the drug.

Altering Levodopa Administration

The most common strategy to try to reduce levodopa-induced dyskinesia is to give smaller doses of levodopa more frequently, trying to keep the doses within the controversial therapeutic window discussed above. This change will, at a minimum, shorten the duration of dyskinesia with each dose of medication, which in itself may make the dyskinesia more acceptable to the patient. However, concomitantly, the duration of antiparkinsonian effect of the drug is also shortened and the response to each dose of the drug may become more unpredictable because the plasma drug concentrations produced by the smaller doses are closer to the minimum effective concentration.[37] Nevertheless, this strategy is worth trying, although it benefits only a minority of patients.

Dopamine Agonists

In patients that have developed dyskinesia during levodopa therapy, dopamine agonists can also induce dyskinesia. However, they appear to have less propensity to induce dyskinesia than does levodopa. For that reason, trying to provide more of the dopaminergic stimulation with a dopamine agonist and less with levodopa may reduce dyskinesia. In a few patients, it is possible to substitute dopamine agonists almost entirely for the levodopa with a marked reduction in dyskinesia and acceptable control of the parkinsonism.

In patients receiving both dopamine agonists and levodopa, the dyskinesia tends to occur in relation to the levodopa administration and not the dopamine agonist administration.

Drugs to Suppress Dyskinesia

A wide variety of drugs have been tried in an attempt to suppress levodopa-induced dyskinesia without loss of the antiparkinsonian efficacy. In general, the benzodiazepines, GABAergic drugs,[81,82] and other sedative agents have been without efficacy. However, dyskinesia is often exacerbated by stress and anxiety, and effective treatment of these symptoms may secondarily reduce dyskinesia. Cholinergic agonists[83] and dopamine antagonists[84,85] reduce dyskinesia but concomitantly increase the parkinsonism. At this point in time, there appears to be no pharmacological manner in which to separate the dyskinetic and antiparkinsonian effects of the levodopa.

Thalamotomy

A ventrolateral thalamotomy will, in addition to its effects on tremor and rigidity, reduce or abolish contralateral levodopa-induced dyskinesia.[6,28,29] Occasionally, thalamotomy has been used for just this purpose, surgical suppression of severe dyskinesia permitting administration of adequate levodopa to control other parkinsonian disability. A particularly appropriate patient for this procedure would be one with disabling unilateral levodopa-induced dyskinesia.

Drug Holidays

Abstinence from levodopa and dopamine agonists for days to weeks ("drug holiday") will reduce or abolish many of the adverse side effects of the dopaminergic drugs, including peak dose dyskinesia, diphasic dyskinesia, "off" dystonia, and myoclonus but concomitantly severe and unrelenting parkinsonism reappears.[86–90] The reintroduction of levodopa at lower doses than prior to the holiday will often produce an equivalent or better antiparkinsonian effect,[86–88] an apparent resensitization to the drug. The duration of this beneficial effect is controversial, some reporting it largely gone at a year[89] and others finding it will persist for at least 2 years.[90] Peak dose dyskinesia appears to be less consistently improved by drug holidays than other adverse effects.[86,88] Because of this, plus the morbidity and mortality associated with drug holidays,[87–90] dyskinesia alone would generally not justify a drug holiday.

Continuous Dopaminergic Stimulation

A variety of methods are available to produce more continuous dopaminergic stimulation in patients with marked motor fluctuations ("wearing-off" and "on-off"). These include: (1) controlled release preparations of levodopa[91]; (2) continuous duodenal delivery of levodopa[92] or levodopa methyl ester[93]; (3) continuous subcutaneous administration of lisuride[94] or apomorphine[95] by "insulin pump"; (4) continuous intravenous administration of levodopa[96] or levodopa ester.[97] These methods may produce constant or varying dopaminergic stimulation throughout the day. Most studies discontinue treatment while the patients are asleep; lisuride and apomorphine are often given in combination with low doses of oral levodopa and the patients can titrate the rate of administration or add boluses of agonist. Thus, with the exception of continuous levodopa,[96] the patients receive continuous but varying dopaminergic stimulation or intermittent constant stimulation. The effect of these various techniques of "continuous dopaminergic stimulation" on dyskinesia vary. Generally, these methods produce more "on" time, which is associated with "on" or "peak dose" dyskinesia being present a greater portion of the day and a corresponding reduction in "off" dystonia. With subcutaneous lisuride,[94] dyskinesia was unchanged or increased in severity with months of continuous therapy; with intravenous levodopa for days, there was an increase in the threshold to induce dyskinesia.[96] Overall, continuous stimulation has not decreased peak dose or diphasic dyskinesia.

A different question, the effect of continuous rather than intermittent administration of dopaminergic drugs on the induction of dyskinesia in patients not previously treated with levodopa, is currently being studied using controlled release levodopa for the "continuous" therapy. This is based on the suggestion that "continuous" therapy simulates the normal physiological state of tonic activity of nigrostriatal dopaminergic neurons in contrast to the intermittent or pulsatile stimulation caused by our current use of standard formulations of levodopa.

Diphasic Dyskinesia

Diphasic dyskinesia, dyskinesia that occurs at the beginning and the end of each dose cycle, is generally most prominent as the effects of a dose wear off. Utilizing larger doses of levodopa or scheduling the doses closer together can prevent the interdose exacerbation of dyskinesia until the end of the day when the patient stops or reduces the levodopa intake.[9] Although this strategy clearly works in the short run, most investigators have found that it is ineffective over the long haul because of increasing peak dose dyskinesia, repeated breakthrough of the diphasic dyskinesia despite further levodopa dosage adjustments, or other toxicity.[22,98] Furthermore, there is the impression that if the patients are kept "on" and free of the diphasic swings throughout the day, the dyskinesia may be even more severe as they "come down" at the end of the day than if it occurred with each dose throughout the day. Dopamine agonists may be of some benefit in reducing the severity of the diphasic dyskinesia but rarely completely control it.[98] Surprisingly, continuous infusions of levodopa will not control diphasic dyskinesia that continues to reappear despite further increases in the infusion rate.[99] The same pattern of breakthrough is described with subcutaneous apomorphine.[95]

"Off" Dystonia

"Off" dystonia is most prominent in the morning when the patient has been without medication overnight, and this is the reason that "off" dystonia was initially described as "early morning dystonia." It frequently is precipitated by the patient trying to get out of bed and walk to the bathroom. Timing of the first dose of the day of levodopa may prevent or reduce this painful dyskinesia. Some patients find that if they have the medicine at the bedside, take it upon awakening, and wait for 15 to 30 minutes before getting out of bed, they may avoid the dystonia. A dose of drug taken during the night will also reduce this dystonia. The controlled release preparations of Sinemet[R] or Madopar[R], which provide more sustained plasma levels of levodopa, will also reduce "off" dystonia as will the other techniques for continuous dopaminergic stimulation discussed. Dopamine agonists are also frequently efficacious in reducing "off" dystonia. Finally, anecdotal reports suggest that lithium or baclofen may also be effective in controlling the symptoms. "Off" dystonia is the most successfully treated of the three major forms of levodopa-induced dyskinesia.

Future Trends

Manipulation of Other Pathways within the Basal Ganglia

The models of normal and disordered basal ganglia function (Figs. 1–3) suggest that manipulation of other neurotransmitter systems and pathways within the basal ganglia may compensate for the loss of the dopaminergic nigrostriatal tract activity. The obvious importance of the subthalamic nucleus in models of hypokinetic and hyperkinetic movement disorders is attracting particular attention. The subthalamic nucleus receives direct glutamatergic input from cortex and has glutamatergic projections to the globus pallidus interna and substantia nigra reticulata. Rapidly accumulating information about glutamatergic receptors and drugs to manipulate them will make this an active area of investigation.[100] A number of pathways within the basal ganglia use GABA as a neurotransmitter (see Fig. 1) with the result that GABAergic agents may have relatively nonspecific or nonselective properties. However, the GABAergic neurons can be divided into subpopulations identified by their co-transmitters. For example, GABAergic neurons projecting from the putamen directly to the globus pallidus have substance P as a co-transmitter; the GABAergic neurons projecting from the putamen to the external segment of the globus pallidus have enkephalin as a co-transmitter. Pharmacological methods of selectively influencing these subpopulations of GABAergic neurons by taking advantage of the co-transmitter specificity may prove useful in manipulating basal ganglia function. Finally, it should be noted that there are other loops within the basal ganglia and thalamus, such as through the pedunculopontine nucleus or through the centromedian nucleus of the thalamus, for which no function is recognized but which may be as important as the substantia nigra compacta or the subthalamic nucleus in modulating basal ganglia function.

Induction of Dyskinesia

The fact that dyskinesia does not occur with the first doses of levodopa but is induced by chronic treatment with levodopa suggests that it may be possible to avoid the development of dyskinesia. The antiparkinsonian effects of levodopa are often mild at the initiation of therapy and increase with continued therapy, suggesting that the antiparkinsonian effect of levodopa may be induced as well. Determining how repeated exposure to dopaminergic agents gradually augments the antiparkinsonism and dyskinetic response to each dose of medication will be another important area of investigation. This apparent sensitization is often attributed to an increase in the number of dopamine receptors, but most studies have found normal striatal D_1 and D_2 receptor densities in levodopa-treated parkinsonian patients with dyskinesia.[101] It is more likely that the increased sensitivity to the dopaminergic agents represents changes that occur in the transduction of dopamine receptor occupancy into changes in neuronal function or changes in multineuronal feedback loops. This induction may be very dependent upon the degree of dopaminergic denervation of the striatum, the profile of dopamine receptor subtype activation produced by the drug and the interdose intervals. Defining the contribution of these variables to induction of dyskinesia may have a very important impact on the manner in which dopaminergic drugs are used in patients. Clinically, studies are underway to see if lower doses of levodopa, more continuous dopaminergic stimulation via controlled release preparations, and different combinations of D_1 and D_2 stimulation by various agonists will alter the induction of dyskinesia.

Pharmacologically Separating Dyskinetic and Antiparkinsonian Effects of Dopaminergic Agents

There are currently three dopamine receptor subtypes characterized by molecular cloning, and pharmacological evidence suggests that there may be at least several more receptor subtypes.[102] To date, efforts to attribute dyskinesia to activation of the D_1 or D_2 receptor subtypes has been unsuccessful,[25,68] but other receptor subtypes will undoubtedly emerge as will agents with more selectivity for the receptor subtypes. Although the basic classification of the dopamine receptors is based on whether they activate or inhibit adenylate cyclase, it is known that there are other effectors for the dopamine receptor including phospholipase C and potassium channels.[102] Drugs directed at these specific effector systems may allow more selectivity and conceivably produce an antiparkinsonian effect without dyskinesia. A final potential method of achieving more specificity within the dopaminergic system may come from manipulating the co-transmitters present in dopamine neurons. Cholecystokinin, which is colocalized with dopamine in a subpopulation of dopaminergic neurons is being looked at in this manner.[103]

Acknowledgment: I thank Michelle Leaver for her patience and skill in preparing this manuscript.

References

1. Cotzias GC, Van Woert MH, Schiffer LM. Aromatic amino acids and modification of parkinsonism. N Engl J Med 1967; 276:374–379.
2. Birkmeyer W, Hornykiewicz O. The effect of L-3,4-dihydroxyphenylalanine (= dopa) on akinesia in Parkinson's syndrome. Klin Wochenschr 1961; 73:787–788.
3. Cotzias GC, Papavasiliou PS, Gellene R. Modification of parkinsonism: chronic treatment with L-dopa. N Engl J Med 1969; 280:337–345.
4. Barbeau A, Mars H, Gillo-Joffroy L. Adverse clinical side effects of levodopa therapy: recent advances in Parkinson's disease. In: McDowell FH, Markham CH (eds), Contemporary Neurology Series, Philadelphia, FA Davis Co., 1971, pp 204–237.
5. Markham CH. Choreoathetoid movement disorder induced by levodopa. Clin Pharmacol Ther 1971; 12(Part 2):340–343.
6. Mones RJ, Elizan TS, Siegel JS. Analysis of L-dopa-induced dyskinesias in 51 patients with parkinsonism. J Neurol Neurosurg Psych 1971; 34:668–673.
7. Tolosa ES, Martin WE, Cohen HP, Jacobsen RL. Patterns of clinical response and plasma dopa levels in Parkinson's disease. Neurology 1975; 25:177–183.
8. Muenter MD, Sharpless NS, Tyce GM, Darley FL. Patterns of dystonia (I-D-I" and "D-I-D") in response to L-dopa therapy for Parkinson's disease. Mayo Clin Proc 1977; 52:163–173.
9. Lhermette F, Agid Y, Signoret JL. Onset and end-of-dose levodopa-induced dyskinesias. Arch Neurol 1978; 35:261–263.
10. Melamed E. Early-morning dystonia: a late side effect of long-term levodopa therapy in Parkinson's disease. Arch Neurol 1979; 36:308–310.
11. Nausieda PA, Weiner WJ, Klawans HL. Dystonic foot response of parkinsonism. Arch Neurol 1980; 37:132–136.
12. Schwab RS, Amador LP, Lettvin JY. Apomorphine in Parkinson's disease. Trans-Am Neurol Assoc 1951; 76:251–253.
13. Cotzias GC, Papavasiliou PS, Fehling C, Kaufman B, Mena I. Similarities between neurological effects of L-dopa and of apomorphine. N Engl J Med 1970; 282:31–33.

14. Cotzias GC, Papavasiliou PS, Tolosaes Mendez JS, Bell-Midura M. Treatment of parkinson's disease with aporphines: possible role of growth hormone. N Engl J Med 1976; 294:567–572.
15. Calne DB, Teychenne PF, Leigh PN, Bamji AN, Greenacre JK. Treatment of parkinsonism with bromocriptine. 1974; 2:1355–1356.
16. Lees AJ, Stern GM. Sustained bromocriptine therapy in previously untreated patients with Parkinson's disease. J Neurol Neurosurg Psychiatry 1981; 44:1020–1023.
17. Rinne UK. Combined bromocriptine-levodopa therapy early in Parkinson's disease. Neurology 1985; 35:1196–1198.
18. Burns RS, Chieuh CC, Markey SP, Ebert MH, Jacobowitz, Kopin IJ. A primate model of parkinsonism. Proc Natl Acad Sci USA 1983; 80:4546–4550.
19. Purves SJ. Paralysis agitans: with an account of a new symptom. Lancet 1889; 2:1258–1260.
20. Klawans HL, Goetz C, Bergen D. Levodopa-induced myoclonus. Arch Neurol 1975; 32:331–334.
21. Lang AE, Johnson K. Akathisia in idiopathic Parkinson's disease. Neurology 1987; 37:477–481.
22. Marsden CD, Parkes JD, Quinn N. Fluctuations of disability in Parkinson's disease: clinical aspects. In: Marsden CD, Fahn S (eds), Movement Disorders, London, Butterworths, 1981, pp 96–122.
23. Nutt JG, Woodward WR. Levodopa pharmacokinetics and pharmacodynamics in fluctuating parkinsonian patients. Neurology 1986; 36:739–744.
24. Hardie RJ, Lees AJ, Stern GM. On-off fluctuations in Parkinson's disease: a clinical and neuropharmacological study. Brain 1984; 107:487–506.
25. Clarke CE, Boyce S, Robertson RG, Sambrook MA, Crossman AR. Drug-induced dyskinesia in primate rendered hemiparkinsonian by intracarotid administration of 1-methyl-4-phenyl-1,2,3,6-tetrahydropyridine (MPTP). J Neurol Sci 1989; 90:307–314.
26. Poewe WH, Lees AJ, Stern GM. Dystonia in Parkinson's disease: clinical and pharmacological features. Ann Neurol 1988; 23:73–78.
27. Horstink M, Zylmans J, Pasman J, Berger H, Van't Hof M. Severity of Parkinson's disease is a risk factor for peak-dose dyskinesia. J Neurol Neurosurg Psychiatry 1990; 53:224–226.
28. Narabayashi H, Yokochi F, Nakajima Y. Levodopa-induced dyskinesia and thalamotomy. J Neurol Neurosurg Psychiatry 1984; 47:831–839.
29. Hashes RC, Polgar JG, Weightman D, et al. L-dopa in parkinsonism and the influence of previous thalamotomy. Br Med J 1971; 1:7–13.
30. Weiner WJ, Goetz CG, Nausieda PA, Klawans HL. Respiratory dyskinesias: extrapyramidal dysfunction and dyspnea. Ann Intern Med 1978; 88:327–331.
31. Zupnick HM, Brown LK, Miller A, Moros DA. Respiratory dysfunction due to L-dopa therapy for parkinsonism: diagnosis using serial pulmonary function tests and respiratory inductive plethysmography. Am J Med 1990; 89:109–114.
32. Ilson J, Braun N, Fahn S. Respiratory fluctuations in Parkinson's disease. Neurology 1983; 33(Suppl 2):113.

33. Vincken WG, Gauthier SG, Dollfus RE, Hanson RE, Darauay CM, Cosio MG. Involvement of upper-airway muscles in extrapyramidal disorders. N Engl J Med 1984; 311:438–442.
34. Jankovic J, Casabona J. Coexistent tardive dyskinesia and parkinsonism. Clin Neuropharmacol 1987; 10:511–521.
35. Mouradian MM, Juncos JL, Fabbrini G, Schlegel J, Bartko JJ, Chase TN. Motor fluctuations in Parkinson's disease: central pathophysiological mechanisms. Part II. Ann Neurol 1988; 24:372–378.
36. Mouradian MM, Heuser IJE, Baronti F, Fabbrini G, Juncos JL, Chase TN. Pathogenesis of dyskinesias in Parkinson's disease. Ann Neurol 1989; 25:523–526.
37. Nutt JG, Woodward WR, Carter JH, Gancher ST. Effect of chronic therapy on the pharmacodynamics of levodopa: relation to on-off phenomenon. Neurology 1990; 40(Suppl):292.
38. Boyce S, Clarke CE, Luquin R, Peggs D, Robertson RG, Mitchell IJ, Sambrook MA, Crossman AR. Induction of chorea and dystonia in parkinsonian primates. Mov Disord 1990; 5:3–7.
39. Bedard PJ, Di Paolo T, Falardeau P, Boucher R. Chronic treatment with L-dopa, but not bromocriptine induces dyskinesia in MPTP-parkinsonian monkeys: correlation with [^{3}H]spiperone binding. Brain Res 1986; 379:294–299.
40. Schneider JS. Levodopa-induced dyskinesias parkinsonian monkeys: relationship to extent of nigrostriatal damage. Pharmacol Biochem Behav 1989; 34:193–196.
41. Gancher ST, Nutt JG, Woodward WR. Response to brief levodopa infusions in parkinsonian patients with and without motor fluctuations. Neurology 1988; 38:712–716.
42. Nutt JG, Woodward WR, Carter JH, Trotman TL. Influence of fluctuations of plasma large neutral amino acids with normal diets on the clinical response to levodopa. J Neurol Neurosurg Psychiatry 1989; 52:481–487.
43. Lesser RP, Fahn S, Snider SR, Cote LJ, Isgreen WP, Barrett RE. Analysis of the clinical problems in parkinsonism and the complications of long-term levodopa therapy. Neurology 1979; 29:1253–1260.
43a. Quinn N, Critchley P, Marsden CD. Young onset Parkinson's disease. Mov Disord 1987; 2:73–91.
44. Sweet RD, McDowell FH. Five years' treatment of Parkinson's disease with levodopa: therapeutic results and survival of 100 patients. Ann Intern Med 1975; 83:456–463.
45. Barbeau A. High-level levodopa therapy in severly akinetic parkinsonian patients: twelve years later. In: Rinne UK, Klinger M, Stamm G (eds), Parkinson's Disease: Current Progress, Problems and Management, Amsterdam/NY, Elsevier, 1980, pp 229–239.
46. Tanner C. Drug-induced movement disorders (tardive dyskinesia and dopa-induced dyskinesia). In: Vinken P, Bruyn GW, Klawans HL (eds), Extrapyramidal Disorders, Handbook of Clinical Neurology, Vol. 5, Amsterdam, Elsevier Science, 1986, pp 185–204.
47. Pederzoli M, Girotti F, Scigliano G, Aiello G, Carella F, Caraceni T. L-Dopa long-term treatment in Parkinson's disease: age-related side effects. Neurology 1983; 33:1518–1522.

48. Quinn NP, Marsden CD. Menstrual-related fluctuations in Parkinson's disease. Mov Disord 1986; 1:85–87.
49. Chase TN, Holden EM, Brody JA. Levodopa-induced dyskinesias: comparison in parkinsonism-dementia and amyotrophic lateral sclerosis. Arch Neurol 1973; 29:328–330.
50. Langston WJ, Ballard P. Parkinsonism induced by 1-methyl-4-phenyl-1, 2,3,6-tetrahydropyridine (MPTP): implications for treatment and the pathogenesis of Parkinson's disease. Can J Neurol Sci 1984; 11:160–165.
51. Lang AE, Meadows JC, Parkes JD, Marsden CD. Early onset of the "on-off" phenomenon in children with symptomatic parkinsonism. J Neurol Neurosurg Psych 1982; 45:823–825.
52. Goodwin FK, Murphy DL, Brodie KH, Bunney WE. L-dopa, catecholamines, and behavior: a clinical and biochemical study in depressed patients. Biol Psychiatry 1970; 2:341–366.
52a. Lang AE, Birnbaum A, Blair RDG, Kierans C. Levodopa dose-related fluctuations in presumed olivopontocerebellar atrophy. Movement Disorders 1986; 1:93–102.
52b. Fearnley JM, Lees AJ. Striatonigral degeneration: a clinicopathological study. Brain 1990; 113:1823–1842.
53. Sassin JF, Taub S, Weitzman ED. Hyperkinesia and changes in behavior produced in normal monkeys by L-dopa. Neurology 1972; 22:1122–1125.
54. Mones RJ. Experimental dyskinesias in normal rhesus monkey. Adv Neurol 1973; 1:665–669.
55. Paulson GW. Dyskinesias in monkeys. Adv Neurol 1973; 1:647–650.
56. Ng LKY, Gelhard RE, Chase TN, MacLean PD. Drug-induced dyskinesia in monkeys: a pharmacologic model employing 6-hydroxydopamine. Adv Neurol 1973; 1:651–655.
57. Boyce S, Rupniak NMJ, Steventon MJ, Iverson SD. Characterization of dyskinesias induced by L-dopa in MPTP-treated squirrel monkeys. Psychopharmacology 1990; 102:21–27.
58. Fahn S, Calne DB. Considerations in the management of parkinsonism. Neurology 1978; 28:5–7.
59. Poewe WH, Lees AJ, Stern GM. Low-dose L-dopa therapy in Parkinson's disease: a six-year follow-up study. Neurology 1986; 36: 1528–1530.
60. Albin RL, Young AB, Penney JB. The functional anatomy of basal ganglia disorders. Trends Neurosci 1989; 12:366–375.
61. Crossman AR. A hypothesis on the pathophysiological mechanisms that underlie levodopa or dopamine agonist-induced dyskinesia in Parkinson's disease: implications for future strategies in treatment. Movement Disorders 1990; 5:100–108.
62. Alexander GE, Crutcher MD. Functional architecture of basal ganglia circuits: neural substrates of parallel processing. Trends Neurosci 1990; 13:266–271.
63. DeLong MR. Primate models of movement disorders of basal ganglia origin. Trends Neurosci 1990; 13:281–285.
64. Bergman H, Wickmann T, DeLong MR. Reversal of experimental par-

kinsonism by lesions of the subthalamic nucleus. Science 1990; 249:1436–1438.

65. Parenti M, Flauto C, Parati E, Vescovi A, Groppetti A. Differential effect of repeated treatment with L-dopa on dopamine D_1 and D_2 receptors. Neuropharmacology 1986; 25:331–334.

66. Juncos JL, Engber TM, Susel Z, et al. Continuous and intermittent levodopa administration differentially affect basal ganglia function. Ann Neurol 1989; 25:473–478.

67. Stoessl AJ, Mak E, Calne DB. (+)-4-Propyl-9-hydroxynaphylhoxazine (PHNO), a new dopaminomimetic, in treatment of parkinsonism. Lancet 1985; 2:1330–1331.

68. Temlett JA, Quinn NP, Jenner PG, et al. Antiparkinsonian activity of CV 208–243, a partial D_1 dopamine receptor agonist, in MPTP-treated marmosets and patients with Parkinson's disease. Mov Disord 1989; 4:261–265.

69. Braun A, Chase TN. Behavioral effects of chronic exposure to selective D_1 and D_2 dopamine receptor agonists. Eur J Pharmacol 1988; 147:441–451.

70. Morelli M, Di Chiara G. Agonist-induced homologous and heterologous sensitization to D_1 and D_2-dependent contraversive turning. Eur J Pharmacol 1987; 141:101–107.

71. Sokoloff P, Giros B, Martres MP, Bouthenet ML, Schwartz JC. Molecular cloning and characterization of a novel dopamine receptor (D_3) as a target for neuroleptics. Nature 1990; 347:146–150.

72. Post RM. Minireview: intermittent versus continuous stimulation: effect of time interval on the development of sensitization or tolerance. Life Sci 1980; 26:1275–1282.

73. Castro R, Abreu P, Calzadilla CH, Rodriguez M. Increased or decreased locomotor response in rats following repeated administration of apomorphine depends on dosage interval. Psychopharmacology 1985; 85:333–339.

74. Nelson LR, Ellison G. Enhanced stereotypies for repeated injections but not continuous amphetamines. Neuropharmacology 1978; 17:1081–1084.

75. Winkler JD, Weiss B. Effect of continuous exposure to selective D_1 and D_2 dopaminergic agonists on rotational behavior in supersensitive mice. J Pharmacol Exp Ther 1989; 249:507–516.

76. Chase TN, Baronti F, Fabbrini G, Heuser IJ, Juncos JL, Mouradian MM. Rationale for continuous dopaminomimetic therapy of Parkinson's disease. Neurology 1989; 39(suppl 2):7–10.

77. Stromberg U. Dopa effects on motility in mice: potentiation by MK 485 and dexchlorpheniramine. Psychopharmacologia 1970; 18:58–67.

78. Vaccheri A, Rossella Dall'Olio LR, Gandolfi O, Montanaro N. Involvement of different dopamine receptors in rat diphasic motility response to apomorphine. Psychopharmacology 1986; 89:265–268.

79. Rubenstein M, Gershanik O, Stefano FJE. Postsynaptic bimodal effect of sulpiride on locomotor activity induced by pergolide in catecholamine-depleted mice. Arch Pharmacol 1988; 337:115–117.

80. McHale DM, Sage JI, Sonsalla PK, Vilagliano D. Complex dystonia of

Parkinson's disease: clinical features and relation to plasma levodopa profile. Clin Neuropharmacol 1990; 13:164–170.

81. Price PA, Parkes JD, Marsden CD. Sodium valproate in the treatment of levodopa-induced dyskinesias. J Neurol Neurosurg Psychiatry 1978; 41:702–706.

82. Nutt J, Williams A, Plotkin F, et al. Treatment of Parkinson's disease with sodium valproate: clinical, pharmacological and biochemical observations. J Can Neurol Sci 1979; 6:337–343.

83. Tarsy D, Leopold N, Sax D. Physostigmine in choreiform movement disorders. Neurology 1974; 24:28–34.

84. Klawans HL, Weiner WJ. Attempted use of haloperidol in the treatment of L-dopa-induced dyskinesias. J Neurol Neurosurg Psychiatry 1974; 427–430.

85. Lees AJ, Lander CM, Stern GM. Tiapride in levodopa-induced involuntary movements. J Neurol Neurosurg Psychiatry 1979; 42:380–383.

86. Sweet RD, Lee JE, Spiegel HE, McDowell F. Enhanced response to low doses of levodopa after withdrawal from chronic therapy. Neurology 1972; 22:520–525.

87. Direnfeld LK, Feldman RG, Alexander MP, Kelly-Hayes M. Is L-dopa drug holiday useful? Neurology 1980; 30:785–788.

88. Weiner WJ, Koller WC, Perlik S, Nausieda PA, Klawans HL. Drug holiday and management of Parkinson's disease. Neurology 1980; 30:1257–1261.

89. Mayeux R, Stern Y, Mulvey K, Cote L. Reappraisal of temporary levodopa withdrawal ("drug holiday") in Parkinson's disease. N Engl J Med 1985; 313:724–728.

90. Kaye JA, Feldman RG. The role of L-dopa holiday in the long- term management of parkinson's disease. Clin Neuropharmacol 1986; 9:1–13.

91. Cederbaum JM, Kutt H, McDowell FH. A pharmacokinetic and pharmacodynamic comparison of Sinemet CR (50/200) and standard Sinemet (25/100). Neurology 1989; 39(Suppl 2):38–44.

92. Sage JI, Trooskin S, Sonsalla PK, Heikkila R, Duvoisin RC. Long-term duodenal infusion of levodopa for motor fluctuations in parkinsonism. Ann Neurol 1988; 24:87–89.

93. Ruggieri S, Stocchi F, Carta A, Catarci M, Agnoli A. Jejunal delivery of levodopa methyl ester. Lancet 1989; 2:45–46.

94. Obeso JA, Luquin MR, Maamonde J, Martinez Lase JM. Subcutaneous administration of lisuride in the treatment of complex motor fluctuations in Parkinson's disease. J Neurol Transm 1988; 27(Suppl):17–25.

95. Lees AJ. The on-off phenomenon. J Neurol Neurosurg Psychiatry 1989; (special suppl):29–37.

96. Mouradian RM, Heuser IJE, Baronti F, Chase TN. Modification of central dopaminergic mechanisms by continuous levodopa therapy for advanced Parkinson's disease. Ann Neurol 1990; 27:18–23.

97. Juncos JL, Mouradian MM, Fabbrini G, Serrati C, Chase TN. Levodopa methyl ester treatment of Parkinson's disease. Neurology 1987; 37:1242–1245.

98. Fahn S. Fluctuations of disability in Parkinson's disease: pathophysi-

ology. In: Marsden CD, Fahn S (eds), Movement Disorders, London, Butterworths, 1981, pp 123–134.

99. Quinn N, Parkes D, Marsden CD. Control of on/off phenomenon by continuous intravenous infusion of levodopa. Neurology 1984; 34:1131–1136.

100. Klockgether T, Turski L. NMDA antagonists potentiate antiparkinsonian actions of L-dopa in monoamine-depleted rats. Ann Neurol 1990; 28:539–546.

101. Pierot L, Desnos C, Bleu J, et al. D_1 and D_2-type dopamine receptors in patients with Parkinson's disease and progressive supranuclear palsy. J Neurol Sci 1988; 86:291–306.

102. Carron MG, Andersen PH, Gingrich JA, Bates MD, et al. Dopamine receptor subtypes] beyond the D_1/D_2 classifications. Trends Pharmacol Sci 1990; 11:231–236.

103. Boyce S.s, Rupniak NM, Steventon M, Iverson SD. CCK-8S inhibits L-dopa-induced dyskinesias in parkinsonian squirrel monkeys. Neurology 1990; 40:717–718.

11

Movement Disorders and Dopaminomimetic Stimulant Drugs

William J. Weiner, M.D.,
Juan Sanchez-Ramos, M.D., Ph.D.

Introduction

This chapter will focus on movement disorders induced by drugs that affect dopaminergic activity within the central nervous system. Drugs used to treat Parkinson's disease (e.g., levodopa, dopamine receptor agonists) and their effects on the motor system are discussed in Chapter 10. The four agents that will be reviewed here are amphetamine, methylphenidate, pemoline, and cocaine. Discussion will focus very briefly on the central pharmacological activities of these drugs. This will be followed by review of reports relating each of these agents to the induction of abnormal movements and to whether or not the use of these agents will alter movement abnormalities that are already present in such disorders as Parkinson's disease, choreiform disorders, Tourette's syndrome, and dystonia.

Amphetamine, one of the most potent sympathomimetic amines, was first synthesized in 1887. It was not until the 1930s that amphet-

Lang AE, Weiner WJ (editors): *Drug-Induced Movement Disorders*, Mount Kisco, NY, © Futura Publishing Co., Inc., 1992.

315

amine was introduced into clinical practice as a nasal decongestant (an inhaler) and as an appetite suppressant. Reports of self-stimulation and abuse occurred in the same decade. The CNS stimulant effects of amphetamine are primarily related to its release of biogenic amines from storage sites in nerve terminals. Amphetamine affects the dopaminergic system by releasing newly synthesized cytoplasmic dopamine, inhibiting dopamine reuptake, and at high doses, inhibition of monoamine oxidase (MAO). Amphetamine's ability to induce spontaneous repetitive behaviors is thought to be related to the release of newly synthesized dopamine from storage sites in the striatum.

Amphetamine and cocaine have very similar psychostimulant properties and induce a sense of increased wakefulness, alertness, a decreased sense of fatigue, elevation of mood, increased initiative, increased confidence, increased concentration, elation, and euphoria. In fact, under laboratory conditions, experienced drug users often cannot distinguish between amphetamine and cocaine. Cocaine has been used for centuries by the inhabitants of the highlands of Peru primarily to induce a sense of well-being. In the late nineteenth century, cocaine's local anesthetic properties were recognized. Freud was particularly impressed by its CNS actions, and his overenthusiasm for the drug has been widely publicized. Cocaine today is at the center of the illegitimate drug abuse problems in the United States.

The central nervous system effects of cocaine are produced by an increase in the synaptic concentration of dopamine. Cocaine inhibits dopamine uptake mechanisms, particularly in the cells that originate in the ventral tegmentum which project to the nucleus accumbens, ventral pallidum, and the frontal cortex. In short, cocaine affects the dopaminergic mesocortical, mesolimbic, and mesostriatal pathways.

Methylphenidate is a piperidine derivative that is structurally related to amphetamine. It is generally recognized as a mild CNS stimulant with more prominent effects on mental rather than motor activities. These CNS effects are mediated by release of dopamine from storage vesicles. The evidence to support the statement that methylphenidate releases dopamine from storage vesicles and not from the newly synthesized dopamine pool comes from animal studies indicating that the effect of methylphenidate on dopamine can be blocked by reserpine but not by alphamethylparatyrosine. This drug has been used widely in the treatment of attention deficit disorder (ADD).

Pemoline, another CNS stimulant, not structurally related to methylphenidate, is also widely used to treat ADD. Its CNS effects are also related to release of dopamine within the CNS.

Amphetamine-Induced Abnormal Movements

Of the drugs discussed in this chapter, the most information is available on amphetamine. After the introduction of amphetamine into clinical practice, there followed a long period of time during which amphetamine was readily prescribed by physicians for a variety of ailments. It was considered safe and effective and it was not until the 1960s that concern began to be raised regarding the potential problems associated with indiscriminate widespread amphetamine use.[1,2] Amphetamine psychosis, which can be indistinguishable from paranoid schizophrenia and various degrees of amphetamine dependence, have now been well described. In this chapter, the effect of amphetamine on the motor system is considered. In particular, the acute and chronic effects of amphetamine on both "normal" and diseased central nervous systems will be discussed.

Stereotyped Behavior

Single high doses or repeated low doses of amphetamine administered to various animals produce a motor phenomenon described as amphetamine-induced stereotyped behavior. The stereotyped behavior produced in various species varies in its behavioral manifestations; for example, a chewing, gnawing behavior occurs in rats, a repetitive chewing behavior occurs in guinea pigs, strange head movements occur in cats, and repetitive pecking is seen in pigeons. Amphetamine induces stereotyped behavior through dopaminergic mechanisms in the basal ganglia.[3-5] In humans, the response to amphetamine with regard to the induction of stereotyped behavior is much more varied. In fact, in an extensive review of the effects of amphetamine in humans, no definite mention is made of this phenomenon when the results of a single standard dose of amphetamine are considered. However, this review suggests that doses exceeding an individual's tolerance do produce intoxication syndromes that may be accompanied by stereotyped behavior.[6] Whether this is really an intoxication or a dose-response relationship is unclear and perhaps semantic.

Stereotyped behavior is considered to be present in animals when certain behavioral repertoires are repeated over and over again without any obvious goal or reinforcement. In more extreme instances, a single behavior or activity is performed continuously and dominates the animal's behavior. In guinea pigs with fully developed amphetamine-induced stereotyped behavior, the animals will chew repetitively at the bars or grid of the cage without moving, and often even loud noises will not disrupt this activity. This type of stereotyped behavior occurs in unlesioned intact animals receiving high doses of amphetamine. In human beings who are intravenous amphetamine abusers, certain behavioral abnormalities that resemble stereotyped behavior are seen. These behaviors have been variously described and include compulsive shoe shining, nail polishing to the point of producing finger ulcerations, repetitive sorting of objects in a handbag, manipulation of the interiors of a watch, days and nights spent rebuilding a car with unrelated parts, and hours spent trying to dismantle and repair items that are in perfect working order.[7,8] Additional descriptions of this behavior include cleaning rooms and drawers, washing dishes, perpetual hair dressing, distinctive and repetitive walking patterns, and sitting in a tub and bathing all day long.[64] This behavior has been called punding.[9] Attempts to disrupt this stereotyped behavior often elicit anxiety, and despite its inane quality, amphetamine abusers often describe the behavior as pleasurable. Punding is usually not recognized by abusers as a sign worthy of mentioning, and a history of its occurrence has to be specifically sought.[7] Some have suggested that these disorganized and perseverative behaviors are exaggerations of individual personality characteristics. However, in almost every patient who develops punding, paranoid symptoms occur sooner or later.[61] Individuals exhibiting this behavior have also been described as withdrawn, giving the impression of absentmindedness. It has also been noted that the punding act is consistent and the same for each amphetamine addict. In fact, witnessed observations of addict "punding" have also included descriptions of questionable psychotic behavior at the same time, including visual and tactile hallucinations and paranoid delusions.[64,65] Similar behaviors have been described in children treated with either racemic amphetamine or d-amphetamine for various behavioral disorders. This report describes undesirable side effects of these drugs to include "accentuation of tic-like motor activities such as nail biting, hair pulling, nose picking, and the like."[13]

Earlier descriptions of stereotyped behavior secondary to amphetamine abuse also exist. In patients with amphetamine psychosis, stereotyped behavior has been described by Bonhoff and Lewrenz[10] and by Connell.[11] Tatetsu and colleagues[12] also describe two patients with amphetamine psychosis who immediately after hospitalization made "incomprehensible, odd, and very unnatural movements." The movements were further described as constant, identical, and energetically repeated. When methamphetamine was administered (30 mg, IV) these movements became greatly enhanced. In these cases, stereotyped behavior was associated with amphetamine psychosis. The previous reports do not necessarily associate these two phenomenon. Although there is not much information available on patients who develop stereotyped behavior in the absence of psychosis, there is no evidence that any pre-existing central nervous system or basal ganglia abnormality need be present for the appearance of these stereotypies in amphetamine abusers.

Dyskinesias

Amphetamine administration is also associated with the induction of dyskinesias, particularly chorea (Table 1). There may be individuals who are "predisposed" to this phenomenon who develop dyskinesia after each dose of amphetamine. These individuals may have pre-existing damage to the basal ganglia (e.g., birth injury, viral infection, anoxia associated with anesthesia) which is not severe enough to produce clinical signs but which alters the response of the caudate putamen to stimulants capable of affecting the dopaminergic system. In addition, as indicated in Table 1, chronic high-dose amphetamine use alone can cause dyskinesias. These subjects presumably were "normal" (i.e., no previous neurological findings or history) prior to the use of stimulants and did not respond acutely with the development of a movement disorder. However, the chronic use of stimulants (particularly amphetamine) resulted in choreoathetoid movements. This raises the possibility that chronic amphetamine administration may alter subsequent dopaminergic behavioral

Table 1

Amphetamine and Dyskinesias

Reference	Age	Sex	Previous Neurological History	Previous Abnormal Movements	Psychosis Associated	Type of Movement	Abuse Pattern	Outcome
52	21	female	0	0	yes	choreoathetoid	chronic intermittent	resolved in 24 hours
52	25	female	0	0	no	choreoathetoid	intermittent needle tracks seen	resolved in 6 hours
52	30	male	0	0	no	rolling of arms, tongue protrusions, writhing of body	chronic long term	resolved in 3 hours
53	27	male	0	0	no	chorea—face & extremities	high dose IV	persistent abnormal movements despite abstinence
53	20	male	0	0	no	chorea—head & neck, ballismus—arms	high dose IV chronic	resolved
53	30	male	0	0	no	chorea—generalized	IV high dose chronic	resolved

53	35	male	0	0	no but stereo-typed behavior present	chorea—generalized	chronic oral	movements decreased but not resolved
54	8	male	organic brain syndrome mixed seizures hyperactivity	0	no	choreoathetoid—mouth, tongue, extremities	oral 15 mg b.i.d. 8 weeks	resolved
55	8	male	learning disability hyperkinetic	mild choreo-athetoid	no	increased choreoathetoid	oral 5 mg b.i.d. 3 months	resolved in 12 hours
55	3	female	seizure disorder mental retardation	0	no	choreo-athetoid generalized	oral 2.5 mg for 1 week	resolved in 12 hours
55	5	male	temper tantrum short attention span hyperactivity	0	no	grimacing dyskinetic movements, mouth	oral 1 dose 5 mg	resolved in 8 hours
55	51	female	narcolepsy	0	no	spasmodic torticollis	oral 20 mg/day years	resolved when medication discontinued

response (e.g., as in amphetamine-induced stereotyped behavior in animals) and eventually result in chorea. In fact, chronic use of high doses of amphetamine has been reported to produce a long-lasting depletion of dopamine in the caudate nucleus.[12a] Given the extensive use of amphetamine at various times in the population and the rarity of case reports of amphetamine-induced chorea, this probably is an infrequent occurrence.

Cocaine can also induce stereotypic behaviors, but this depends on dosing frequency and route of administration. Smoking of cocaine paste (60–80% cocaine sulfate) by young people in Peru has been associated with a variety of psychopathological states including stereotypic behaviors (e.g., bruxism, repeated touching of the face, licking of lips). In monkeys who chronically self-administer intravenous cocaine, stereotypic behaviors are elicited that are so intense that self-mutilation can result. By contrast, cocaine ingested by chewing the coca leaf for decades rarely results in psychosis or chronic toxicity in the natives of Peru and Bolivia.

Amphetamine, Cocaine, Methylphenidate, and Pemoline in Movement Disorders

Parkinson's Disease

The enhancement of the dopaminergic system by amphetamine and older literature reporting that amphetamine induced improvement in postencephalitic parkinsonism led to interest in the use of amphetamine in Parkinson's disease. In the late 1930s, there were several reports that suggested that benzedrine, 20 to 60 mg/day, alone and in combination with atropine, provided significant changes in patients' condition. Most of these reports suggested that the positive changes were in the "subjective" sphere. Patients described increased energy, decreased fatigue, decreased somnolence, and increased well being. These reports include the description of a bedridden patient who, when treated with amphetamine, was able to dress himself, and of another "helpless" patient who was able to start feeding himself. Most of the reports were unable to document much in the way of objective changes, but there are descriptions of decreased tremor, decreased rigidity, and decreased salivation.

These papers suggest that positive changes were seen in 50% to 93% of patients with postencephalitic parkinsonism treated with amphetamine. It is of interest that the authors also commented that oculogyric crises were improved or abolished in almost all of the patients.[14-17] In 1961, exploiting the effect of methylphenidate on the dopaminergic system, Halliday and Nathan[18] reported on its use in the treatment of Parkinson's disease. They noted that some patients had increased freedom of movement and decreased rigidity, but that tremor was not affected. However, they concluded that only one-half of the patients felt better while taking methylphenidate and that they were unsure that this "feeling better" was related to methylphenidate's antiparkinsonian effects.

Parkes et al.[19] examined the effect of both l- and d-amphetamine in idiopathic Parkinson's disease. These patients continued to take their antiparkinsonian medications including levodopa, amantadine, and anticholinergics, and l- or d-amphetamine (l, 50 mg/day and d, 15 mg/day) was introduced on an outpatient basis. Both l- and d-amphetamine produced a slight reduction (17–20%) in total disability, tremor, akinesia, and rigidity. As a result of side effects induced by amphetamine and because of the mild nature of clinical improvement, it was concluded that neither isomer was of value in routine treatment.

The failure of amphetamine or methylphenidate to induce more improvement in Parkinson's disease or to induce more dopaminergically induced dyskinesias in these patients may relate to the mechanism of action of these drugs. Amphetamine and methylphenidate require intact synthesis and storage of dopamine. If the dopamine system is already badly damaged or depleted as in Parkinson's disease, a drug that releases stores of dopamine might not prove very effective.

Amphetamine or methylphenidate is almost never employed in the treatment of Parkinson patients today. The beneficial motor effects are minimal. Most physicians do not use these agents to treat the hypersomnolence of Parkinson's disease, fearing the anorectic and potential encephalopathic side effects. This latter problem has not been fully studied.

Choreiform Disorders

It has been proposed that the severity of choreiform disorders, regardless of etiology, are affected by manipulation of the striatal dopaminergic system. In particular, drugs that enhance dopaminergic activity are thought to enhance chorea, whereas drugs that block dopamine receptors or deplete central nervous system dopamine often ameliorate chorea.[20] Intravenous amphetamine has been reported to enhance chorea in patients with Huntington's disease, Sydenham's chorea, and chorea associated with systemic lupus erythematosus (SLE). In all of these patients, some pre-existing dysfunction of the striatum could be assumed from their diagnosis. Of particular interest is that amphetamine did not elicit chorea on the uninvolved side in the patient with SLE and amphetamine also did not cause chorea in "normal" controls. One patient had a history of Sydenham's chorea but had no abnormal movements at the time of the study. Amphetamine in this patient elicited chorea, suggesting that amphetamine's ability to induce or enhance chorea might be related to pre-existing subclinical dysfunction of the basal ganglia.[21] The ability of chronic amphetamine abuse to cause punding or stereotyped behavior in humans has already been discussed and represents a different type of abnormal motor activity than the induction of chorea.

Many of the case reports describing chorea secondary to the administration of methylphenidate or pemoline also raise questions regarding the baseline status of the patient. Palatucci[22] noted the appearance of severe, predominantly choreiform dyskinesias in a 19-year-old male admitted to the hospital with an acute organic brain syndrome, possibly acute schizophrenia. This patient received treatment with neuroleptics for 6 to 7 weeks before being given a single intravenous injection of methylphenidate (40 mg) to make him more responsive to psychotherapeutic maneuvers. Over the next hour, the dyskinesias developed and did not resolve for the next 30 hours. Although there was a striking temporal relationship between the IV administration of methylphenidate and the chorea, the patient had been taking neuroleptics for at least 6 weeks prior to the administration of the drug. Another patient, a 55-year-old woman with manic depressive illness treated for many years with neuroleptics and lithium, stopped her medications and began abusing methylphenidate (30 to 100 mg/day). She developed a generalized choreoathetoid movement disorder.[23] The chronic use of neuroleptics is believed to affect dopamine receptor mechanisms and may predispose individuals to develop chorea (tardive dyskinesia) (see Chapter 5). It is possible that the prior exposure of neuroleptics may have presensitized these patients to the dopaminergic effects of methylphenidate.

In a study of hyperkinetic behavior and learning disorders, Millichap et al.[24] noted the effect of methylphenidate on 30 children, 29 of whom had signs of minimal brain dysfunction (MBD). In one of these 30 patients, methylphenidate administration resulted in difficulty speaking, difficulty moving the lips, and twitching movements of the face. When the dose was decreased but not discontinued, the movements improved. The paper does not make it clear whether the child who developed abnormal movements was one of the 29 with signs of MBD. In another patient with hyperactivity, Weiner et al.[25] reported that following a methylphenidate dosage escalation, the child developed chorea that persisted for 2 years. When methylphenidate was discontinued, the chorea subsided but the hyperactivity returned. These reports of methylphenidate-induced chorea occurred in children with MBD and other predisposing CNS factors. Weiner et al. suggested, on the basis of the ability of chronic methylphenidate administration to alter the threshold for the appearance of stereotyped behavior in guinea pigs, that doses below the threshold for the induction of chorea could eventually lead to alterations in the dopaminergic system which would result in the development of chorea.[25]

Whether pemoline can induce chorea or other abnormal movements in normal individuals remains in doubt. In the cases reported by Bonthala and West[26] and by Singh et al.,[27] the two patients had been treated with neuroleptics prior to the administration of pemoline. In addition, one of the patients was retarded and had seizures and hyperactivity. Nausieda et al.[28] reported a single patient (age 2 years) who overdosed on pemoline and developed a choreiform disorder associated with an encephalopathy. The patient's neurological condition resolved and returned to normal over 38 hours. This child was reported to be normal prior to the overdose incident. The authors concluded that chronic administration of pemoline should be used with caution and may result in similar side effects to those seen with the chronic administration of amphetamine.

We have seen an additional patient who, following a crack cocaine binge, presented to the emergency room with a generalized choreiform disorder. After hospitalization and withdrawal of all medications, the choreiform disorder resolved over a period of 2 to 3 days. When this occurred, the patient had a multifocal tic disorder, which apparently had been present since she was a young child. Before further evaluation of this patient could be carried out, she left the hospital against medical advice.

Tics

The relationship between stimulants and tics has been extensively evaluated. Methylphenidate is commonly used to treat attention deficit hyperactivity disorder (ADHD). ADHD is often associated with Gilles de la Tourette syndrome (GTS) and it may be the earliest and isolated manifestation of this condition in many patients. This association probably accounts for the increased awareness of stimulant-induced tics that may either present de novo or as an exacerbation of a pre-existing tic disorder (e.g., in patients with overt GTS). The ability of methylphenidate to increase dopaminergic activity in the CNS is the proposed mechanism by which this and other stimulants may precipitate or exacerbate tics. The pathophysiology of GTS (a genetic disorder) may involve abnormalities of dopaminergic transmission in the basal ganglia.[29,30] A greater knowledge of the prevalence of the Tourette gene in the asymptomatic general population, which some believe is very high, is necessary before we can readily interpret the potential for stimulant medication to induce tics.

Although there had been isolated previous reports of facial tics induced by methylphenidate in children with MBD,[31,32] it was in 1973 that Meyerhoff and Snyder[33] described an increase in tics in a GTS patient treated with stimulants. In 1974, Golden[34] reported the first case of methylphenidate-induced GTS in a 9-year-old who was being treated for hyperkinetic behavior. Despite improvement in the hyperkinetic behavior 8 weeks following the initiation of methylphenidate treatment, the child suddenly developed "full-blown" GTS. Discontinuation of the drug resulted in return to baseline motor status. Denckla et al.[35] reported that 1.3% of a large population of patients (1,520) with minimal brain dysfunction treated with methylphenidate developed transient tics. Of the 20 cases identified, 14 developed new onset of motor tics and 6 experienced an exacerbation of their pre-existing tics during methylphenidate administration. Although a relationship was acknowledged between tics and methylphenidate treatment, the nature of the relationship is presented as obscure even though a linkage to the dopaminergic system is mentioned. The authors concluded that tics related to methylphenidate administration appear to be rare and may point to a specific susceptibility possibly related to personality profile.

The study of Denckla et al.[35] remains very useful in documenting that methylphenidate treatment in MBD children only rarely elicits tics. The relationship to personality profile has for the most part been discarded in favor of neurochemical explanations, although these often also fall short of explaining the phenomenon. Although there is no further large population study to dispute the 1.3% incidence of methylphenidate-induced tics, it should be noted that the incidence may in fact be higher since Denckla et al. relied in part on phone follow-ups from the parents. Phone conversations and family member interviews are often most unreliable in trying to establish the presence or absence of abnormal movements in a given patient.

Several additional case reports document that methylphenidate can exacerbate GTS symptomatology, particularly vocal or motor tics.[36,37] In addition, Bremness and Sverd[38] reported another case of a child with hyperactivity aggressive syndrome treated with methylphenidate who developed full-blown GTS.

Further support for a relationship between stimulants and tics is found in several case series that assess the use of stimulants in patients with GTS. Golden[39] reviewed his patient records and solicited information from the Tourette Syndrome Association to further investigate the relationship between stimulants and GTS. He found that 17 of 32 (53%) GTS patients who had been exposed to stimulants (primarily methylphenidate and amphetamine) experienced marked accentuation of tics. There were no apparent clinical differences between those whose symptomatology was exacerbated and those who were not affected by stimulants except the latter group tended to be older. Lowe et al.[40] identified 15 of 100 GTS patients who were treated with stimulants and who experienced an exacerbation of their tics. In many of their patients, a family history of GTS or other tic disorders was present, and the authors stressed that a positive family history of tics may predispose the patient to stimulant-induced tics. It should be noted that in many of their patients the tics did not appear immediately after the introduction of stimulant treatment but occurred months to years later. Bachman,[41] in a retrospective review of his patient records, found 14 of 64 GTS patients who had been treated with stimulants. In three treated with methylphenidate there was worsening of tics, in one treated with amphetamine tics improved, and in the remaining 10 patients there was no change in tic frequency. Erenberg et al.[42] found similar results after reviewing the records of 200 GTS patients; 48 patients had been treated with stimulants (42 with methylphenidate, 13 with pemoline, and 5 with amphetamine). Thirty-nine of their patients had pre-existing tics, and stimulants increased tic severity in 11, produced no change in 26, and decreased tics in 2. Where a comparison could be made, various stimulant treatments had no different effects on the tics. These children with GTS were being treated for ADHD, and it should be noted that in 22 of 39 patients behavior improved. The authors conclude that in patients with ADHD and GTS, a cautious trial of stimulants may be of benefit in terms of managing the overall clinical situation. Nine patients in their study were treated with stimulants prior to the onset of tics. Only four of the patients were still receiving stimulants when the tics began. The delay in onset of tic symptomatology from the time of stimulant treatment raises the question of whether the stimulants are actually precipitating the tics or whether the appearance of tics in some of these children with ADHD simply represents the normal evolution of the ADHD-GTS syndrome (Table 2).

Price et al.[43] identified 34 of 170 (20%) GTS patients who had been treated with stimulants prior to age 18. Fifty percent of these patients reported worsening of their tics. Of considerable interest is the finding that in six monozygotic twin pairs there was 100%

Table 2

Delay in Onset of New Tics While Receiving Stimulant

Reference	N	Duration of Treatment Before Tic Onset
Bachman[41]	1	Promptly
Bremness and Sverd[38]	1	10 weeks
Denckla et al.[35]	14 of 1,475	Days to months
Erenberg et al.[42]	4	Weeks to months
Golden[34]	1	8 weeks
Golden[39]	2	Immediately to within days
Lowe et al.[40]	6	Months to years
Mitchell and Matthews[47]	1	8 weeks
Pascual-Leone and Dhuna[51]	2	Immediate after increase dosage
Pollack et al.[36]	1	6 months
Rapoport et al.[59]	5	8 weeks to 1 year
Cohen et al.[60]	1	6 months

Modified from Erenberg et al.[42]

concordance for GTS and complete discordance for prior stimulant use. The authors suggest that stimulant treatment may not substantially increase the risk for prematurely exacerbating tics in many individuals. On the other hand, their data do reveal a close temporal relationship in some GTS patients between stimulant treatment and an exacerbation of tics. Therefore, they also conclude that there may exist the real danger of worsening tics in some patients with GTS. It has been proposed that lack of complete concordance in monozygotic twin pairs for GTS suggests that cerebral development up to 15 years of age may play a role in the phenotypic expression of the disorder. Leckman et al.[44] have proposed that chronic stress and exposure to stimulants may be environmental factors capable of precipitating the expression of the phenotype. However, the twin data of Price et al.[43] suggest that stimulants are not one of these factors, although the number of patients is small.

Careful analysis of individual patients challenged with stimulants does not always demonstrate that these drugs increase pre-exiting tics (Table 3). However, Feinberg and Carroll[45] studied two patients with GTS in whom oral administration of amphetamine definitely resulted in increased tics. In a later study, Caine et al.[46] administered oral d-amphetamine, l-amphetamine, and haloperidol to six patients with GTS. Their report is described as a "labor-intensive" investigation of the effects of these drugs on GTS. The patients experienced a heterogeneous array of responses to these agents, which the authors felt precluded them from making any inferences regarding the neurochemistry of GTS. They did report that d-amphetamine appeared to be more consistently potent in increasing tic frequency in their patients. Overall, the authors believe that amphetamine increases tics in some but not all patients with GTS.

Pemoline, which is also used to treat ADHD, has been implicated in the induction of tics. In the clearest case, Bachman[41] reported a 9-year-old child with ADHD treated with pemoline who promptly developed tics. Pemoline was discontinued after 2 months of treatment, but the tics persisted. During subsequent years, the child developed fluctuating motor and vocal tics and the diagnosis of GTS was made. Although the tics were induced by pemoline and never resolved, it is most likely that this child had incipient GTS, which was precipitated by pemoline. Mitchell and Matthews[47] reported a 10-year-old who had previously been treated with thioridazine (no movement disorder reported) for hyperactivity who was started on pemoline and developed motor tics. When pemoline was

Table 3

Increase in Existing Tics While Receiving Stimulant Drugs

Reference	N	Duration Before Tic Increase
Bachman[41]	3 of 14	Not stated
Caine et al.[46]	2 of 6	Immediate
Denckla et al.[35]	6 of 45	Days to months
Erenberg et al.[42]	11 of 39	Days to months
Factor et al.[50]	1	Immediate
Feinberg and Carroll[45]	2	Immediate
Fras and Karlavage[37]	3	Not stated
Golden[39]	13 of 25	Not stated
Lowe et al.[40]	9	Not stated
Meyerhoff and Snyder[33]	1	Days
Pascual-Leone and Dhuna[51]	2 of 2	Immediate
Price et al.[43]	5 of 12	Months to years
Mesulam[49]	1	Immediate
Rapoport et al.[59]	2 of 6	Days to weeks
Cohen et al.[60]	4 of 20	Not stated
Sleator[48]	1	Days

stopped the tics resolved, and when the child was rechallenged with pemoline the tics recurred. In this case, it is possible that prior exposure to thioridazine may have sensitized dopaminergic neurons to the subsequent effects of pemoline treatment. Sleator[48] reported a 6-year-old with GTS, also treated previously with thioridazine, who developed an exacerbation of tics when pemoline was introduced. This child had the same response to methylphenidate.

Cocaine, which potentiates dopaminergic neurotransmission by blocking reuptake of dopamine, has also been reported to induce tics. Mesulam[49] and Factor et al.[50] both reported single patients with GTS who experienced increased severity of their tics when using cocaine. The increase in tic severity was immediate to 20 minutes later and lasted 1 to 5 hours. Pascual-Leone and Dhuna[51] reported two additional GTS patients who experienced a marked increase in severity of both motor and vocal tics following the use of cocaine and cocaine as "crack." In one of these patients, the increased tics did not resolve for 4 days. This duration of cocaine-induced tics is difficult to explain. These same authors also reported new onset of multifocal tics in two additional patients who were habitual cocaine abusers.[51] In both of these patients, the onset of the movement disorder occurred during binges of cocaine use. In both of these patients there was no previous history of tics, no family history of tics, and in both patients the resolution of the tic disorder occurred over weeks to months. In the latter two patients, CT and EEG were normal and there was no history to suggest prior central nervous system insult. These two patients are particularly interesting. If both were "truly" neurologically normal, then chronic cocaine use alone may be sufficient to induce tic disorders possibly related to its ability to cause dopaminergic supersensitivity as documented in animal models of stereotyped behavior.

Dystonia, Myoclonus, and Tremors

The use of stimulants in patients with various other movement disorders is an infrequent occurrence. In the last several years, there have been a series of reports indicating that cocaine abuse is associated with acute dystonic reactions. Kumor et al.[52] reported that six of seven cocaine abusers administered haloperidol in a research setting developed acute dystonic reactions. These patients had not used cocaine for at least 10 days prior to the administration of haloperidol. The acute dystonia developed within 22 hours of the first haloperidol dosage in four patients and within 3 hours of the second haloperidol dosage in two. The acute dystonia was severe enough to require parenteral administration of diphenhydramine or benztropine, which promptly resolved the movement disorder in all cases. Choy-Kwong and Lipton[53] noted in a study of consecutive patients admitted to a psychiatric hospital and treated with neuroleptics that prior history of cocaine abuse was associated with a threefold increased risk of dystonic reactions. These reports have served to alert clinicians that prior history of cocaine abuse may predispose to acute and slightly delayed dystonic reactions when these patients are treated with neuroleptics. Kumor[54] described a single patient who first developed an acute dystonic response to haloperidol and who, when administered cocaine 5 days later, also developed an acute dystonic response. The pathogenesis of acute dystonia is not completely understood (see Chapter 2); however, based on these reports, altered neurotransmitter and/or receptor function has been implicated.

Acute dystonic reactions have also been reported in cocaine abusers not exposed to neuroleptics. Shortly after cocaine use, one patient developed focal dystonic movements that lasted 45 minutes.[55] In another single case report, a 15-year-old girl admitted to a psychiatric service developed acute generalized dystonia 16 hours after admission. She had not been treated with neuroleptics and it was postulated that the dystonia was associated with cocaine withdrawal.[56] It should be noted that in these patients in whom dystonia was associated with cocaine use with or without neuroleptic use, there was no prior history of a movement disorder. Recent animal studies indicate that even in unlesioned animals, chronic cocaine administration can produce a relative deficiency of dopamine.[57]

Scharf[58] reported a 26-year-old woman who was a chronic intermittent cocaine abuser who developed opsoclonus-myoclonus the morning after she used intranasal cocaine. She was "normal" when she went to bed but awoke with generalized severe myoclonic jerks involving both the trunk and limbs. In addition, she had opsoclonus and complained of the inability to keep her eyes still. She was treated with lorazepam, valproic acid, and clonazapam with moderate success. MRI, CT, and EEG were normal. The movement disorder completely resolved over 4 weeks, and follow-up 12 months later revealed no neurological abnormalities. The author ascribed the onset of this dramatic myoclonus opsoclonus syndrome to cocaine use since none of the other well-known causes were present.

Excluding the questionable role of stimulants in the treatment of parkinsonian tremor, there are no specific reports of the effect of stimulants on tremor. It is well known that stimulants alone may be associated with increased postural tremor in the upper extremities, but this has not been specifically studied. The enhancement of a postural, physiological tremor is often related to the sympathomimetic effects of stimulants, particularly via stimulation of peripheral adrenergic receptors.

Severe tremors (no further description) are reported by IV amphetamine abusers to be danger signs that occur after several days of abuse and are considered to be a signal to terminate a "run."[61] Tremulous behavior associated with frequent startling in response to minimal stimulation has been reported as a sign of cocaine intoxication in a 2-week-old infant.[62] However, in a study of jitteriness (defined as rhythmic tremors of equal amplitude around a fixed axis) in full-term neonates, maternal marijuana use during pregnancy and soon before delivery but not cocaine use was associated with increased jitteriness. Cocaine's effect on jitteriness did not reach statistical significance.[63]

Conclusions

Amphetamine, methylphenidate, pemoline, and cocaine all affect the dopaminergic system. In those movement disorders in which the dopaminergic system is altered, the use of stimulants tends to enhance (usually but not always) dopaminergic effects. Minor improvement in parkinsonian states, increase in tics, and chorea all conform to this general hypothesis.

Amphetamine can produce altered motor behavior in chronic abusers as detailed in the discussion of punding. It is of interest that there is little to suggest that punding is induced by methylphenidate, pemoline, or cocaine. The lack of punding-like behavior associated with chronic cocaine abuse is most curious. This may relate to dose and route of administration. Alternatively, although there are no reports indicating the existence of cocaine-induced punding, it may be that this behavior is so commonplace among abusers that it does not warrant mention. Whether or not cocaine elicits punding clearly needs further study.

The question of whether or not stimulants can induce other abnormal movements (e.g., chorea, tics, dystonia) in subjects who have absolutely no pathological or chemical predisposing factors is not entirely resolved. In most instances, the "normal" individual who develops a movement disorder is found to have a history or subtle neurological findings suggestive of prior CNS insult. Examples of this type of clinical setting include delayed motor development, prior exposure to neuroleptics, history of encephalitis, and history of extensive systemic surgical procedures. In these situations, which comprise the majority of these rare events, it may well be that the previous history "predisposed" the patient (the basal ganglia) to develop an acute movement disorder when exposed to those drugs that alter central neurotransmitter and receptor function.

There are some patients who develop stimulant-induced movement disorders despite the complete absence of any obvious predisposing factors. Since our society has had long-standing and widespread abuse of various substances, particularly amphetamine and cocaine, the incidence of stimulant-induced movement disorders in a "normal" individual must be extremely low. We continue to favor the hypothesis that even in these patients there is some pre-existing undetermined abnormality that predisposes them to the development of a movement disorder. There is little evidence in humans to suggest that chronic exposure alone, in an otherwise healthy nervous system, can eventually result in an abnormal movement disorder.

References

1. Connell PH. Clinical manifestation and treatment of amphetamine type of dependence. JAMA 1966; 196:718–723.
2. Editorial. Addiction to amphetamine. Br J Med 1963; 2:399–400.
3. Randrup A, Munkuad I. Stereotyped activities produced by amphetamine in several animal species and man. Psychopharmacologia (Berlin) 1967; 11:300–310.
4. Randrup A, Munkuad I. Special antagonism of amphetamine- induced abnormal behavior. Psychopharmacologia (Berlin) 1965; 7:416–422.
5. Klawans HL, Hitri A, Nausieda PA, Weiner WJ. Animal models of dyskinesia. In: Hanin I, Usdin E (eds), Animal Models in Psychiatry and Neurology, Oxford/New York, Pergamon Press, 1977.
6. Gunne LM. Effects of amphetamine in humans. In: Martin WR (ed), Drug Addiction 2: Amphetamine, Psychogenic, and Marijuana Dependents, Berlin, Springer-Verlag, 1977, pp 247–275.
7. Rylander G. Preludin-narkomamer fran klinisk och medicinsk-kriminologisk synpunkt. Svenska Lak-Tidn 1966; 63:4973–4979.
8. Kramer JC, Fishman VS, Littlefield DC. Amphetamine abuse: pattern and effects of high doses taken intravenously. JAMA 1967; 201:305–309.
9. Rylander G. Psychosis and the punding and choreiform syndromes in addiction to central stimulant drugs. Psychiatry Neurol Neurochir (Amsterdam) 1972; 75:203–212.
10. Bonhoff G, Lewrenz H. Uber Weckamine (Pervitin und Benzedrin). Monograph, Gesamtgeb Neurol Psychiat 1954; 77:1–144.
11. Connell PH. Amphetamine Psychosis, Maudsley monograph #5, London, Chapman & Hall, 1958, Thesis, University of London, 1957, case #20.
12. Tatetsu S, Goto A, Fujiwara T. The methamphetamine-psychosis (Kakuseizai Cudohku), Tokyo, Igaku Shoin, 1956.
12a. Ellinwood EH, Jr. Amphetamine/anorectics. In: Dupont RL, Goldstein A, O'Donnell J (eds), Handbook on Drug Abuse, Washington, DC, National Institute on Drug Abuse, U.S. Government Printing Office, 1979, pp 221–231.
13. Bradley C. Benzedrine and Dexedrine in the treatment of children's behavior disorders. Pediatrics 1950; 5:24–37.
14. Davis PL, Stewart WB. The use of benzedrine sulfate in postencephalitic parkinsonism. JAMA 1938; 110:1890–1892.

15. Solomon P, Mitchell RS, Prinzmetal M. The use of benzedrine sulfate in postencephalitic Parkinson's disease. JAMA 1937; 108:1765–1770.
16. Finkelman I, Shapiro LB. Benzedrine sulfate and atropine in treatment of chronic encephalitis. JAMA 1937; 109:344–346.
17. Matthews RA. Symptomatic treatment of chronic encephalitis with benzedrine sulfate. Am J Med Sci 1938; 195:448–452.
18. Halliday AM, Nathan PW. Methylphenidate in Parkinsonism. Br Med J 1961; 1:1652–1655.
19. Parkes JD, Tarsy D, Marsden CD, Bovill KT, et al. Amphetamines in the treatment of Parkinson's disease. J Neurol Neurosurg Psychiatry 1975; 38:232–237.
20. Weiner WJ, Lang AE. Movement Disorders: A Comprehensive Survey, Mt. Kisco, New York, Futura Publishing, 1989.
21. Klawans HL, Weiner WJ. The effect of d-amphetamine on choreiform movement disorders. Neurology 1974; 24:312–318.
22. Palatucci DM. Iatrogenic dyskinesias: a unique reaction to parenternal methylphenidate. J Nervous Mental Dis 1974; 159:73–76.
23. Extein I. Methylphenidate-induced choreoathetosis. Am J Psychiatry 1979; 135:252–253.
24. Millichap JG, Aymat F, Sturgis LH, Larsen KW, Egan RA. Hyperkinetic behavior and learning disorders. Am J Dis Child 1968; 116:235–244.
25. Weiner WJ, Nausieda PA, Klawans HL. Methylphenidate-induced chorea: case report and pharmacologic implications. Neurology 1978; 28:1041–1044.
26. Bonthala C, West A. Pemoline-induced chorea and Gilles de la Tourette's syndrome. Br J Psychiatry 1983; 143:300–302.
27. Singh BK, Singh A, Chusid E. Chorea in long-term use of pemoline. Ann Neurol 1983; 13:218.
28. Nausieda PA, Koller WL, Weiner WJ, Klawans HL. Pemoline-induced chorea. Neurology 31:356–360, 1981.
29. Cohen DJ, Shaywitz BA, Young JG, et al. Central biogenic anime metabolism in children with the syndrome of chronic multiple tics of GTS: norepinephrine, serotonin, and dopamine. J Am Acad Child Psychiatry 1979; 18:320–341.
30. Butler IJ, Koslow S, Seifert W, et al. Biogenic amine metabolism in Tourette's syndrome. Ann Neurology 1979; 6:37–39.
31. Weiss G, Minde K, Douglas V, Werry J, Sykes D. Comparison of the effects of chlorpromazine, dextroamphetamine, and methylphenidate on the behavior and intellectual function of hyperactive children. CMA 1971; 104:20–22.
32. Winsberg BG, Press M, Bialer I, Kupietz S. Dextroamphetamine and methylphenidate in the treatment of hyperactive/aggressive children. Pediatrics 1974; 53:236–241.
33. Meyerhoff JH, Snyder SH. Gilles de la Tourette's disease and minimal brain dysfunction: amphetamine isomers reveal catecholamine correlate in an affected patient. Psychopharmacologia 1973; 29:211–220.
34. Golden GS. Gilles de la Tourette's syndrome following methylphenidate administration. Dev Med Child Neurol 1974; 16:76–78.

35. Denckla MB, Bemporad JR, Mackay MC. Tics following methylphenidate administration. JAMA 1976; 235:1349–1351.
36. Pollack MA, Cohen NL, Friedhoff AJ. Gilles de la Tourette's syndrome: Familial occurrence and precipitation by methylphenidate therapy. Arch Neurol 1977; 34:630–632.
37. Fras I, Karlavage J. The use of methylphenidate and imipramine in Gilles de la Tourette's disease in children. Am J Psychiatry 1977; 134:195–197.
38. Bremness AB, Sverd J. Methylphenidate-induced Tourette's syndrome: case report. Am J Psychiatry 1979; 136:1334–1335.
39. Golden GS. The effect of CNS stimulants on Tourette's syndrome. Ann Neurol 1977; 2:69–70.
40. Lowe TL, Cohen DJ, Detlor J, Kremenitzer MW, Shaywitz BA. Stimulant medications precipitate Tourette's syndrome. JAMA 1982; 247:1729–1731.
41. Bachman DS. Pemoline-induced Tourette's disorder: a case report. Am J Psychiatry 1981; 138:1116–1117.
42. Erenberg G, Cruse RP, Rothner AD. Gilles de la Tourette's syndrome: effects of stimulant drugs. Neurology 1985; 35:1346–1348.
43. Price RA, Leckman JF, Pauls DL, Cohen DJ, Kidd KK. GTS: tics and CNS stimulants in twins and non-twins. Neurology 1986; 36:232–237.
44. Leckman JF, Cohen DJ, Price RA, Minderaa RB, Anderson GM, Pauls DL. The pathogenesis of GTS: a review of data and hypotheses. In: Shah AB, Shah NS, Donald AG, (eds), Movement Disorders, New York, Plenum Press, 1985.
45. Feinberg M, Carroll BJ. Effects of dopaminergic agonists and antagonists in Tourette's disease. Arch Gen Psychiatry 1979; 36:979–985.
46. Caine ED, Ludlow CL, Polinsky RJ, Ebert MH. Provocative drug testing in Tourette's syndrome: d- and l- amphetamine and haloperidol. J Am Acad Child Psychiatry 1984; 23:147–152.
47. Mitchell E, Matthews KL. Gilles de la Tourette's disorder associated with pemoline. Am J Psychiatry 1980; 137:1618–1619.
48. Sleator EK. Deleterious effects of drugs used for hyperactivity on patients with Gilles de la Tourette syndrome. Clin Pediatr 1980; 19:453–454.
49. Mesulam MM. Cocaine and Tourette's syndrome. N Engl J Med 1986; 315:398.
50. Factor SA, Sanchez-Ramos JR, Weiner WJ. Cocaine and Tourette's syndrome. Ann Neurol 1988; 23:423–424.
51. Pascual-Leone A, Dhuna A. Cocaine-associated multifocal tics. Neurology 1990; 40:999–1000.
52. Kumor K, Sherer M, Jaffe J. Haloperidol-induced dystonia in cocaine addicts. Lancet 1986; 2:1341–1342.
53. Choy-Kwong M, Lipton RB. Cocaine withdrawal dystonia. Neurology 1990; 40:863–864.
54. Kumor K. Cocaine withdrawal dystonia. Neurology 1990; 40:863.
55. Merab J. Acute dystonic reaction to cocaine. Am J Med 1988; 84:564.
56. Choy-Kwong M, Lipton RB. Dystonia related to cocaine withdrawal: a case report and pathogenic hypothesis. Neurol 1989; 39:996–997.

57. Robertson MW, Leslie CA, Bennett JP. Apparent synaptic dopamine deficiency induced by withdrawal from chronic cocaine treatment. Brain Res 1991; 538:337–339.
58. Scharf D. Opsoclonus-myoclonus following the intranasal usage of cocaine. J Neurol Neurosurg Psychiatry 1989; 52:1447–1448.
59. Rapoport JL, Nee L, Mitchell S, et al. Hyperkinetic syndrome and Tourette syndrome. In: Friedhoff AJ, Chase TN (eds), Advances in Neurology, Vol. 35, Gilles de la Tourette Syndrome, New York, Raven Press, 1982, pp 423–426.
60. Cohen DJ, Detlor J, Shaywitz BA, et al. Interaction of biological and psychological factors in the natural history of Tourette syndrome: a paradigm for childhood neuropsychiatric disorders. In: Friedhoff AJ, Chase TN (eds), Advances in Neurology, Vol. 35, Gilles de la Tourette Syndrome, New York, Raven Press, 1982, pp 31–40.
61. Kramer JC, Fischman VS, Littlefield DC. Amphetamine abuse: patterns and effects of high doses taken intravenously. JAMA 1967; 201:305–309.
62. Chasnoff IJ, Lewis DE, Squires L. Cocaine intoxication in a breast-fed infant. Pediatrics 1987; 80:836–838.
63. Parkes S, Zuckerman B, Bauchner H, Frank D, Vinci R, Cabral H. Jitteriness in full-term neonates: prevalence and correlates. Pediatrics 1990; 85:17–23.
64. Lees AJ. Tics and Related Disorders, Edinburgh, Churchill Livingstone, 1985.
65. Schiorring E. Changes in individual and social behavior induced by amphetamine and related compounds in monkeys and man. In: Ellenwood EH, Kilbey, MM (eds), Cocaine and Other Stimulants, New York, Plenum Press, 1977, pp 481–522.

12

Miscellaneous Drug-Induced Movement Disorders

Anthony E. Lang

Introduction

The purpose of this chapter is to discuss the movement disorders induced by a broad range of other drugs not considered in previous chapters. The list of medications reported to cause movement disorders seems unending. As indicated in Chapter 1, the literature is filled with individual case reports that suggest an etiological relationship between a certain drug and a specific movement disorder. In the case of many of the less well documented or uncommon associations that will be reviewed here, the true cause and effect relationship between drug and movement disorder may be rather tenuous. Concomitant drugs, diseases (including subclinical brain diseases/damage), or interactions between these and the implicated agent must all be regularily considered.

The following sections discuss a variety of drug-induced movement disorder syndromes organized by general category of medications causing the abnormal movements. Although alcohol is not a

Lang AE, Weiner WJ (editors): *Drug-Induced Movement Disorders,* Mount Kisco, NY, © Futura Publishing Co., Inc., 1992.

pharmaceutical, its common usage and association with a variety of different movement disorders justifies its inclusion in this chapter.

Alcohol

Movement disorders associated with alcoholism have been recently reviewed in detail.[1] Certain idiopathic movement disorders may be markedly improved by small amounts of alcohol, and this response occasionally may lead to alcoholism. This alcohol responsiveness is particularly evident in many patients with essential tremor, essential myoclonus, and autosomal-dominant myoclonic dystonia. Chronic inflammatory and fibrotic liver disease complicating chronic alcohol abuse may be severe enough to result in hepatic encephalopathy. This is commonly manifested in part by *asterixis*, characterized by brief, irregular lapses in posture ("negative myoclonus") best demonstrated as coarse, flexion/extension movements of the extended wrists in the outstretched hands. These lapses are associated with involuntary 50–200 ms periods of absent electrical activity in any skeletal muscle of the body that is maintained tonically active.[2] The more common tremulousness of hepatic encephalopathy (*metabolic tremor*) may simply be a less pronounced manifestation of the same disorder in which the pauses in voluntary muscle activity are briefer, less pronounced, and do not occur simultaneously in all muscles of the limb.[2,3]

A more common form of tremor associated with alcohol is the so-called *alcoholic tremor* usually seen during periods of alcohol withdrawal. This is a postural tremor of the arms that may spread to other structures when severe, resulting in titubation, facial, tongue, and laryngeal involvement.[4,5] Alcoholic tremor often persists weeks after discontinuation of alcohol consumption although the amplitude usually diminishes. How long it persists remains uncertain although some alcoholics free of alcohol for over 1 year still demonstrated the tremor in one study.[4] It is said that two types of postural tremor can be differentiated in alcoholics: the first with an alternating EMG pattern in antagonist muscles at a frequency greater than 8 Hz, while the second has synchronous bursts of EMG activity in antagonist muscles and a frequency of less than 8 Hz.[6] Both of these EMG patterns can also be seen in the same patient with essential tremor.[7] The exact pathophysiology of alcoholic tremor is not understood. There may be multiple influencing factors, possibly the most important being an enhancement of physiological tremor by the elevation of circulating levels of catecholamines during alcohol withdrawal.[8] Treatment of choice for alcoholic tremor is abstinence from alcohol. In severe cases, propranolol or short-term use of benzodiazepines may be helpful. In the differential diagnosis of alcoholic tremor, one must consider the abuse of other substances by these same individuals. Withdrawal of opiates, barbiturates, or benzodiazepines[9–11] and the use of amphetamines and other stimulants[12] may cause a similar postural tremor. The metabolic tremor of liver failure should also be considered.

Alcoholic cerebellar degeneration may be accompanied by different types of tremors. Occasionally, tremor resembling a *parkinsonian resting tremor* occurs in the upper limbs, especially when the hands are placed in certain positions.[13] A better characterized form of tremor seen in association with alcoholic cerebellar degeneration is a *3-Hz leg tremor*. This peculiar slow tremor is produced by synchronous extension/flexion of hip girdle muscles, best demonstrated when the patient stands with feet together and knees half bent producing a slow "bobbing" of the body.[14] Alternatively, it can be seen when the patient lies on the back with legs elevated and with knees and hip joints flexed to 90 degrees, causing a typical kicking movement.[15,16] This poorly recognized form of tremor may affect gait, contributing to the disability of the accompanying cerebellar ataxia. Abstinence from alcohol may result in a decrease in the intensity of the leg tremor. However, it usually persists long after cessation of drinking. This form of tremor may be much more common than generally appreciated. In a group of alcoholics with radiologically diagnosed cerebellar atrophy, studied with a sway platform, all showed a slow 3-Hz leg tremor[17] and a 3-Hz component occurred in 45 of 78 chronic alcoholics during measurement of postural sway.[18] The pathophysiology of this type of tremor is not understood although it is logical to assume that the superior vermis, which is sensitive to alcoholic cerebellar toxicity, might play a role.

A variety of basal ganglia movement disorders may occur in alcoholics with cirrhosis complicated by portosystemic shunts with resulting *acquired hepatocerebral degeneration*.[19] These include various forms of tremor, chorea, dystonia, and parkinsonism as well as myoclonus and cerebellar ataxia. Distinct from these disturbances, a small number of patients have been described who demonstrate transient basal ganglia dysfunction associated with alcohol abuse or withdrawal. *Transient parkinsonism* has been reported in 12 cases.[20–23] These patients have been chronic alcoholics of both sexes over the age of 50 years with little or no evidence of significant liver dysfunction. A few days after their last drink, and less commonly, while intoxicated, patients have developed features of classic parkinsonism with bradykinesia, resting tremor, limb rigidity, flexed posture, and slow, shuffling gait. Additional signs of alcohol withdrawal and alcoholism including postural tremor, ataxia, and confusion have often been concurrent. Recovery is usually complete within several days to 2 months, although residual, milder parkinsonian signs have been described in some. Short courses of biperiden[22] and levodopa[20] have been partially successful in a small number of patients.

Investigations have been unrevealing, although one patient demonstrated bilateral basal ganglia calcification on CT scan.[20] It has been hypothesized that the effects of alcohol on dopamine transmission might result in parkinsonism in susceptible individuals, for example, those with subclinical idiopathic Parkinson's disease. However, follow-up of a small group of alcoholics who previously demonstrated transient parkinsonism failed to reveal any clinical evidence of a parkinsonian state 10 years after their original presentation.[24]

Transient choreoathetotic dyskinesias have also been described in a small number of chronic alcoholics during heavy alcohol abuse[25] or more often, within 10–14 days of cessation of drinking.[25,26] The predominant abnormal movements include orolingual dyskinesias with twisting and pursing of the mouth, protrusion of the tongue, and facial grimacing. Some patients also demonstrate neck and arm choreoathetosis with legs being uncommonly affected. A small number of patients demonstrating an alcohol withdrawal-related parkinsonian syndrome have also developed dyskinesias later during alcohol withdrawal.[20,23] Most patients seem unaware of the involuntary movements and some have demonstrated bizarre behavior including paranoid ideation, delusions and hallucinations. As in the case of transient parkinsonism associated with alcohol withdrawal, investigations in these uncommon patients with transient dyskinesias are usually unrevealing (aside from abnormalities commonly found in nondyskinetic alcoholics). One case coming to autopsy had changes compatible with subacute Wernicke's encephalopathy combined with a slight generalized fibrillary gliosis.[26] The significance of these changes is uncertain, given the frequency of Wernicke's encephalopathy in alcoholics without movement disorders. No specific treatment is usually required in these patients since the dyskinesias are typically self-limited, resolving in a few weeks. Chlorpromazine reduced the severity of the abnormal movements in one patient.[26]

The pathophysiology of transient parkinsonism and dyskinesias is not certain. There is particular interest in the possible role of the nigrostriatal dopamine system, given the similarity between these movement disorders and those caused by drugs that influence dopamine transmission. Further support is the finding that acute alcohol intoxication may predispose to the development of short-lived akathisia and dystonia in young adults (ages 20–30) on chonic neuroleptic therapy.[27] However, the influence of alcohol on dopaminergic function is complex. In experimental animals, alcohol both decreases striatal dopamine release[22] and striatal dopamine-induced adenylate cyclase activity.[28] However, prolonged use of alcohol or alcohol withdrawal may induce functional dopamine receptor supersensitivity, both in experimental animals[29] and in humans.[30] The exact mechanisms by which alcohol alters dopamine-mediated transmission are not known. One possible explanation, which is interesting in light of recent hypotheses related to cell death in Parkinson's disease, involves the ability of alcohol to cause lipid peroxidation in the nigrostriatal system.[23] This may be especially important in alcoholics whose antioxidant capabilities are reduced.[31] However, one might have expected these effects to be particularly evident in those predisposed by underlying basal ganglia dysfunction (e.g., subclinical Parkinson's disease). However, this has not proven to be the case in the small number of patients who were followed for several years after their initial movement disorder presentation. On the other hand, the discovery of basal ganglia calcification in one case[20] emphasizes the need to remain vigilant to the presence of underlying predisposing factors. The importance of possible effects of alcohol on numerous other neurotransmitter systems including gamma amino butyric acid (GABA) and enkephalins must also be considered.

Anticonvulsant-Induced Movement Disorders

The most common movement disorder caused by toxic levels of anticonvulsant drugs is cerebellar ataxia. Nystagmus and dysarthria often accompany the syndrome of gait and limb ataxia. Occasionally, asterixis and even spontaneous myoclonic jerks also may be seen. Uncommonly, a chronic permanent cerebellar syndrome has been described following long-term phenytoin use.[32] Asterixis may be seen in the absence of other signs of toxicity, especially in the case of pre-existing focal neurological damage. Here, unilateral asterixis is often present.[3]

Rarely, anticonvulsants induce other abnormal involuntary movement disorders. Phenytoin, carbamazepine, and less often, a variety of other anticonvulsants have been reported to cause generalized chorea, choreoathetosis, orofacial dyskinesia, hemichorea, hemiballism, and dystonia. These movements are usually continuous while the patient is awake. However, paroxysmal dyskinesias have also been described.[33] Pre-existing choreic disorders may be exacerbated. De novo tics or worsening of pre-existing tics have been recently described with carbamazepine therapy. Akathisia has been rarely reported with anticonvulsant drugs. Phenytoin-induced parkinsonism has been described.[34,35] Finally, a postural tremor is commonly recognized with valproate therapy (rarely with other anticonvulsants). Here too, there may be an exaggeration of an underlying pre-existing essential or physiological tremor. The following sections will discuss these movement disorders in greater detail.

Choreoathetosis and Dystonia

The most common hyperkinetic movement disorder induced by anticonvulsants is chorea or choreoathetosis. Less often, movements may be bizarre, of wider amplitude, and even ballistic in nature.[36] Most, but not all patients experiencing this complication have been on polypharmacy. Phenytoin[37-39] and carbamazepine[40-42] account for the majority of these cases. Smaller numbers have been described with numerous other anticonvulsants including ethosuximide,[43,44] methsuximide,[43] keto-carbamazepine,[41] phenobarbital,[45-47] primidone,[48] and sulthiame.[37] Most (but not all) cases of phenytoin- or carbamazepine-induced choreoathetosis or dystonia demonstrate additional features of drug toxicity, including cerebellar ataxia, altered level of consciousness, and elevated plasma drug levels. The age of the patient, type or duration of epilepsy, and duration of anticonvulsant therapy seem to be unrelated to the development of the dyskinesias in most cases. Usually, the movement disorders occur in patients chronically treated with the causative agent. Less often, patients develop dyskinesias on initial exposure. Occasional examples of chorea have occurred with intravenous phenytoin treatment for status epilepticus.[39,49,50] The hyperkinetic movement disorder usually resolves with declining plasma levels of the causative drug. Occasional examples have recovered spontaneously despite maintenance of the drug. Others resolve over hours or days, while a small number have persisted for weeks or months after the drug was withdrawn.[37,51] In the case of phenytoin-induced dyskinesias, Kurata et al.[39] have pointed out that the abnormal movements usually occur at plasma levels greater than 20 μg/mL and decline and vanish as phenytoin disappears from the plasma.[37,38,49,50–59] Dyskinesias occurring with therapeutic levels of phenytoin are well recognized.[37,38,49,50,60–62] In some of these patients, this may be associated with reduced protein binding, resulting in toxic-free fraction levels despite maintenance of therapeutic levels.[63] This has not been found in other patients[33] in whom the contribution of underlying cerebral pathology may have been greater.

Pre-existing cerebral pathology, commonly involving the basal ganglia, seems to predispose many patients to the development of these dyskinesias.[37,38,59,60,64] In their review of the literature, Nausieda and colleagues[38,64] found a prior history of chorea, or previous use of neuroleptic therapy (plus or minus tardive dyskinesia) in a large proportion of cases of phenytoin-induced dyskinesias. Other examples emphasizing the importance of predisposing factors include one case with "localized encephalomalacias" in the striatum on postmortem examination[60] and another with enhancing basal ganglia calcifications on CT scan.[47] Both of these patients lacked other features of toxicity and had therapeutic anticonvulsant plasma levels (phenytoin and phenobarbital, respectively). The occurrence of hemichorea[37,55,65] is probably further support for the importance of pre-existing cerebral pathology in the predisposition of these movement disorders.

Management of anticonvulsant-induced dyskinesias obviously requires recognition of this rare complication of commonly used medications. When chorea is severe, short-term use of an antidopaminergic drug may suppress the abnormal movements.[59] When dystonia is the predominant hyperkinesia, anticholinergic drugs may reduce the severity of the movements. In the case of acute dystonia, parenteral anticholinergics may completely abate the dyskinesia. The dosage of the causative drug should be reduced or the offending agent should be withheld. In the case of polypharmacy, plasma levels should be used to guide therapeutic decisions. In the majority of patients, the movement disorders resolve rapidly with this approach. In the rare examples of prolonged or persistent abnormal involuntary movements, severe underlying brain damage has always been present. At times it is impossible to determine whether the anticonvulsant contributed to the syndrome or whether the association was simply coincidental. In view of the high incidence of predisposing brain disease, the treating physician should always consider and pursue the possibility of underlying, unsuspected structural or functional alterations of the basal ganglia.

The pathophysiological mechanisms accounting for anticonvulsant-induced dyskinesias remain unknown. Interactions with dopamine receptors[37,66] as well as anticholinergic effects[67,68] have been emphasized in the case of phenytoin. Rare examples of phenytoin-induced parkinsonism[34,35] may be support for the former. However, clinical and pharmacological differences between phenytoin and neuroleptic-induced dyskinesias[37,64] indicate that dopamine receptor blockade is probably not the sole explanation for these cases. Although phenytoin alone or in combination with chlorpromazine produces behavioral supersensitivity in response to the dopamine agonist apomorphine, there are no accompanying dopamine D_2 receptor density or affinity changes.[69] Different pharmacological mechanisms may underlie cases of carbamazepine-induced dyskinesias. This drug is chemically related to tricyclic antidepressants, which are also known to cause orofacial dyskinesias (see Chapter 8). Both dopaminergic[70] and cholinergic[42] mechanisms have been emphasized to account for carbamazepine-induced dyskinesias. The support for overlapping or similar mechanisms for different drugs comes from cases developing dyskinesias with both phenytoin and carbamazepine, given on separate occasions.[60] Here again, the importance of predisposing basal ganglia pathology cannot be overemphasized. The involvement of other neurotransmitters such as GABA in these and other anticonvulsant-induced movement disorders remains uncertain.

Special mention should be made of *ethosuximide-induced dyskinesias*. This complication has typically been an acute idiosyncratic reaction occurring early in treatment, in contrast to the usual dose-related association with most other anticonvulsants. Although these patients have generally demonstrated chorea, the hyperkinesia has behaved clinically and pharmacologically like neuroleptic-induced acute dystonic reactions. The movements have often occurred shortly after the first dose of ethosuximide and have abated rapidly after withdrawal or with parenteral diphenhydramine. Several of the patients reported with carbamazepine-induced dyskinesias have also had clinical features (i.e., onset early in the treatment course, oculogyric crises, opisthotonus, other dystonia) resembling acute dystonic reactions,[70–72] although one case treated with intravenous diphenhydramine did not respond.[70]

Akathisia

Akathisia, or a subjective inner restlessness, which often causes the patient to move about in order to ease the discomfort, has been described in a small number of patients treated with anticonvulsants, particularly carbamazepine[73] and ethosuximide.[43] As in the case of neuroleptic-induced akathisia, this side effect has occurred early in the course of treatment and has resolved on dose reduction or drug withdrawal. The single case of carbamazepine-associated akathisia is relatively well documented.[73] However, it is not clear whether the two children said to have akathisia and generalized chorea induced by ethosuximide truly had akathisia or whether their "restlessness" was simply part of or due to the choreiform movements.

Tics

Carbamazepine has also been reported to cause tics in a small number of patients. Neglia et al. first reported this association in 1984 in three children.[74] Two of these patients with pre-existing tics experienced an exacerbation following the institution of carbamazepine while the third developed the tics de novo. Plasma levels were in the therapeutic range. Despite discontinuing the drug, all three had persistent tics and two required haloperidol for tic control. Kurlan and collegues[75] have recently reported three further patients. One with Huntington's disease developed phonic and motor tics 2 weeks after beginning 300 mg of carbamazepine for depression. The tics resolved 4 weeks after the drug was discontinued. A second patient with Alzheimer's disease and neuroleptic-induced tardive dyskinesia and akathisia developed multiple motor tics and grunting a few days after discontinuing neuroleptics and beginning carbamazepine 200 mg daily. The tics "lessened considerably" over 8 weeks after both discontinuation of the carbamazepine and re-institution of haloperidol. A final young patient with Tourette's syndrome experienced a marked exacerbation of his tics after an EEG abnormality was treated with carbamazepine and phenytoin. The tics improved on withdrawal of anticonvulsants and initiation of haloperidol. This combined experience suggests that patients with pre-existing movement disorders (particularly Tourette's syndrome) are predisposed to this uncommon complication of carbamazepine. Other drugs capable of causing or exacerbating tics include chronic neuroleptic administration ("tardive Tourette's syndrome" – most often following neuroleptic withdrawal; see Chapter 6) and stimulant therapy including methylphenidate, pemoline, and cocaine (see Chapter 11). In addition, a single patient has been reported experiencing an exacerbation of tics following sudden withdrawal of chronic opiate therapy.[76] The mechanism underlying carbamazepine-induced tics remains uncertain, particularly in view of the diverse neurochemical effects of the drug.[77] In keeping with the central dopaminergic properties of other drugs reported to induce tics, Kurlan and colleagues have suggested that dopaminergic effects of carbamazepine may be critical. These include the enhancement presynaptic release of dopamine by striatal neurons,[78] an increase in ventricular CSF levels of dopamine,[79] and the potentiation of apomorphine-induced stereotypy.[80]

Tremor

Mild drug-induced asterixis is occasionally mistaken for a postural tremor. Rare examples of postural tremor have been described with carbamazepine[81] and phenytoin.[35] In these patients, additional clinical features of toxicity were present as well. On the other hand, shortly after *valproic acid* was introduced in the 1970s, it was recognized that a significant proportion of patients treated with this drug developed tremor. Approximately 20–25% of patients on chronic valproic acid therapy are found to have this complication, particularly if accelerometric recordings are carried out.[82] Half of these (10% of all patients) may be symptomatic from the tremor.[83] Tremor usually begins within 3 to 14 months of starting therapy,[84,85] although many patients experience it within the first month of treatment.[82] The tremor, which is usually present in the arms, is a postural or action variety, brought out during postural maintenance and worsened at the end-points of action. Some patients also demonstrate a resting component, and occasionally titubation of the head, neck and trunk also may occur.[82] The frequency of the tremor ranges between 6 and 15 Hz.[82] Clinically, the appearance is similar to essential tremor or enhanced physiological tremor. Indeed, some patients give a prior history of milder tremor or a family history of essential tremor without having noticed tremulousness in themselves before the introduction of valproic acid. Valproate-induced tremor typically occurs in patients taking doses over 750 mg daily with therapeutic blood levels. There is no apparent correlation between the severity of the tremor and valproate blood levels. However, patients note a reduction in the severity of the tremor when doses are withheld or missed, and we have seen patients lacking tremor while taking one formulation of valproic acid, who developed symptomatic tremor when the formulation was changed (possibly due to greater bioavailability of the second drug).

Most patients with valproate tremor probably do not require treatment. As in the case of essential tremor, symptomatic patients may benefit from the addition of propranolol. Karas and colleagues[83] found that propranolol (up to 100 mg daily) was the most effective drug for reducing tremor, while amantadine was moderately effective in a small number of patients, and cyproheptadine, diphenhydramine, and benztropine were ineffective. Uncommonly, patients have to be withdrawn from valproic acid because of the tremor.

The pharmacological mechanism underlying valproate-induced tremor is unknown. The association with essential tremor and response to propranolol suggests a pharmacological link to this disorder. However, the anatomical and biochemical basis of essential tremor are not known. Karas et al. have emphasized that valproic acid interacts with a number of neurotransmitter systems including GABA, dopamine, acetylcholine, and serotonin.[82] Further research is clearly needed in this area. Advances in the understanding of valproate-induced tremor may provide important insights into the pathophysiology of essential tremor.

Recently, a syndrome of valproate-induced parkinsonism-dementia has been reported.[85a] Strikingly, this was said to be present in 92% of 36 patients treated with valproate for over 12 months. Cognitive and personality changes (present in most) and parkinsonism (present in 77%) usually improved after varying periods of drug withdrawal. It is surprising that this association has not been recognized previously. Further confirmatory reports are required.

Oral Contraceptives

In 1966, Fernando[86] described the first case of chorea complicating oral contraceptive therapy. Since then, there have been approximately 30 additional cases reported. Chorea has occurred equally with high- and low-dose hormonal preparations. Most patients have been young, nulliparous women with an average age of 22 years (range 15–40). In over 80%, the movement disorder has evolved subacutely, beginning on average 12 weeks after starting oral contraceptive therapy. More prolonged exposure has been described in a small proportion of cases with one patient taking oral contraceptives for 3 years. However, 2 months before chorea began, she had interrupted the treatment for a period of 4 weeks.[87] In contrast to most other drug-induced dyskinesias, the distribution of oral contraceptive-induced chorea is frequently unilateral. Approximately 60% of patients have had pure hemichorea with the remainder generalized, often evolving from hemichorea and remaining asymmetrical.

The majority of patients developing chorea as a complication of oral contraceptives have a history of pre-existing abnormalities of the basal ganglia. Forty-six percent have had previous rheumatic fever, usually (30%) with Sydenham's chorea. Other predisposing factors have been a history of chorea gravidarum (with or without a past history of rheumatic fever), chorea secondary to Henoch-Schonlein purpura, systemic lupus erythematosis, cyanotic heart disease, neonatal anoxia, and migraine. The chorea induced by oral contraceptives in these patients usually mimics the nature and distribution of the movement disorder experienced earlier in life. In approximately three quarters of the patients, chorea occurs in isolation. Mild nonspecific abnormalities such as irritability, subtle personality changes, and increased forgetfulness have been seen in a small proportion. In three of the 30 cases reviewed by Galimberti,[88] chorea began abruptly and was associated with hemiparesis. This course, which occurred in the oldest patient reported in the literature with oral contraceptive-induced chorea (40 years old), suggests a possible vascular etiology. Another patient[89] had experienced an exacerbation of migraine before the onset of chorea.

Oral contraceptive-induced chorea seems to persist as long as the inciting agent is continued. Once the hormone therapy is withdrawn, chorea usually resolves spontaneously and completely within an average of 4 to 5 weeks (range 1–8 weeks). Occasional patients have been described with mild residual chorea with cyclic worsening of the movements during the week prior to menses.[90,91] However, it is likely that chorea had been a manifestation of pre-existing static encephalopathy in these cases.[88] Chorea has reccurred in the majority of individuals who were later rechallenged with oral contraceptives.[87] Patients with a past history of chorea induced by oral contraceptives may later develop chorea during pregnancy (chorea gravidarum) and vice versa. However, this is not a universal experience.

Patients should be managed by withdrawal of the oral contraceptive. In the case of severe, disabling chorea, dopamine antagonist therapy may be necessary for a short time using either a dopamine receptor blocker, such as haloperidol, or a presynaptic dopamine depletor such as reserpine or tetrabenazine. In view of the link with rheumatic fever, some authors have suggested the use of prophylactic penicillin;[92] however, there is little evidence to support this need.

The pathophysiology of oral contraceptive-induced chorea remains obscure. The estrogenic component of oral contraceptives is most likely the important causative factor in chorea induced by these agents. This is supported by a case of chorea recurrently induced with a combination pill (ethinyl estradiol 50 μg and norethindrone 1 mg) but not by progestin alone.[93] Another patient, with a past history of spontaneous right hemichorea, two episodes of chorea gravidarum, and a left caudate infarct of uncertain age, developed generalized chorea at the age of 61 within 3 weeks of starting to use a topical vaginal cream containing conjugated estrogen.[93a] Vascular, immunological and neurotransmitter mechanisms have all been proposed. The occurrence of sudden onset hemichorea associated with hemiparesis in a small number of cases might support an ischemic mechanism possibly induced by the effects of oral contraceptives on coagulation and central capillary tone.[90,92,94,95] Gamboa et al.[96] have proposed an immunological etiology with estrogen inducing a reactivation of subclinical rheumatic disease. In accord with an immunological hypothesis, Buge et al.[97] described the presence of antiestrogen antibodies in one patient, and circulating immune complexes containing antibodies to ethinyl estradiol have been detected in some women receiving oral contraceptives who may be at greater risk of thromboembolic complications.[98] A case of presumed oral contraceptive-induced SLE manifested by chorea (among other things)[99] might further support an immunological basis for the disorder.

However, the neurotransmitter hypotheses are most strongly

favored, particularly in relation to the effects of estrogen (plus or minus progesterone) on dopaminergic mechanisms. But these actions are complex and controversial with both antidopaminergic and dopamine-enhancing effects described. For example, in a guinea pig model, Nausieda et al.[91,100] reported evidence that estrogen had the potential for increasing sensitivity of postsynaptic dopamine receptors. This same group has also found a persistent striatal dopaminergic hypersensivity in patients with previous Sydenham's chorea.[101,102] The combination of these changes may account for the occurrence of chorea in response to oral contraceptives in patients with a past history of rheumatic fever. As well as potentially upregulating dopamine receptors, estrogens may have additional effects on dopamine degradation via the inhibition of monoamine oxidase and the saturation of catechol-O-methyltransferase by catecholestrogens formed through the 2-hydroxylation of estrogens within the CNS.[103] However, other studies[104,105] have found that estrogen treatment (particularly acute) exerts an antidopaminergic effect and that withdrawal of the hormone induces a state of heightened dopaminergic activity. These results may explain the higher incidence of tardive dyskinesia in postmenopausal females as well as the occasional report of the beneficial effect of estrogen treatment in this disorder.[106,107] Premarin treatment has also been reported to increase the severity of parkinsonism and decrease levodopa-induced dyskinesias in some patients with Parkinson's disease.[107,108] On the other hand, a dopamine-enhancing effect of estrogen is supported by the report of Quinn and Marsden, who found that 11 out of 12 premenopausal women with idiopathic Parkinson's disease experienced an increase in the severity of their symptoms for a few days before and during menstruation, a time when estrogen titres are lowered.[109] Further confusing the picture is an interesting patient reported by Robinson et al.[110] in whom a dystonic/ballistic movement disorder was exacerbated when serum estradiol, LH, and FSH levels were lowest and who improved markedly with low-dose (10 mg) ethinyl estradiol treatment. Van Hartesveldt and Joyce have reviewed these confusing and apparently conflicting effects of estrogens on dopaminergic mechanisms.[111] They point out that estrogen may affect the mesolimbic and mesostriatal dopamine systems differently, possibly accounting for different motor behaviors, especially in animal studies. In addition, estrogen may have different effects on pre- and postsynaptic mesostriatal elements. Certain effects of estrogen may be indirect, induced by its metabolites, particularly the catechol-estrogens and prolactin, both of which may reverse an initial suppression of mesostriatal dopamine induced by estrogen itself. Thus, a combination of locus of effect, timing, dosage, metabolism, and other indirect properties probably accounts for the complex interaction of estrogen on human movement disorders. Other neurotransmitter systems may also contribute to oral contraceptive-induced chorea. For example, one suggestion[92] supports a role for estrogen-induced competitive inhibition of pyridoxine-dependent glutamic acid decarboxylase (GAD), the synthesizing enzyme for GABA.

None of the proposed mechanisms provide an adequate explanation for all cases or answers to such questions as (1) why oral contraceptives do not always induce chorea in every patient with a past history of chorea or basal ganglia dysfunction, (2) why oral contraceptive-induced chorea sometimes occurs in patients without any history of these previous problems, (3) why chorea does not occur in men treated with estrogens for carcinoma of the prostate, or (4) why chorea does not occur earlier in the course of Huntington's disease in women.[87]

Calcium Channel Blockers

Flunarizine and Cinnarizine

Cinnarizine (Cz) is a selective calcium entry blocker. Flunarizine (Fz) is a difluorinated derivative of cinnarizine with greater potency and longer plasma half-life than the parent drug. Both agents have additional antihistaminic and serotonin antagonist properties, and because both are piperazine derivatives, with chemical structures resembling trifluoperazine, they also have mild D_2 receptor-blocking effects.[112,113] Cz has been available alone and in several combination preparations in certain Latin American and European countries since the mid-1970s while Fz reached these markets in approximately 1980. Fz has been recently approved in North America for migraine prophylaxis. Both drugs have been used widely for vertigo (both central and peripheral causes), cerebral blood flow disorders, atherosclerotic peripheral vascular disease, migraine prophylaxis, and even epilepsy. Recently, Fz has been reported effective in essential tremor.[114] The most common side effects have included drowsiness and asthenia. In 1984, DeMello-Souza[115] first reported the occurrence of parkinsonism secondary to Fz. Since that time, there have been over 200 cases of movement disorders reported secondary to these drugs. These side effects have included rare acute dystonic reactions and acute akathisia, parkinsonism, orofacial tremor, tardive dyskinesia, and tardive akathisia. Depression has been a common feature in these cases.

Movement disorder side effects occur more commonly due to Fz,[116] probably because it is 2.5 to 15 times more potent than Cz.[117] These side effects occur at the usual therapeutic doses of both drugs (Fz mean 13.2 mg, range 10–50 mg; Cz mean 152.1 mg, range 50–225 mg[118]). There does not seem to be a correlation between the severity of the movement disorder or depression with the dose.[119] As with neuroleptic drugs, acute dystonic reactions and acute akathisia have occurred within hours or days of beginning the drug. The other movement disorder complications have been delayed from 1 to 120 months after the initiation of the causative drug treatment.[118] Women outnumber men by approximately 2:1 or more. These side effects have been rare in patients under the age of 50 (usually acute dystonic reactions, acute akathisia, or isolated tremor). Most patients have been in their mid- to late 60s or older. A recent report suggests that two important predisposing factors to Cz-induced parkinsonism are aging and a history of essential tremor in patient or immediate family members.[119a] It is difficult to determine how common these side effects are. However, one group of investigators[120] found that Fz-induced parkinsonism accounted for the majority of cases of drug-induced parkinsonism seen in their neurology clinic between May 1985 and October 1986. The clinical features of these drug-induced movement disorders are entirely the same as those complicating the neuroleptic antipsychotic drugs (see Chapters 2–7). Parkinson's disease may worsen when patients are exposed to either agent.[121] Several patients with pure drug-induced parkinsonism have been misdiagnosed as having Parkinson's disease. Usually therapy with levodopa, anticholinergics or bromocriptine has been ineffective.[118] The responses of the other movement disorder syndromes to drug intervention has not been documented.

All patients with parkinsonism (including the rabbit syndrome) induced by Cz or Fz have recovered essentially completely within 1–40 weeks of drug withdrawal. It has been suggested that rigidity improves more rapidly than tremor.[120] Depression has also resolved in all patients upon drug withdrawal, and this usually occurs more rapidly than the improvement in parkinsonism. Examples of acute dystonia and acute akathisia have resolved spontaneously, usually despite the patient continuing to take the causative agent. As in the case of neuroleptic-related side effects, tardive dyskinesia has often shown less complete recovery and in some cases the movements remain persistent longer than 2 years after drug withdrawal. Micheli and colleagues have found that tardive akathisia has had the worst prognosis, persisting in one third of their cases (three out of nine, all with additional orofacial dyskinesia).[118] Where tardive orofacial dyskinesia or akathisia has resolved, it has taken between 15 days and 8 months.[118,121]

The pathophysiological mechanism(s) underlying Fz- and Cz-induced movement disorders remain uncertain. The marked similarity between this movement disorder side effect profile and that of other dopamine receptor blockers strongly favors the principal cause being their ability to block D_2 receptors. On the other hand, Micheli and colleagues argue that Cz and Fz have radically dissimilar tridimensional structures from trifluoperazine and much less D_2 receptor-blocking capabilities.[118] They propose that the calcium entry blocking effects may also be important. By impairing calcium channel opening, these drugs could interfere with the release of neurotransmitters at the presynaptic terminal. Indeed, Cz and Fz, as well as nifedipine, have been shown to be capable of reducing striatial dopamine release in rats.[122,123] Differences in the affinity for calcium receptors and blood-brain barrier passage have been proposed to explain why these complications have occurred with Fz and Cz but not other calcium blockers.[118] Alternatively, the dopamine receptor blocking properties of Fz and Cz may be amplified by their potential to inhibit dopamine release through calcium channel blockade. Obviously, further work needs to be done in this area. The potential contribution of pre-existing basal ganglia dysfunction due to vascular disease, age, or other factors remains uncertain.

Other Calcium Entry Blockers

Movement disorders have only rarely been described complicating the use of other calcium antagonists. The mechanism of action of these drugs in causing the various movement disorders is uncertain. All of the patients described have had one or more systemic diseases and have been taking several other medications. The importance of drug-drug and drug-disease interactions in the causation of the movement disorders is not known.

Pedro-Botet et al. described myoclonus involving the upper limbs and face within a week of *nifedipine* 40 mg per day, resolving in 3 days after the drug was stopped.[124] Another patient was reported with generalized, symmetrical 6 per second myoclonic movements beginning 10 days after starting 40 mg of nifedipine and resolving 24 hours after the drug was discontinued.[125] A "fine tremor" in the arms has been reported occurring after 1 month of nifedipine 30 mg.[126] As little as a single oral dose of 10 mg has been found to enhance both physiological tremor (by 56%) and essential tremor (by 71%) while verapamil 80 mg had no effect in the same essential tremor patients.[126a] Finally, nifedipine has resulted in a prolonged oculogyric crisis in a single autistic patient taking concomitant neuroleptic drugs.[127]

Verapamil has occasionally been associated with abnormal movements, possibly in part due to its known effects on dopaminergic systems.[128] One patient with pre-existing orofacial tardive dyskinesia developed severe generalized chorea within 4 days of the addition of verapamil 120 mg t.i.d. to stable lithium therapy. Chorea resolved 3 to 4 days after verapamil was discontinued.[129] Hicks and Abraham[130] described a patient treated with verapamil 80 mg four times daily for a period of 10 months. Subsequently, the patient developed a combination of myoclonus involving the arms and legs and dystonia affecting the neck and torso. Verapamil was discontinued and diltiazem was substituted. The movements subsided over the following 3 weeks. The fact that changing to diltiazem led to clearing of the movements argues against the importance of calcium-channel blocking properties to the cause of the movements.

Diltiazem has been reported to cause akathisia that recurred upon re-exposure of the drug.[131] Diltiazem-induced parkinsonism has also been described in a single patient who was also taking several other medications.[132] Although symptoms improved after diltiazem withdrawal and increased again upon rechallenge, the patient continued to demonstrate persistent residual cogwheel rigidity possibly suggesting underlying basal ganglia dysfunction.

Antihistaminics, Anticholinergics, and Antiserotoninergics

Many, but not all of the drugs discussed in the following section have some degree of overlapping properties in their ability to antagonize the effects of histamine, acetylcholine, and serotonin. A number of other drugs with anticholinergic properties, most notably the tricyclic antidepressants and some neuroleptics, are discussed in detail in other chapters of the text.

Antihistaminics

A small number of cases have been reported in which abnormal involuntary movements have occurred after prolonged use of *antihistaminic decongestants* such as chlorpheniramine, brompheniramine, phenindramine, and mebhydroline.[133–135] The abnormal movements have included orofacial dyskinesias, blepharospasm, tic-like bobbing of the head, a 3-per-second tremor of mandible and soft palate, cranial-cervical dystonia, and involuntary semi-purposeful movements of the hands. The course of these movements has varied from patient to patient with spontaneous improvement followed by incomplete[133] or complete[135] remission occurring within several weeks of drug withdrawal. Haloperidol treatment was used briefly in two patients.[135] In addition to the dyskinesias occurring with more chronic therapy described above, diphenhydramine (Benadryl) has been described to cause an acute dystonic reaction.[136] Oxatomide, an H_1 antihistaminic, anti-allergy agent, has also been reported to cause acute dystonic reactions in children, followed in some by a period of 2–3 days of impaired consciousness, mimicking encephalitis.[137]

The pathophysiology of these dyskinesias is uncertain. The ethanolamine antihistaminics are structurally related to the phenothiazines. These drugs, particularly diphenhydramine, are frequently used in the treatment of neuroleptic-induced acute dystonic reactions. Their efficacy in this disorder, and possibly a significant contributing factor to the dyskinesias described above, may relate to their potent anticholinergic properties. Primary or secondary effects on dopaminergic mechanisms are suggested by the report of Thach et al.[133] in which CSF dopamine turnover was found to be reduced in two patients, compared to normals.

A small number of cases of movement disorders induced by H_2 *receptor blockers* have been described. Most cases have involved cimetidine. Here, the abnormal movements have included postural and action tremor,[138] dystonic reactions,[139] parkinsonism, confusion, and cerebellar dysfunction (with "orofacial dyskinesia and marked twitching" after benztropine was used to treat the parkinsonism)[140] and chorea.[141,142] In one patient, both cimetidine and ranitidine, given at different times, resulted in chorea which began shortly after starting the drug (1 month and 5 days, respectively) and resolved spontaneously shortly after the drug was discontinued. Since these H_2 receptor antagonists have anticholinesterase activity on the brain at therapeutic levels (rather than anticholinergic effects) and no action on dopaminergic or adrenergic receptors, Lehmann suggests that H_2 receptors in the brain may be implicated in the origin of these abnormal movements.[142]

Anticholinergics

Anticholinergic drugs have been widely used in the treatment of Parkinson's disease for over a century with the synthetic agents utilized since the late 1940s.[143] Occasionally these drugs have the ability to cause orofacial dyskinesia or generalized chorea in parkinsonian patients.[144–146] More often they can exaggerate levodopa-induced dyskinesias.[147] In addition, it is well recognized that anticholinergics may exacerbate tardive dyskinesia,[148] and there has been some concern regarding the ability of these agents to predispose patients to this complication of neuroleptic drugs.[149]

Patients with various forms of dystonia are commonly exposed to the highest doses of anticholinergics used in clinical medicine. These patients occasionally obtain a very gratifying response from this treatment. However, much higher doses are usually required than are used in Parkinson's disease (e.g., 15–80 mg or more of trihexyphenidyl in dystonia versus 6 mg per day in parkinsonism). We have occasionally seen chorea developing as a side effect of this treatment,[150] and Nomoto et al. described five such patients who developed chorea with a mean dose of 31.7 mg of trihexyphenidyl daily (15–60 mg daily).[151] All patients had generalized chorea, which was disabling in two of the five. They had been treated on average for 3 years with anticholinergics (8 months to 9 years), and there was an inverse relationship between the age of the patient and dosage causing the side effect. All patients had experienced more common anticholinergic side effects at lower doses than those resulting in chorea. The abnormal movements markedly improved or resolved with a reduction in dosage. Four of the five patients had obtained an improvement in dystonia. The authors noted that occasional patients with idiopathic dystonia experience an increase in the amplitude of mobile spasms resulting in wilder and more uncontrolled movements on taking critical doses of trihexyphenidyl. This might be secondary to anticholinergic-induced chorea becoming superimposed on the dystonia.

The mechanism whereby anticholinergics result in these involuntary movements remains somewhat speculative. Acetylcholine is an important interneuronal neurotransmitter in the striatum. Anticholinergic drugs potentiate a variety of dopaminergic actions in the brain while cholinergic agents have the opposite effect.[152]

Cyproheptadine is a drug that combines antihistaminic, antiserotoninergic, and anticholinergic properties. This drug has been reported to cause "akathisia" in one patient[153] and recently cyproheptadine overdosage has resulted in short-lived, generalized chorea.[154] Myoclonic jerks persisted after the chorea subsided and other more common clinical features of anticholinergic toxicity (tachycardia, dry skin and mucous membranes, hallucinations) all resolved with the use of intravenous physostigmine. *Methysergide* has resulted in prominent akathisia in a single patient.[155] It is uncertain whether this side effect relates to the serotonin antagonist properties of the drug or to its effects on dopaminergic systems; the parent compound is a dopamine antagonist, while its metabolite, methergine, is a dopamine agonist.[155] *Trazadone*, an anxiolytic-antidepressant has anti-serotonin effects as well as possibly dopamine antagonist properties due to its propylpiperazine ring structure. Rare cases of parkinsonism[156] and chorea with myoclonus[157] have been described due to this drug. *Buspirone* is another anxiolytic that binds to 5-HT1A receptors, blocks presynaptic dopamine receptors, and may have additional effects on GABA systems. One patient with azotemia and a previous stroke has been reported to develop generalized myoclonus, unilateral shoulder dystonia, and akathisia after 5 days of buspirone treatment. The symptoms resolved rapidly on drug withdrawal and short-term clonazepam therapy.[158] Other cases of recurrent akathisia,[159] persistent dystonia,[160] and oral dyskinesia[161] have also been attributed to buspirone.

Antidepressant drugs represent one of the largest group of agents with mixed effects on acetylcholine, serotonin, and other monoamine systems. These are discussed in detail in Chapter 8 of this volume.

Benzodiazepines

Movement disorders have been reported in a small number of patients taking various benzodiazepines, including diazepam, flurazepam, chlorazepate, lorazepam, and midazolam. Most of these patients have been on other drugs, particularly neuroleptics or tricyclic antidepressants. Despite this, in some the benzodiazepine has been the principal offending agent[162] while in most, these drugs have appeared to exacerbate a pre-existing or covert tardive dyskinesia.[163,164] The abnormal movements have usually been orofacial dyskinesias similar to classic tardive dyskinesia, developing at variable intervals of days to many weeks after beginning the benzodiazepines and resolving within a few days of drug withdrawal. Acute dystonic reactions responsive to diphenhydramine have occasionally been described secondary to diazepam.[165] In one case of acute intense akathisia and lingual dyskinesia after a single intravenous 5-mg dosage of midazolam, the "acute dystonia" was rapidly abolished after the intravenous administration of the benzodiazepine antagonist flumazenil.[166] Finally, high doses of diazepam (140–400 mg/d) used in schizophrenic patients previously withdrawn from neuroleptics have been reported to cause drug-induced parkinsonism.[167] Classic parkinsonian signs began within 1–8 weeks of starting diazepam, were resistant to anticholinergic therapy, and resolved 1–3 weeks after drug withdrawal.

The pathophysiological mechanisms underlying benzodiazepine-induced movement disorders are unknown. These are rare complications, most often occurring in pharmacologically predisposed patients. The central chemical effects of benzodiazepines are complex, involving interactions with a variety of neurotransmitters including GABA, glycine, norepinephrine, and serotonin.[168] Adding to the confusion is the fact that a beneficial therapeutic effect in neuroleptic-induced tardive dyskinesia is seen far more often with benzodiazepines than is the rare occurrence of an exacerbation of this movement disorder.

Antimicrobials

Central nervous system side effects of *antibiotics*, particularly the penicillins and cephalosporins, are well recognized. A toxic encephalopathy with seizures is the usual manifestation occurring with high doses of these medications, particularly given to patients with compromised renal function. Isolated myoclonus is also not uncommon. An acute, reversible parkinsonian syndrome has been reported in a single patient treated with cephaloridine 4 gm/day, beginning on the 16th day of therapy and resolving within 3 days of drug withdrawal.[169] Four patients with AIDS treated with trimethoprim-sulfamethoxazole for 3–8 days were reported to develop resting and/or postural tremors as well as a variety of other neurological features including apathy, hallucinations, ataxia, ankle clonus, and skin rash. All of these symptoms resolved within 2–3 days of discontinuing the drug.[170] Transient[171] and permanent[172] parkinsonism (levodopa-responsive) have been reported with intraventricular amphotericin-B treatment for cryptococcal meningitis. The role of the drug versus the complications of the fungal infection, including obstructive or communicating hydrocephalus, in these rare cases remains uncertain.

Antiviral agents may cause a broad range of neurotoxicity. The importance of additional contributing factors such as hepatic and renal dysfunction as well as the underlying primary viral infection should not be underestimated. With respect to movement disorder side effects, adenine arabinoside (vidarabine) seems to have a propensity to cause tremor that is sometimes generalized and quite severe. Mild tremor may be a forewarning of more serious, life-threatening neurotoxic side effects. When present in its extreme form, tremor is usually associated with pronounced encephalopathic features, occasionally resulting in death (see ref. 173 for review).

Antimalarials deserve special mention. Dyskinesias similar to neuroleptic-induced acute dystonic reactions have been described with a variety of 4-aminoquinolines such as chloroquine, hydroxychloroquine, amidiaquine, and cycloquine[174–177] These dyskinesias respond to anticholinergics or antihistaminics in a similar fashion to neuroleptic-induced acute dystonic reactions and remit rapidly upon withdrawal of the antimalarial agent. A single case of a chloroquine-induced acute dystonic reaction occurring despite concomitant diphenhydramine has suggested a possible adverse pharmacodynamic interaction between chloroquine and metronidazole.[177] The authors of this report proposed that chloroquine causes acute dystonic reactions by reducing dopamine via inhibition of neuronal calcium uptake for exocytosis through its interaction with neuronal membrane phospholipids. They suggested that metronidazole may have potentiated this action through its effects in lowering synaptosomal calcium. Others[175] have implicated a direct effect of antimalarial drugs on nigrostriatal dopamine receptors.

Miscellaneous Drugs

There are numerous descriptions of movement disorders occurring with a wide variety of other drugs. These are usually individual case reports often lacking substantive information that might definitively prove a cause and effect relationship between the drug and the movement disorder. It is impractical to provide an extensive discussion of any of these. The following section and Table 1 will briefly review this literature.

Table 1
Miscellaneous Drugs Causing Movement

Drug Name Dosage and Duration	Number of Patients	Drug Category	Possible Biochemical Effects Causing the Movement Disorder
Digoxin 0.25 mg × 1 mo (3 days after OR for aortic dissection in one case)	2	Cardiac glycoside	?
Captopril 25 mg/d × several days	1	Antihypertensive ACE inhibitor	?
Pindolol* 2.5–60 mg for 1–72 hr	6	Antihypertensive beta blocker	Partial beta agonist
Procaine IM injections	1	Local anesthetic	?
Perhexiline 300 mg/d × 1–2 mo	2	Antianginal	?
Oxymetholone 200–300 mg/d for 1 yr	1	Anabolic steroid (in this case used in the treatment of aplastic anemia)	?
Ketamine (0.5 cc IV (abuse)	1	Anesthetic	?
Betel nuts	2	Active ingredient arecholine	Cholinergic
Flecainide	1	Benzamide class 1c antiarrhythmic	?Dopamine antagonist

* The combination of pindolol and clopamide has been reported to cause parkinsonism in two patients. However, this report completely lacks any support for a cause and effect relationship.[242]

Disorders (not discussed elsewhere)**

Nature of the Abnormal Movements	Additional Features	Outcome	Reference No.
Facial, L arm and leg chorea	Renal failure; Plasma level = 4.2 nmol/L (N = 1.2–2.6)	Incomplete resolution over 7 days	231
Generalized chorea	Fatigue, confusion; Level 34 μg/L (1.2–2.6)	Responded to haloperidol; remitted	232
Parkinsonism	Nil	Resolved after D/C	233
Postural arm tremor, jaw tremor	Nil	Resolved 24–72 hr after D/C	234, 235
Also worsens essential tremor			236
Parkinsonism	Earlier symptoms suggestive of acute dystonic reaction and akathisia	Resolved; initially responsive to Artane not L-dopa	237
Parkinsonism	Peripheral neuropathy in one case. Previous metoclopramide-induced parkinsonism in one	Resolved in 2 mo after D/C	238
Chorea of R arm and leg, grimacing, tongue movements	Confused, morbid thoughts	Resolved in 2 mo after D/C, thioridazine treatment used	239
Acute dystonic reaction	Nil	Resolved with diphenhydramine	240
Precipitation of neuroleptic-induced parkinsonism	Red staining of teeth	Resolved over 4–7 d after D/C	241
Oromandibular dystonia	Nil	Persisted >1½ years total (~1 year after drug withdrawal)	243

** Very few of these represent unequivocal cause and effect relationships. Indeed, in some (e.g., oxymetholone) the relationship between the drug and the movement disorder is somewhat questionable, and other causes (e.g., cerebral ischemia) might better explain the clinical picture.

A number of *nonsteroidal anti-inflammatory drugs* (NSAIDs) have been reported to cause a variety of movement disorders. For example, acute dystonic reactions have been described with mefenamic acid[178] and the combination of indomethacin and azapropazone.[179] Mefenamic acid (combined with alcohol and diazepam) has also been described as causing an acute generalized dyskinesia with dystonic features responsive to benztropine[180] and ibuprofen has caused bilateral ballistic movements.[181] NSAIDs have also been variably reported to exacerbate or improve parkinsonism.[182,183] Although other cases of movement disorders secondary to NSAIDs have not been formally reported, Wood and colleagues found that several reports of "extrapyramidal disorders" and "tremor" were listed with the Committee on Safety of Medicines of the United Kingdom.[179] The origin of these rare complications of NSAIDs remains unknown.

Amiodarone is a di-ionated benzofurane derivative, used in the treatment of cardiac arrhythmias. Tremor is an occasional side effect of this drug. This is usually a bilateral 6–10 Hz postural and action tremor of the arms, which is similar to essential tremor. Werner and Olanow[184] described a coarse, parkinsonian resting tremor in the left leg in a single patient treated for a period of 4 days with 1.2 to 1.6 gm daily. The tremor resolved within 5 days of drug withdrawal and returned again on re-exposure. Review of the literature reveals a variety of uncommon examples of movement disorders occurring in patients exposed to this drug including myoclonus,[185,186] hemiballism, dyskinesias of the extremities,[187] and orofacial dyskinesias.[188] The contribution of the drug to these side effects remains uncertain given the concurrent use of other medications and the presence of significant cardiovascular disease in all cases. Werner and Olanow reviewed nine cases of parkinsonian features due to amiodarone.[184] They suggest that the reversibility of symptoms relates to the duration of treatment and that some patients exposed for prolonged periods of time may develop persistent parkinsonian features. It is difficult to interpret the one case exposed to amiodarone for a period of 24 months who had persistent parkinsonian features and was found to have depigmentation of the substantia nigra at autopsy.[189] Clearly, further data on the central effects of this agent are required.

A number of *antineoplastic chemotherapeutic agents* have occasionally been reported to cause movement disorders. Unfortunately, many of these are poorly described or are mentioned only briefly in larger population studies. The role of concomitant medications or

illnesses is usually uncertain. The mechanism(s) by which chemotherapeutic drugs induce these movement disorders is usually unknown. Several of them result in peripheral neuropathy, which may
account for tremor or athetotic-like movements and cerebellar dysfunction which may cause additional tremor. These problems are
exemplified by reports of abnormal movements complicating hexamethylmelamine. Respiratory and orofacial dyskinesia reported in
one case was almost certainly entirely due to the concomitant prochlorperazine[190] while tremor has probably resulted from peripheral
nerve damage.[191] The validity of a single reported case of parkinsonism is uncertain.[192] Vincristine in one case given with prednisone
resulted in bilateral arm athetosis as well as depression, agitation,
gait ataxia, later followed by fever, inappropriate ADH secretion,
leukopenia, and paralytic ileus. All of these manifestations resolved
over a 5-day period.[193] In another case, vincristine given with adriamycin resulted in a poorly described Parkinson-like syndrome, persisting until death, which occurred shortly thereafter.[194] Slightly
better documented is a case of recurrent acute dystonic reactions
from etoposide, a derivative of podophyllotoxin.[195] Diphenhydramine successfully prevented further reactions. The cyclophospha-
mide analogue ifosfamide was implicated in another patient who
also received etoposide and cisplatin.[195a]

Finally, one of the more convincing cases of chemotherapy inducing a movement disorder is that of a 64-year-old woman receiving
cytosine arabinoside for acute myelomonocytic leukemia. After a
second course of high-dose (72 gm over 6 days) treatment for relapse,
this patient developed severe parkinsonism which initially progressed to a bed-bound state and which was resistant to antiparkinsonian therapy. Over a period of 12 weeks, the patient experienced
a spontaneous, complete resolution of neurological symptoms and
signs.[196] The underlying mechanism of this rare complication is completely unknown. We have seen a similar patient who developed
severe parkinsonism combined with the more common cerebellar
syndrome that occurs in 10–20% of patients within 5 to 7 days of
onset of therapy.[197]

Despite a variety of central biochemical effects, *opiate derivatives* rarely result in movement disorder side effects. The meperidine
analogue, 1-methyl-4-phenyl-1,2,3,6-tetrahydropyridine induces a
permanent parkinsonian syndrome. However, this has little to do
with the opiate properties of the "synthetic heroin" parent compound
(MPPP). Rather, MPTP is metabolized to a potent neurotoxin

(MPP +) with selective effects on dopaminergic neurons, especially those of the substantia nigra pars compacta.

Myoclonus is the most common movement disorder reported secondary to opiate drugs. Meperidine may result in stimulus-sensitive and action myoclonus, particularly in patients with chronic renal failure.[198,199] This myoclonus may or may not be associated with confusion and other encephalopathic features. One report emphasizes the painful nature of the myoclonus, which may help differentiate meperidine-associated myoclonus from that occurring in uremic encephalopathy.[199] Myoclonus has been both extremely sensitive[198] and resistant[199] to clonazepam therapy. It is generally believed that meperidine-induced myoclonus occurring in renal failure patients is secondary to the accumulation of the metabolite normeperidine. In view of this potential complication of meperidine, it may be more appropriate to use morphine or codeine when narcotic analgesia is required in uremic patients despite their depressant effects. On the other hand, chronic high-dose narcotic treatment in cancer patients with morphine, meperidine, methadone, or oxycodone may also result in myoclonus.[200] Concomitant neuroleptic and nonsteroidal anti-inflammatory drug therapy may increase the risk of this side effect,[200] and it has been argued that these opiates simply increase the likelihood of neuroleptic-induced side effects.[201] This may explain why others find that morphine-induced myoclonus is extremely uncommon.[202] The argument for an opiate-neuroleptic interaction is supported by a report that suggests that heroin addiction predisposes to acute dystonic reactions secondary to the neuroleptic sulpiride[203] (see Chapter 11 re cocaine addiction predisposing to acute dystonic reactions). Other movement disorders include transient chorea reported with methadone therapy in one patient[204] and reversible parkinsonism described in a single patient taking meperidine.[205] The pharmacological mechanisms underlying these extremely uncommon cases are not known. Narcotics have a variety of effects on central dopaminergic systems, some of which are similar to those of neuroleptic drugs. It is likely that these are indirect, possibly secondary to effects on opiate receptors, in part related to the enkephalinergic pathways from the striatum to the external globus pallidus. Finally, although intraspinal administration of morphine is known to cause myoclonus in animals, there is only a single case report of such a side effect in man.[206] However, the term "myoclonus" was used inappropriately since this patient experienced "spasms" in the upper legs and lower abdomen lasting 5–10 seconds each (i.e., far too long for myoclonus) and occurring at 30–40 second intervals. These periodic dystonic spasms (earlier literature might have classified the movement disorder as spinal or segmental myoclonus) necessitated spinal anesthesia for relief.

Alpha-methyldopa is a competitive inhibitor of dopa decarboxylase, the enzyme essential for the conversion of dopa to dopamine. In addition, the drug is metabolized to a false neurotransmitter, alpha-methylnorepinephrine, which theoretically may compete with dopamine at postsynaptic striatal dopamine receptors.[207] Despite concern raised by these biochemical properties, parkinsonism due to alpha-methyldopa is rather uncommon. There are a small number of reports of de novo, reversible parkinsonism, or worsening of pre-existing Parkinson's disease in patients treated with this agent.[208–210] It has also been suggested that idiopathic cranial dystonia may predispose to severe alpha-methyldopa-induced parkinsonism while the dystonic movements may improve,[211] although this has not been our experience. Parkinsonism induced by alpha-methyldopa has usually occurred in individuals in their sixth decade after treatment with a dose of 1–2 gm/day for a period of 3–8 weeks. Once the drug is withdrawn, signs have resolved rapidly, usually within a few days to weeks. Dopamine agonist properties have also been proposed[212] and these may account for the rare example of dyskinesias reported with alpha-methyldopa.[213]

Disulfiram (tetraethylthiuramdisulfide), used in the treatment of chronic alcholism, has occasionally been reported to cause movement disorders. Rare examples of transient choreoathetosis after accidental intake in children[214,215] and transient parkinsonism with chronic treatment[216–218] or overdose[219] have been described. Persistent movement disorders, usually combining dystonia and akinesia[216,220–222] have also been reported. A recently described patient demonstrated a slowly progressive course following the acute encephalopathic period with the evolution of severely disabling dystonia.[222] Imaging has usually demonstrated cystic necrosis of the globus pallidus (probably accounting for the akinesia) and the putamen (possibly resulting in dystonia).[222] The exact cause of disulfiram-induced transient or persistent movement disorders is uncertain. The role of concomitant alcohol intake is unclear. Considerable evidence supports a critical role for carbon disulfide, an important metabolite of disulfiram. Multiple other contributing factors may exist, including hypotension, acidosis and the effects of inhibition of dopamine-beta-hydroxylase on basal ganglia neurotransmitter systems.[222]

Cyclosporin A is an immunosuppressant, often used in organ transplantation therapy, which selectively inhibits helper T-cells. Indirect neurological toxicity relates to hepatic and renal dysfunction caused by the drug. Symptoms of organ rejection can sometimes be confused with side effects of the medication. Direct neurological complications include tremor, seizures, ataxia, leukoencephalopathy, cortical blindness, paraparesis or quadraparesis, mental status changes, and peripheral neuropathy.[223] Occasionally, tremor is one component of an encephalopathic process dominated by cerebellar ataxia. Isolated postural tremor is probably the most common neurological side effect, occurring in anywhere from 20% to 39% of cases.[224,225] This may simply be an exaggerated physiological tremor due to activation of the sympathetic nervous system.[226] Tremor is usually not very disabling and its presence or severity diminishes with time. For example, in one study of renal transplant recipients, tremor was present in 20% at 3 months after transplantation, 12% after 4 months, 10% at 1 year, and in none 3 years post-transplantaion.[225] Recently, three patients have been described who developed akinetic mutism on the third day of intravenous cyclosporin treatment after liver transplantation.[227] One had oculogyric upward deviation of the eyes and another had severe orofacial dyskinesia, choreoathetosis in the arms, and a resting tremor in all limbs. Two patients subsequently were found to have evidence for central pontine myelinolysis in the absence of fluctuations in serum sodium or other risk factors for this disorder.

A variety of other drugs are known to cause a postural tremor. In most cases this is due to an exaggeration of normal physiological tremor as is seen with sympathomimetic agents (e.g., beta agonists), bronchodilators (e.g., xanthines), thyroid hormone, glucocorticoids, anabolic steroids, hypoglycemic agents, procainamide, and caffeine. Several others, including lithium, tricyclic antidepressants, amphetamines, levodopa and dopamine agonists, neuroleptics, sodium valproate, and amiodarone are discussed elsewhere in this volume.

A final emphasis should be made regarding the potential for underlying cerebal pathology to predispose to drug-induced movement disorders. Several examples have already been discussed here and elsewhere in the text. Mention should also be made of the potential for the pathology and neurochemical defects of Alzheimer's disease to predispose to movement disorders induced by various drugs.

For example, physostigmine has been reported to cause myoclonus in some patients, possibly due to an alteration in the interaction between cholinergic and either serotoninergic or dopaminergic neurotransmitter systems.[228] Bethanechol, a cholinergic agonist given intraventricularly, has induced parkinsonism, possibly indicating pre-existing asymptomatic nigral dopaminergic deficiency (e.g., due to concomitant Parkinson's disease or other brainstem pathology).[229] Finally, baclofen has resulted in chorea in a single patient with Alzheimer's disease.[230]

Acknowledgments: Special thanks to Mrs. Jill Lennox and Mrs. Shelley Malton for assistance in typing the manuscript and Dr. T. Curran for helpful comments.

References

1. Neiman J, Lang AE, Fornazzari L, Carlen PL. Movement disorders in alcoholism. Neurology 1990; 40:741–746.
2. Leavitt S, Tyler HR. Studies in asterixis. Arch Neurol 1964; 10:360–368.
3. Young RR, Shahani BT. Asterixis: One type of negative myoclonus. Adv Neurol 1986; 43:137–157.
4. Koller W, O'Hara R, Durus W, Bauer J. Tremor in chronic alcoholism. Neurology 1985; 35:1660–1662.
5. Rondot P, Jedynak CP, Ferrey G. Pathological tremors: nosological correlates. Prog Clin Neurophysiol 1978; 5:95–113.
6. Lefebbre-D'Amour M, Shahani BT, Young RR. Tremor in alcoholic patients. Prog Clin Neurophysiol 1978; 5:160–164.
7. Shahani BT, Young RR. Physiological and pharmacological aids in the differential diagnosis of tremor. J Neurol Neurosurg Psychiatry 1976; 39:772–783.
8. Carlsson C, Hagendal J. Arterial noradrenaline levels after ethanol withdrawal. Lancet 1967; 2:889.
9. Jaffe JH. Drug addiction and drug abuse. In: Gilman A, Goodman LS, Rall TW, Murad F (eds), The Pharmacological Basis of Therapeutics, New York, Macmillan Publishing, 1985, pp 532–581.
10. Wikler A. Diagnosis and treatment of drug dependence of the barbiturate type. Am J Psychiatry 1968; 125:758–765.
11. MacKinnon GL, Parker WA. Benzodiazepine withdrawal syndrome: a literature review and evaluation. Am J Drug Alcohol Abuse 1982; 9:19–33.
12. Martin WR, Sloan JW, Sapira JD, Jasinski DR. Physiologic, subjective and behavioural effects of amphetamine, metamphetamine, ephedrine, pentrazine and methylphenidate. Man Clin Pharmacol Ther 1971; 12:245–258.

13. Adams RD, Victor M. "Alcoholic" cerebellar degeneration. In: Principles of Neurology, 4th ed, New York, McGraw-Hill Information Services, 1989, p 837.
14. Silverskiold BP. Romberg's test in the cerebellar syndrome occurring in chronic alcoholism. Acta Neurol Scand 1969; 45:292–302.
15. Silverskiold BP. A 3-sec leg tremor in a cerebellar syndrome. Acta Neurol Scand 1977; 55:385–393.
16. Rosenhamer HJ, Silverskiold BP. Slow tremor and delayed brainstem auditory evoked responses in alcoholics. Arch Neurol 1980; 37:293–296.
17. Scholz E, Diener HC, Dichgans J, Langohr HD, Schied W, Schupmann A. Incidence of peripheral neuropathy and cerebellar ataxia in chronic alcoholics. J Neurol 1986; 233:212–217.
18. Torvik A, Lindboe CF, Rogde S. Brain lesions in alcoholics. J Neurol Sci 1982; 56:233–248.
19. Victor M, Adams RD, Cole M. The acquired (non-Wilsonian) type of chronic hepatocerebral degeneration. Medicine (Baltimore) 1965; 44:345–396.
20. Carlen PL, Lee MA, Jacob MA, Livshits O. Parkinsonism provoked by alcoholism. Ann Neurol 1981; 9:84–86.
21. Lang AE, Marsden CD, Obeso JA, Parkes JD. Alcohol and Parkinson disease. Ann Neurol 1982; 12:254–256.
22. Shen WW. Extrapyramidal symptoms associated with alcohol withdrawal. Biol Psychiatry 1984; 19:1037–1043.
23. Nieman J, Borg S, Wahlund L-O. Parkinsonism and dyskinesiaa during ethanol withdrawal. Br J Addict 1988; 83:437–439.
24. Shandling M, Carlen PL, Lang AE. Parkinsonism in alcohol withdrawal: a follow-up study. Mov Disord 1990; 5:36–39.
25. Fornazzari L, Carlen PL. Transient choreiform dyskinesias during alcohol withdrawal. Can J Neurol Sci 1982; 9:89–90.
26. Mullin PJ, Kershaw PW, Bolt JMW. Choreoathetotic movement disorder in alcoholism. Br Med J 1970; 4:278–281.
27. Lutz EG. Neuroleptic-induced akathisia and dystonia triggered by alcohol. JAMA 1976; 236:2422–2423.
28. Lai H, Carino MA, Horito A. Effects of ethanol on central dopamine functions. Life Sci 1980; 27:299–301.
29. Liljequist S. Changes in the sensitivity of dopamine receptors in the nucleus accumbens and in the striatum induced by chronic ethanol administration. Acta Pharmacol Toxicol 1978; 43:19–28.
30. Balldin J, Alling C, Gottfries CG, Lindstedt G, Langstrom G. Changes in dopamine receptor sensitivity in humans after heavy alcohol intake. Psychopharmacology (Berlin) 1985; 86:142–146.
31. Tanner AR, Bantock I, Hinks L, Lloyd B, Turner NR, Wright R. Decreased selenium and vitamine E levels in the alcoholic populations: possible relationship to hepatic injury through increased lipid peroxidation. Dig Dis Sci 1986; 31:1307–1312.
32. Reynolds EH, Trimble MR. Adverse neuropsychiatric effects of anticonvulsant drugs. Drugs 1985; 29:570–581.
33. Dravet C, Dalla BB, Mesdjian E, Galland MC, Roger J. Phenytoin-

induced paroxysmal dyskinesias. In: Oxley J, Janz D, Meinardi H (eds), Anti-epileptic Therapy: Chronic Toxicity of Anti-epileptic Drugs, New York, Raven Press, 1983, pp 229–235.

34. Goni M, Jimenez M, Feijoo M. Parkinsonism induced by phenytoin. Clin Neuropharmacol 1985; 8:383–384.

35. Prensky AL, DeVivo DC, Palkes H: Severe bradykinesia as a manifestation of toxcity to ani-epileptic medications. J Pediatr 1974; 78:700–704.

36. Critchley EMR, Phillips M. Unusual idiosyncratic reactions to carbamazepine. J Neurol Neurosurg Psychiatry 1988; 51:1238.

37. Chadwick D, Reynolds EH, Marsden CD. Anticonvulsant-induced dyskinesias: a comparison with dyskinesias induced by neuroleptics. J Neurol Neurosurg Psychiatry 1976; 39:1210–1218.

38. Nausieda PA, Koller WC, Weiner WJ, Klawans HL. Clinical and experimental studies of phenytoin-induced hyperkinesias. J Neural Trans 1979; 45:219–305.

39. Kurata K, Kido H, Kobayashi K, Yamaguchi N. Long-lasting movement disorder induced by intravenous phenytoin administration for status epilepticus. Clin Neuropharmacol 1988; 11:467–471.

40. Joyce RP, Gunverson CH. Carbamazepine-induced orofacial dyskinesia. Neurology 1980; 30–1333–1334.

41. Bimpong-Buta K, Froescher W. Carbamazepine-induced choreoathetoic dyskinesias. J Neurol Neursurg Psychiatry 1982; 45:560–567.

42. Jacome D. Movement disorder induced by carbamazepine. Neurology 1981; 31:1059–1060.

43. Ehyai A, Kilroy A, Fenichel G. Dyskinesia and akathisia induced by ethosuximide. Am J Dis Child 1978; 132:527–528.

44. Kischberg GI. Dyskinesia-An unusual reaction to ethosuximide. Arch Neurol 1975; 32:137–113.

45. Lightman SL. Phenobarbital dyskinesia. Postgrad Med J 1978; 54:114–115.

46. Strandjord RE, Johannessen SI. Involuntary movements in patients with organic brain lesions treated with anti-epileptic drugs. In: Gardner-Thorpe C, Janz D, Meinardi H, et al. (eds), Anti-epileptic Drug Monitoring, Tunbridge Wells, Pitman, 1977, pp 89–103.

47. Wiznitzner M, Younkin D. Phenobarbital-induced dyskinesia in a neurologically impaired child. Neurology 1984; 34:1600–1601.

48. Schmidt D. Die behandlung der epilepsien mit hilfe der blutspiegelbestimmung van antiepileptika. Nervenartz 1977; 48:183–196.

49. Mauguiere F, Dalery J, de Villard R, Courjon J. Transient hyperkinesia after a single intravenous perfusion of diphenylhydantoin. Eur Neurol 1979; 18:116–123.

50. Howrie DL, Crumrine DK. Phenytoin-induced movement disorder associated with intravenous administration for status epilepticus. Clin Pediatr (Phila) 1985; 24:467–469.

51. Ahmad S, Laidaw J, Houghton GW, Richens A. Involuntary movements caused by phenytoin intoxication in epileptic patients. J Neurol Neurosurg Psychiatry 1975; 38:225–231.

52. Kooiker DL, Sumi SM. Movement disorder as a manifestation of diphenylhydantoin intoxication. Neurology 1974; 24:68–71.

53. McLellan DL, Swash M. Choreo-athetosis and encephalopathy induced by phenytoin. Br Med J 1974; 2:204–205.
54. Rosenblum E, Rodichok L, Hanson PA. Movement disorder as a manifestation of diphenylhydantoin toxicity. Pediatrics 1974; 64:364–366.
55. Shuttleworth E, Wise G, Paulson G. Choreoathetosis and diphenylhydantoin intoxication. JAMA 1974; 230:1170–1171.
56. Chalhub EG, DeVivo DC. Phenytoin-induced choreoathetosis. J Pediatr 1976; 39:1210–1218.
57. Zinsmeister S, Marks RE. Acute athetosis as a result of phenytoin toxicity in a child. Am J Dis Child 1976; 130:75–76.
58. Opida CL, Korthals JK, Somasundara M. Bilateral ballism in phenytoin intoxication. Ann Neurol 1978; 3:186.
59. Lazaro RP. Involuntary movements induced by anticonvulsant drugs. Mount Sinai J Med 1982; 49:274–281.
60. Rasmussen S, Kristensen M. Choreoathetosis during phenytoin treatment. Acta Med Scand 1977; 201:239–241.
61. Yoshida M, Yamada S, Osaki Y, Nakanishi T. Phenytoin-induced orofacial dyskinesia: a case report. J Neurol 1985; 231:340–342.
62. Filloux F, Thompson JA. Transient chorea induced by phenytoin. J Pediatr 1987; 110:639–641.
63. Tomson T. Choreoathetosis induced by ordinary phenytoin levels explained by high free fraction? A case report. Ther Drug Monit 1988; 10:239–241.
64. Nausieda PA, Koller WC, Klawans HL, et al. Phenytoin and choreic movements. N Engl J Med 1978; 298:1093.
65. Luhdorf K, Lund M. Phenytoin-induced hyperkinesia. Epilepsia 1977; 18:409–15.
66. Mendez JS, Cotzias GC, Mena I, Papavasiliou PS. Diphenylhydantoin blocking of levodopa effects. Arch Neurol 1975; 32:44–46.
67. Agrawal S, Bhargara V. Effect of drugs on brain acetylcholine level in the rat. Indian J Med Res 1964; 52:1179–1182.
68. Eadie MJ, Tyrer JH. Anticonvulsant Therapy: Pharmacological Basis, Edinburgh, Churchill Livingston, 1974, p 74.
69. Sethi KD, Hitri A, Diamond BI. Phenytoin potentiation of neuroleptic-induced dyskinesias. Mov Disord 1990; 5:325–327.
70. Crosley CJ, Swender PT. Dystonia associated with carbamazepine administration: experience in brain-damaged children. Pediatrics 1979; 63:612–615.
71. Berchou RC, Rodin EA. Carbamazepine-induced oculogyric crisis. Arch Neurol 1979; 63:612–615.
72. Jacome D: Carbamazepine-induced dystonia. JAMA 1979; 241:2263.
73. Schwarch G, Gosenfeld L, Gilderman A, Jiwesh J, Ripple RE. Akathisia associated with carbamazepine therapy. Am J Psychiatry 1986; 143:1190–1191.
74. Neglia JP, Glaze DG, Zion TE. Tics and vocalizations in children treated with carbamazepine. Pediatrics 1984; 73:841–844.
75. Kurlan R, Kersun J, Behr J, et al. Carbamazepine-induced tics. Clin Neuropharmacol 1989; 12:298–302.
76. Lichter D, Majunmdar L, Kurlan R. Opiate withdrawal unmasks Tourette's syndrome. Clin Neuropharmacol 1988; 11:559–564.

77. Post RM. Mechanisms of action of carbamazepine and related anticonvulsants in affective illness. In: Melzer HY (ed), Psychopharmacology: The Third Generation of Progress, New York, Raven Press, 1987, 567–576.
78. Barros HM, Braz S, Leite JR. Effect of carbamazepine on dopamine release and reuptake in rat striatal slices. Epilepsia 1986; 27:361–366.
79. Kawalik S, Levitt M, Barkai A. Effects of carbamazepine and antidepressant drugs on endogenous catecholamine levels in the cerebroventricular compartment of the rat. Psychopharmacology (Berlin) 1984; 83:169–171.
80. Barros HM, Leite JR. Effects of acute and chronic carbamazepine administration on apomorphine-elicited stereotypy. Eur J Pharmacol 1986; 123:345–349.
81. Hajnsek F, Sartorius N. A case of intoxication with Tegretol. Epilepsia 1964; 5:371–375.
82. Karas BJ, Wilder BJ, Hammond EJ, Bauman AW. Valproate tremors. Neurology 1982; 32:428–432.
83. Karas BJ, Wilder BJ, Hammond EJ, Bauman AW. Treatment of valproate tremors. Neurology 1983:33:1380–1382.
84. Price DJI. The advantages of sodium valproate in the neurosurgical practice. In: Legg NJ (ed), Clinical and Pharmacological Aspects of Sodium Valproate (Epilim) in the Treatment of Epilepsy, Tunbridge Wells, England, MCS Consultants 1976, pp 44–50.
85. Hyman NM, Dennis PD, Sinclair KGA. Tremor due to sodium valproate. Neurology (NY) 1979; 29:1177–1180.
85a. Armon C, Miller P, Carwile S, Brown E, Edinger JD, Paul RG, Shin C. Valproate-induced parkinsonism-dementia syndrome: clinical features. Mov Disord 1991; 6:269.
86. Fernando SJM. An attack of chorea complicating oral contraceptive therapy. Practitioner 1966; 197:210–212.
87. Leys D, Destee A, Petit H, Warot P. Chorea associated with oral contraception. J Neurol 1987; 235:46–48.
88. Galimberti D. Chorea induced by the use of oral contraceptives: report of a case and review of the literature. Ital J Neurol Sci 1987; 8:383–386.
89. Gautier JC, Rosa A, Lhermitte F. Accidents vasculaires cerebreaux et contraceptifs oraux. Rev Neurol 1974; 130:217–236.
90. Riddoch D, Jefferson M, Bickerstaff ER. Chorea and the oral contraceptives. Br Med J 1971; 4:217–218.
91. Nauseida PA, Koller WG, Weiner WJ, et al. Chorea induced by oral contraceptives. Neurology 1979; 29:1605–1609.
92. Pulsinelli WA, Hamil RW. Chorea complicating oral contraceptive therapy: case report and review of the literature. Am J Med 1978; 65:557–559.
93. Barber P, Arnold A, Evans G. Recurrent hormone-dependent chorea: Effects of estrogens and progesterone. Clin Endocrinol 1976; 5:291–293.
93a. Caviness JN, Muenter MD. An unusual case of recurrent chorea. Mov Disord 1991; 6:355–357.
94. Lewis PD, Harrison MJ. Involuntary movements in patients taking oral contraceptives. Br Med J 1969; 4:404.

95. Donaldson JO. Movement Disorders. In: Donaldson JO (ed), Neurology of Pregnancy, Philadelphia, WB Saunders Co., 1978, pp 74–87.
96. Gamboa ET, Isaacs G, Harter DH. Chorea associated with oral contraceptive therapy. Arch Neurol 1971; 25:112–114.
97. Buge A, Vincent D, Rancurel G, Cheron F. Hemichoree et contraceptifs oraux. Rev Neurol (Paris) 1985; 141:663–665.
98. Beaumont V, Delplanque B, Lemort N, et al. Blood changes in sex steroid hormone users: circulating immune complexes induced by estrogens and progestogens and their relation to vascular thrombosis. Atherosclerosis 1982; 44:343–353.
99. Mathur AK, Gatter RA. Chorea as the initial presentation of oral contraceptive-induced systemic lupus erythematosis. J Rheumatol 1988; 15:1042–1043.
100. Nausieda PA, Koller WC, Weiner WJ, Klawans HL. Modification of post-synaptic dopaminergic sensitivity by female sex hormones. Life Sci 1979; 25:521–526.
101. Nausieda PA, Grossman BJ, Koller WC, Weiner WJ, Klawans HL. Syndenham chorea: a update. Neurology 1980; 30:31–334.
102. Nausieda PA, Bielanskas LA, Bacon LD, Hagerty M, Koller WC Glantz RN. Chronic dopaminergic sensitivity after Sydenham's chorea. Neurology 1983; 33:750–754.
103. Schipper HM. Sex hormones in stroke, chorea and anticonvulsant therapy. Semin Neurol 1988; 8:181–186.
104. Gordon JH, Diamond BI. Antagonism of dopamine supersensitivity by estrogen: neurochemical studies in an animal model of tardive dyskinesia. Biol Psychiatry 1981; 16:365–371.
105. Euvrard C, Oberlander C, Boissier JR. Antidopaminergic effect of estrogens at the striatal level. J Pharmacol Exp Ther 1980; 214:179–185.
106. Gordon JH, Borison RI, Diamond BI. Estrogen in experimental tardive dyskinesia. Neurology 1980; 30:551–554.
107. Bedard P, Langelier P, Danbova J, et al. Estrogens, progesterone and the extrapyramidal system. Adv Neurol 1979; 24:411–422.
108. Koller WC, Barr A, Biary N. Estrogen treatment of dyskinetic disorders. Neurology (Cleveland) 1982; 32:547–550.
109. Quinn NP, Marsden CD. Menstrual-related fluctuations in Parkinson's disease. Mov Disord 1986; 1:85–87.
110. Robinson RO, Stutchfield P, Hicks B, et al. Estrogens and dyskinesia. Neurology 1984; 34:404.
111. Van Hartesveldt C, Joyce JN. Effects of estrogen on the basal ganglia. Neurosci Biobehav Rev 1986; 10:1–14.
112. Godfrain T, Towse G, Van Nueten JM. Cinnarizine: a selective calcium entry blocker. Drugs Today 1982; 18:27–42.
113. Leysen JE, Gommeren W. Receptor binding profile of flunarizine: Preclinical research report. Janssen Pharmaceutical Research Laboratories, R14950/24, March, 1983.
114. Biary N, Aldeeb SM, Langenberg P. The effect of flunarizine on essential tremor. Neurology 1991; 41:311–312.
115. DeMello-Souza SE. Flunarizina, parkinsonismo e depressao. XI Congresso Brasiliero de Neurologgia, Goiania-Goias Brazil, 1984. Abstracts.

116. Micheli F, Fernandez Pardal M, Gatto M, et al. Flunarizine- and cinnarizine-induced extrapyramidal reactions. Neurology 1987; 37:881–884.
117. Holmes B, Brogden RN, Heel RC, Speight TM, Avery GS. Flunarizine: a review of its pharmacodynamic and pharmacokinetic properties and therapeutic use. Drugs 1984; 27:6–44.
118. Micheli, FE, Fernandez Pardal MM, Giannaula, et al. Movement disorders and depression due to flunarizine and cinnarizine. Mov Disord 1989; 4:139–146.
119. Chouza C, Scaramelli A, Caamano JL, DeMedina O, Aljanati R, Romero S. Parkinsonism, tardive dyskinesia, akathisia and depression induced by flunarizine. Lancet 1986; 1:1303–1304.
119a. Gimenez-Roldan S, Mateo D. Cinnarizine-induced parkinsonism: susceptibility related to aging and essential tremor. Clin Neuropharmacol 1991; 14:156–164.
120. Moretti A, Lucantoni C. Flunarizine-induced parkinsonism: clinical report. Ital J Neurol Sci 1988; 9:295–297.
121. Mangone CA, Herskovits E. Extrapyramidal and depressive reactions with flunarizine and cinnarizine. J Neurol Neurosurg Psychiatry 1989; 52:288–289.
122. Fernandez Pardal MM, Fernandez Pardal J, Micheli F. Effect of flunarizine and nifedipine on the ^{3}H dopamine release by potassium in the rat caudate nucleus. Acta Physiol Phamacol Latinoam 1987; 37:156–158.
123. Fernandez Pardal MM, Fernandez Pardal J, Micheli F. Aggravation of Parkinson's disease by cinnarizine. J Neurol Neurosurg Psychiatry 1988; 51:158–159.
124. Pedro-Botet ML, Bonal J, Caralps A. Nifedipine and myoclonic disorders. Nephron 1989; 51:281.
125. DeMedina A, Biasini O, Rivera A, Sampera A. Nifedipine and myoclonic dystonia. Ann Intern Med 1986; 104:125.
126. Rodger C, Stewart A. Side effects of nifedipine. Br J Med 1978; 276:1619–1620.
126a. Topaktas S, Onur R, Dalkara T. Calcium channel blockers and essential tremor. Eur Neurol 1987; 27:114–119.
127. Singh I. Prolonged oculogyric crisis on addition of nifedipine to neuroleptic medication regime. Br J Psychiatry 1987; 150:127–128.
128. Pickar D, Wolkowitz OM, Doran AR, et al. Clinical and biochemical effects of verapamil: administration to schizophrenic patients. Arch Gen Psychiatry 1987; 44:113–118.
129. Helmuth D, Ljaijevic Z, Ramirez L, Meltzer HY. Choreoathetosis induced by verapamil and lithium treatment. J Clin Psychopharmacol 1989; 9:454–455.
130. Hicks CB, Abraham K. Verapamil and myoclonic dystonia. Ann Intern Med 1985; 103:154.
131. Jacobs MB. Diltiazem and akathisia. Ann Intern Med 1983; 99:794–795.
132. Dick RS, Barold SS. Diltiazem-induced parkinsonism. Am J Med 1989; 87:95–96.
133. Thach BT, Chase TN, Bosma JS. Oral facial dyskinesia associated with

prolonged use of antihistaminic decongestants. N Engl J Med 1975; 293:486–487.

134. Worz R. Spate extrapyramidale hyperkinesen wahrend langzetiger einnahme von mebhydrolin. Dtsch Med Wochenschr 1975; 98:1071–1074.

135. Davis WA. Dyskinesia associated with chronic antihistamine use. N Engl J Med 1976; 294:113.

136. Lavenstein BL, Cantor FK. Acute dystonia. An unusual reaction to diphenhydramine. JAMA 1976; 236:291.

137. Casteels-Van-Daele M, Eggermont E, Casaer P, Van de Cassey W, De Boeck K. Acute dystonic reactions and long-lasting impaired consciousness associated with oxatomide in children. Lancet 1986; 1:1204–1205.

138. Bateman DN, Bevan P, Longley BP, Mastaglia F, Wandless I. Cimetidine induced postural and action tremor. J Neurol Neurosurg Psychiatry 1981; 44:94.

139. Romisher S, Felter R, Dougherty J. Tagamet-induced acute dystonia. Ann Emerg Med 1987; 16:1162–1164.

140. Handler CE, Besse CP, Wilson AO. Extrapyramidal and cerebellar syndrome with encephalopathy associated with cimetidine. Postgrad Med J 1982; 58:527–528.

141. Kushner MJ. Chorea and cimetidine. Ann Intern Med 1982; 96:126.

142. Lehmann AB. Reversible chorea due to ranitidine and cimetidine. Lancet 1988; 2:158.

143. Lang AE, Blair RDG. Anticholinergic drugs and amantidine in the treatment of Parkinson's disease. In: Calne DB, Drugs for the Treatment of Parkinson's Disease, Berlin, Springer-Verlag, 1989, pp 307–323.

144. Fahn S, David E. Orofacio-lingual dyskinesia due to anticholinergic medication. Trans Am Neurol Assoc 1972; 97:277–279.

145. Birket-Smith E. Abnormal involuntary movements induced by anticholinergic therapy. Acta Neurol Scand 1974; 50:801–811.

146. Ware RW, Gubbay SS. Choreiform movements induced by anticholinergic therapy. Med J Aust 1979; 1:465.

147. Birket-Smith E. Abnormal involuntary movements in relation to anticholinergics and levodopa therapy. Acta Neurol Scand 1975; 52:158–160.

148. Klawans HL, Rubovits R. Effect of cholinergic and anticholinergic agents on tardive dyskinesia. J Neurol Neurosurg Psychiatry 1974; 27:941–947.

149. Weiner WJ, Lang AE. Movement Disorders: A Comprehensive Survey, Mount Kisco, NY, Futura Publishing Co., 1989.

150. Lang AE. High-dose anticholinergics in adult dystonia. Can J Neurol Sci 1986; 13:42–46.

151. Nomoto M, Thompson PD, Sheehy MP, Quinn NP, Marsden CD. Anticholinergic-induced chorea in the treatment of focal dystonia. Mov Disord 1987; 2:53–56.

152. Pycock C, Milson J, Tarsy D, Marsden CD. The effect of manipulation of cholinergic mechanisms on turning behaviour in mice with unilat-

eral destruction of the nigro-neostriatal dopaminergic system. Neuropharmacology 1978; 17:175–183.

153. Calmels JP, Sorbette F, Montastruc JL, Albarede JL. Syndromes hyperkinetique iatrogene par antihistaminique. La Nouvelle Presse Med 1982; 30:2296–2297.

154. Samie MR, Ashton AK. Choreoathetosis induced by cyproheptadine. Mov Disord 1989; 4:81–84.

155. Bernick C. Methysergide-induced akathisia. Clin Neuropharmacol 1988; 11:87–89.

156. Albanese A, Rossi P, Altavista MC. Can trazodone induce parkinsonism? Clin Neuropharmacol 1988; 11:180–182.

157. Demuth GW, Breslow RE, Drescher J. The elicitation of a movement disorder by trazodone: case report. J Clin Psychiatry 1985; 46:535–536.

158. Ritchie EC, Bridenbaugh RH, Jabbari B. Acute generalized myoclonus following buspirone administration. J Clin Psychiatry 1988; 49:242–243.

159. Patterson, JF. Akathisia associated with buspirone. J Clin Psychopharmacol 1988; 8:296–297.

160. Boylan, K. Persistant dystonia associated with buspirone. Neurology 1990; 40:1904.

161. Strauss, A. Orodyskinesia associated with buspirone use in an elderly woman. J Clin Psychiatry 1988; 49:322–323.

162. Kaplan SR, Murkofsky C. Oral-buccal dyskinesia symptoms associated with low-dose benzodiazepine treatment. Am J Psychiatry 1978; 135:1558–1559.

163. Rosenbaum AH, De la Fuente JR. Benzodiazepines and tardive dyskinesia. Lancet 1979; 2:900.

164. Sandyk R. Orofacial dyskinesias associated with lorazepam therapy. Clin Pharmacol 1986; 5:419–421.

165. Hooker EA, Danzl DS. Acute dystonic reaction due to diazepam. J Emerg Med 1988; 6:491–493.

166. Stolarek IH, Ford MJ. Acute dystonia induced by midazolam and abolished by flumazenil. Br Med J 1990; 300:614.

167. Suranyi-Cadotte BE, Nestoros JN, Nair NPV, Lal S, Gauthier S. Parkinsonism induced by high doses of diazepam. Biol Psychiatry 1985; 20:451–460.

168. Snyder SH, Enna SJ, Young AB. Brain mechanisms associated with therapeutic actions of benzodiazepines: focus on neurotransmitters. Am J Psychiatry 1977; 134:662–664.

169. Mintz U, Liberman UA, De Vries D. Parkinsonism syndrome due to cephaloridine. JAMA 1971; 216:1200.

170. Borucki MJ, Matzke DS, Pollard RB. Tremor induced by trimethoprim-sulfamethoxazole in patients with acquired immunodeficiency syndrome (AIDS). Ann Intern Med 1988; 109:77–78.

171. Schonheyder H, Thestrup-Pedersen K, Esmann V, Stenderup A. Cryptococcal meningitis: complications due to intrathecal treatment. Scand J Infect Dis 1980; 12:1555–1557.

172. Fisher JF, Dewald J. Parkinsonism associated with intraventricular amphotericin B. J Antimicrob Chemother 1983; 12:97–99.

173. Burdge DR, Chow AW, Sacks SL. Neurotoxic effects during vidarabine therapy for herpes zoster. Can Med Assoc J 1985; 132:392–395.
174. Akindele MO, Odejide AO. Amodiaquine-induced involuntary movements. Br Med J 1975; 38:225–231.
175. Majumdar SK. Mechanism of chloroquine-induced involuntary movements. Br Med J 1977; 1:1350.
176. Umez-Eronini EM, Eronini EA. Chloroquine-induced involuntary movements. Br Med J 1977; 1:945–946.
177. Achumba JI, Ette EI, Thomas WOA, Essein EE. Chloroquine-induced acute dystonic reactions in the presence of metronidazole. Drug Intell Clin Pharm 1988; 22:308–310.
178. Cremona-Barbaro A. Extrapyramidal symptoms following mefenamic acid. J R Soc Med 1983; 76:435.
179. Wood N, Paull HS, Williams AC, Dieppe C. Extrapyramidal reactions to anti-inflammatory drugs. J Neurol Neurosurg Psychiatry 1988; 51:731–732.
180. Redmond AD. Dyskinesia induced by mefanimic acid? J R Soc Med 1981; 74:558–559.
181. Sandyk R, Awerbuch G, Rapcsak SZ. Bilateral ballism induced by ibuprofen in a schizophrenic patient. Postgrad Med J 1987; 63:593–594.
182. Sandyk R, Gillman MA. Acute exacerbation of Parkinson's disease with sulindac. Ann Neurol 1985; 17:104–105.
183. Anderson CB, Larson EJ. Diflunisal in idiopathic Parkinson's disease. Neurology 1984; 34:400–402.
184. Werner EG, Olanow CW. Parkinsonism and amiodarone therapy. Ann Neurol 1989; 25:630–632.
185. Greene HL, Graham EL, Werner JA. Toxic and therapeutic effects of amiodarone in the treatment of cardiac arrhythmias. J Am Coll Cardiol 1983; 2:1114–1128.
186. Fogoros RN, Anderson KP, Winkle RA, et al. Amiodarone: clinical efficacy and toxicity in 96 patients with recurrent, drug-refractory arrhythmias. Circulation 1983; 68(1):88–94.
187. Dailheu-Geoffrey P. Une possibilite therapeutique nouvelle dans l'angina de poitrine: l'amiodarone. Gaz Med France 1971; 78:2114–2120.
188. Palakurthy PR, Iver V, Mechler RJ. Unusual neurotoxicity associated with amiodarone therapy. Arch Intern Med 1987; 147:881–884.
189. LeMaire JF, Autret A, Biziere K, et al. Amiodarone neuropathy: further arguments for human drug-induced neurolipidosis. Eur Neurol 1982; 21:65–68.
190. Murray GB, Greenberg DB. Respiratory dyskinesia associated with hexamethylmelamine. Cancer Treat Rep 1980; 64:355–356.
191. Vogl SE, Pagano M, Davis TE, et al. Hexymethylmelamine and cisplatin in advanced ovarian cancer after failure of alkylating-agent therapy. Cancer Treat Rep 1982; 66:1285–1290.
192. Wilson WL, Bisel HF, Cole D, et al. Prolonged low-dose administration of hexymethylmelamine (NC13875). Cancer 1970; 25:568–570.
193. Carpentieri U, Lockhart LH. Ataxia and athetosis as side effects of chemotherapy with vincristine in non-Hodgkin's lymphoma. Cancer Treat Rep 1978; 62:561–562.

194. Boranic M, Raci F. A Parkinson-like syndrome as side effect of chemotherapy with vincristine and adriamycin in a child with acute leukemia. Biomedicine 1979; 31:124–125.
195. Ascher DP, Delaney RA. Acute dystonia from etoposide. Drug Intell Clin Pharm 1988; 22:41–42.
195a. Anderson NR, Tandon DS. Ifosfamide extrapyramidal neurotoxicity. Cancer 1991; 68:72–75.
196. Luque AF, Selhorst JB, Petruska P. Parkinsonism induced by high-dose cytosine arabinoside. Mov Disord 1987; 2:219–222.
197. Barnett MJ. CNS toxicity of high-dose cytosine arabinoside. Semin Oncol 1985; 22:227–232.
198. Reutens DC, Stewart-Wynn EG. Norpethidine-induced myoclonus in a patient with renal failure. J Neurol Neurosurg Psychiatry 1989; 52:1450–1451.
199. Hochman MS. Meperidine-associated myoclonus and seizures in long-term hemodialysis patients. Ann Neurol 1983; 14:593.
200. Potter JM, Reid DB, Shaw RJ, Hackett P, Hickman PE. Myoclonus associated with treatment with high doses of morphine: a role of supplemental drugs. Br Med J 1989; 299:150–153.
201. Quinn N. Myoclonus associated with high doses of morphine. Br Med J 1989; 299:683–684.
202. McQuay HJ, Gorman DJ, Hanks GW. Myoclonus associated with high doses of morphine. Br Med J 1989; 299:684.
203. DeMaio D, Caponeri MA, Cicchetti V, Mellado C, Schieghi G. Sulpiride and extrapyramidal syndromes in chronic heroin addiction. Neuropsychobiology 1978; 4:36–39.
204. Wasserman S, Yahr MD. Choreic movements induced by the use of methadone. Arch Neurol 1980; 37:727–728.
205. Leiberman AN, Goldstein M. Reversible parkinsonism related to meperidine. N Engl J Med 1985; 312:509.
206. Glavina MJ, Robertshaw R. Myoclonic spasms following intrathecal morphine. Anesthesia 1988; 43:389–390.
207. Carlsson A, Lindquist M. In vivo decarboxylation of α-methyldopa and α-methylmetatyrosine. Acta Physiol Scand 1962; 54:87–94.
208. Groden BM. Parkinsonism occurring with methyldopa treatment. Br Med J 1963; 1:1001.
209. Peaston MJT. Parkinsonism associated with alphamethyldopa therapy. Br Med J 1963; 2:168.
210. Strang RR. Parkinsonism occurring during methyldopa therapy. Can Med Assoc J 1966; 95:928–929.
211. Sechi GP, Demontis G, Rosati G. Relationship between Meige syndrome and alpha-methyldopa-induced parkinsonism. Neurology 1985; 35:1668–1669.
212. Duvoisin RC, Marsden CD. Alphamethyldopamine as a dopaminergic agonist. Adv Neurol 1975; 9:243–298.
213. Yamadori A, Albert ML. Involuntary movement disorder caused by methyldopa. N Engl J Med 1972; 286:610.
214. Manoguerra AS, Kearney TE. Acute disulfiram toxicity. Vet Hum Toxicol 1982; 24:282.

215. Wokittel E. Vergiftung mit Antabus bei einem 10-jährigen Madchen. Arch Kinderheilkd 1960; 161:145–149.
216. Fontan M, Petit H, Delahousse J, Ascher J, Decoulx-Poutignat M. Signes extrapyramidaux d'intoxications aigues ou subaigues par disulfiram ou disulfiram-alcool. Lille Méd 1967; 12:814–817.
217. Kane FJ. Carbon disulfide intoxication from overdosage of disulfiram. Am J Psychiat 1970; 127:690–694.
218. Trillat E, Richet L, Mignen JC. Encéphalopathie subaigue survenue au cours d'un traitement au disulfiram. Ann Méd Psychol 1958; 116:347–351.
219. Aupy M, Latinville D, Bretegnier F, Henry P. Accidents neurologiques inhabituels au disulfiram: apropos de 2 observations. Bordeaux Méd 1981; 14:1101–1104.
220. Lidy C, Priollet P, Pepin B. Syndrome pyramidal et extrapyramidal apparu au decours d'une intoxication aigue par le disulfiram. Nouv Presse Méd 1979; 8:3561.
221. Weissenborn K, Peters J, Heinze HJ, Becker H. Hirninfarkte und Polyradikulitis als Folge von Suizidversuchen mit Disulfiram. Nervenarzt 1986; 57:159–162.
222. Krauss JK, Mohadjer M, Wakhloo AK, Mundinger F. Dystonia and akinesia due to pallidoputaminal lesions after disulfiram intoxication. Mov Disord 1191; 6:166–170.
223. Walker RW, Brochstein JA. Neurologic complications of immunosuppressive agents. Neurol Clin 1988; 6(Suppl 2):261–278.
224. European Multicentre Trial Group. Cyclosporin in cadaveric renal transplantation: one year follow-up of a multicentre trial. Lancet 1983; 2:986–989.
225. Kahan DB, Flechner Sm, Lorber MI, et al. Complications of cyclosporine-prednisone immunosuppression in 402 renal allograft recipients exclusively followed at a single centre for from one to five years. Transplantation 1987; 43:768–769.
226. Moss NG, Powell SL, Falk RJ. Intravenous cyclosporine activates afferent and efferent renal nerves and causes sodium retention in innervated kidneys in rats. Proc Natl Acad Sci USA 1985; 82:8222–8226.
227. Bird GLA, Meadows J, Goka J, Polson R, Williams R. Cyclosporin-associated akinetic mutism and extrapyramidal syndrome after liver transplantation. J Neurol Neurosurg Psychiatry 1990; 53:1068–1071.
228. Mayeux R, Albert M, Genike M. Physostigmine-induced myoclonus in Alzheimer's disease. Neurology 1987; 37:345–346.
229. Harbaugh RE, Roberts DW, Coombs Dw, Saunders RL, Reeder TM. Preliminary report: intracranial cholinergic drug infusion in patients with Alzheimer's disease. Neurosurgery 1984; 15:514–518.
230. Crystal HA. Baclofen therapy may be associated with chorea in Alzheimer's disease. Ann Neurol 1990; 28:239.
231. Wedzicha JA, Gibb WR, Lees AJ, Hoffbrand BI. Chorea in digoxin toxicity. J Neurol Neurosurg Psychiatry 1984; 47:419.
232. Mulder LJMM, Van der Mast RC, Meerwaldt JD. Generalized chorea due to digoxin toxicity. Br Med J 198; 296:1262.
233. Sandyk R. Parkinsonism induced by captopril. Clin Neuropharmacol 1985; 8:197–200.

234. Hod H, Kaplinsky N, Har-Zahav J, Frankl O. Pindolol-induced tremor. Postgrad Med J 1980; 56:346–347.
235. Koller W, Orebaugh C, Lawson L, Potempa K. Pindolol-induced tremor. Clin Neuropharmacol 1987; 10:449–452.
236. Teravainen R, Larsen A, Fogelholm R. Comparison between the effects of pindolol and propranolol on essential tremor. Neurology 1977; 27:439–442.
237. Gjerris F. Transitory procaine-induced parkinsonism. J Neurol Neurosurg Psychiatry 1971; 34:20–22.
238. Gordon M, Gordon AS. Perhexiline maleate as a cause of reversible parkinsonism and peripheral neuropathy. J Am Geriat Soc 1981; 29:259–262.
239. Tilzey A, Heptonstall J, Hamblin T. Toxic confusional state and choreiform movements after treatment with anabolic steroids. Br Med J 1981; 283:349–350.
240. Felser JM, Orban DJ Dystonic reactions after ketamine abuse. Ann Emerg Med 1982; 11:673–675.
241. Deahl M. Betelnut-induced extrapyramidal syndrome: an unusual drug interaction. Mov Disord 1989; 4:330–333.
242. Lervy B. Parkinson's disease on treatment with Viskaldix. J R Coll Gen Pract 1984; 34:184.
243. Miller LG, Jankovic J. Persistent dystonia possibly induced by flecainide. Mov Disord 1992; 7:62–63.

Index

In this index, page numbers followed by "f" designate figures; page numbers followed by "t" designate tables. *See* cross-references designate synonymous terms as used in this text. *See also* cross-references designate related topics or more detailed topic breakdowns.